2004
YEAR BOOK OF
DENTISTRY®

The 2004 Year Book Series

Year Book of Allergy, Asthma, and Clinical Immunology™: Drs Rosenwasser, Boguniewicz, Milgrom, Routes, and Spahn

Year Book of Anesthesiology and Pain Management™: Drs Chestnut, Abram, Black, Lang, Roizen, Trankina, and Wood

Year Book of Cardiology®: Drs Gersh, Cheitlin, Graham, Kaplan, Sundt, and Waldo

Year Book of Critical Care Medicine®: Drs Dellinger, Parrillo, Balk, Bekes, Dries, and Roberts

Year Book of Dentistry®: Drs Zakariasen, Boghosian, Burgess, Hatcher, Horswell, McIntyre, and Zakariasen

Year Book of Dermatology and Dermatologic Surgery™: Drs Thiers and Lang

Year Book of Diagnostic Radiology®: Drs Osborn, Birdwell, Dalinka, Gardiner, Groskin, Levy, Maynard, and Oestreich

Year Book of Emergency Medicine®: Drs Burdick, Cone, Cydulka, Hamilton, Handly, and Quintana

Year Book of Endocrinology®: Drs Mazzaferri, Becker, Kannan, Kennedy, Kreisberg, Meikle, Molitch, Osei, Poehlman, and Rogol

Year Book of Family Practice®: Drs Bowman, Apgar, Dexter, Miser, Neill, and Scherger

Year Book of Gastroenterology™: Drs Lichtenstein, Dempsey, Ginsberg, Katzka, Kochman, Morris, Nunes, Reddy, Rosato, and Stein

Year Book of Hand Surgery®: Drs Berger and Ladd

Year Book of Medicine®: Drs Barkin, Frishman, Klahr, Loehrer, Mazzaferri, Phillips, Pillinger, and Snydman

Year Book of Neonatal and Perinatal Medicine®: Drs Fanaroff, Maisels, and Stevenson

Year Book of Neurology and Neurosurgery®: Drs Gibbs and Verma

Year Book of Nuclear Medicine®: Drs Coleman, Blaufox, Royal, Strauss, and Zubal

Year Book of Obstetrics, Gynecology, and Women's Health®: Drs Mishell, Kirschbaum, and Miller

Year Book of Oncology®: Drs Loehrer, Arceci, Glatstein, Gordon, Morrow, Schiller, and Thigpen

Year Book of Ophthalmology®: Drs Rapuano, Cohen, Eagle, Grossman, Myers, Nelson, Penne, Regillo, Sergott, Shields, and Tipperman

Year Book of Orthopedics®: Drs Morrey, Beauchamp, Peterson, Swiontkowski, Trigg, and Yaszemski

Year Book of Otolaryngology-Head and Neck Surgery®: Drs Paparella, Keefe, and Otto

2004

The Year Book of DENTISTRY®

Editor-in-Chief
Kenneth L. Zakariasen, DDS, MS, MS(ODA), PhD

Associate Dean and Chair, Department of Dentistry, Faculty of Medicine and Dentistry, University of Alberta, Alberta, Canada; Organizational Consultant, Heliomage Organizational Consultants; Private Practice, Madison, Wisconsin

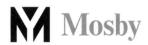 Mosby

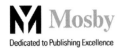

Dedicated to Publishing Excellence

Vice President, Continuity Publishing: Timothy M. Griswold
Developmental Editor: Ali Gavenda
Senior Manager, Continuity Production: Idelle L. Winer
Senior Issue Manager: Pat Costigan
Composition Specialist: Betty Dockins
Illustrations and Permissions Coordinator: Kimberly E. Hulett

Printed in the United States of America
Composition by Thomas Technology Solutions, Inc.
Printing/binding by Sheridan Books, Inc.

Editorial Office:
Elsevier
300 East
170 South Independence Mall West
Philadelphia, PA 19106-3399

International Standard Serial Number: 0084-3717
International Standard Book Number: 0-323-01599-9

Editors

Table of Contents

Journals Represented

Mosby and its editors survey approximately 500 journals for its abstract and commentary publications. From these journals, the editors select the articles to be abstracted. Journals represented in this YEAR BOOK are listed below.

Academy of General Dentistry Impact
American Journal of Dentistry
American Journal of Orthodontics and Dentofacial Orthopedics
Angle Orthodontist
Arthritis and Rheumatism
Australian Dental Journal
British Dental Journal
California Dental Association Journal
Cancer
Cleft Palate-Craniofacial Journal
Community Dentistry and Oral Epidemiology
Compendium of Continuing Education in Dentistry (Compendium)
Dentomaxillofacial Radiology
General Dentistry
Implant Dentistry
International Journal of Oral and Maxillofacial Surgery
International Journal of Prosthodontics
Journal of Clinical Pediatric Dentistry
Journal of Clinical Periodontology
Journal of Cranio-Maxillo-Facial Surgery
Journal of Dental Education
Journal of Dental Research
Journal of Dentistry
Journal of Dentistry for Children
Journal of Endocrinology
Journal of Endodontics
Journal of Esthetic and Restorative Dentistry
Journal of Evidence-Based Dental Practice
Journal of Oral and Maxillofacial Surgery
Journal of Pediatric Hematology/Oncology
Journal of Periodontology
Journal of Prosthetic Dentistry
Journal of Prosthodontics
Journal of the American College of Surgeons
Journal of the American Dental Association
Journal of the Canadian Dental Association (CDA)
Oral Surgery, Oral Medicine, Oral Pathology, Oral Radiology, and Endodontics
Otolaryngology - Head and Neck Surgery
Pediatric Dentistry
Practical Procedures & Aesthetic Dentistry
Quintessence International

STANDARD ABBREVIATIONS

The following terms are abbreviated in this edition: acquired immunodeficiency syndrome (AIDS), cardiopulmonary resuscitation (CPR), central nervous system (CNS), cerebrospinal fluid (CSF), computed tomography (CT), deoxyribonucleic acid (DNA), electrocardiography (ECG), health maintenance organization (HMO), human immunodeficiency virus (HIV), intensive care unit (ICU), intramuscular (IM), intravenous (IV), magnetic resonance (MR) imaging (MRI), ribonucleic acid (RNA), temporomandibular joint (TMJ), and ultrasound (US).

NOTE

The YEAR BOOK OF DENTISTRY® is a literature survey service providing abstracts of articles published in the professional literature. Every effort is made to assure the accuracy of the information presented in these pages. Neither the editors nor the publisher of the YEAR BOOK OF DENTISTRY® can be responsible for errors in the original materials. The editors' comments are their own opinions. Mention of specific products within this publication does not constitute endorsement.

To facilitate the use of the YEAR BOOK OF DENTISTRY® as a reference tool, all illustrations and tables included in this publication are now identified as they appear in the original article. This change is meant to help the reader recognize that any illustration or table appearing in the YEAR BOOK OF DENTISTRY® may be only one of many in the original article. For this reason, figure and table numbers will often appear to be out of sequence within the YEAR BOOK OF DENTISTRY®.

Introduction

The 2004 edition of the YEAR BOOK OF DENTISTRY is fortunate to have back all of last year's editors with the exception of Dr Gerald Harrington. For years, Dr Harrington directed one of the premier endodontic graduate programs in the country at the University of Washington. Several years ago, he retired from the university but graciously agreed to serve as guest editor for the Endodontics section of the YEAR BOOK, which he did for a number of years. I always marveled at the incredible thoroughness, insights, and effort that Dr Harrington put into his work on the Endodontics chapter. This year, Dr Harrington decided to retire from the YEAR BOOK, and I thank him, not only for his superb efforts on behalf of the YEAR BOOK, but also for his incredible contributions to the field of endodontics over a period of many decades. It has been a real privilege to work with him.

The 2004 YEAR BOOK introduces both new chapters and new editors. Joining the superb group of returning editors are Dr Michelle Robinson, Dr Drew Dentino, Dr Denis Lynch, and Mr Charles Moreno. Dr Robinson introduces a new chapter on Dental Informatics, a vitally important area in today's digital world. Dr Robinson brings to the YEAR BOOK not only her expertise as a dentist, but also her extensive experience in directing dental informatics at Marquette University, along with a graduate degree in medical informatics. Dr Drew Dentino directs periodontics at Marquette University and brings extensive clinical and research experience to his role in preparing the chapter on Periodontics. After his specialty training in periodontics, Dr Dentino completed a PhD in periodontal research, which he very actively pursues at Marquette. Dr Denis Lynch is Associate Dean for Academic Affairs, also at Marquette, and is an oral pathologist who holds a PhD in experimental pathology. Dr Lynch is responsible for the chapter on Oral Medicine and Pathology. Mr Charles Moreno is an award-winning dental laboratory technician from California who brings the YEAR BOOK a new chapter on Dental Laboratory Science. Never has the importance of quality in dental laboratory work been more evident than during the esthetic revolution, and I am delighted to be able to bring this chapter to the book to aid our readers in this important discipline.

As is the YEAR BOOK tradition, the editors for 2004 have gone through hundreds and hundreds of articles to select the 294 articles for this year's book. The articles are selected to be helpful to clinicians directly in their practices, and also in simply trying to make some sense of the never-ending continuous change that confronts our profession. Hopefully, the YEAR BOOK, particularly the editors' comments, helps to bring perspective to what can often seem like a fairly chaotic professional world. Please enjoy reading the 2004 edition of the YEAR BOOK OF DENTISTRY.

Kenneth L. Zakariasen, DDS, MS, MS(ODA), PhD

1 General Restorative Dentistry

Introduction

The demand for tooth-colored restorations increases every year. Composite restoratives are steadily replacing the use of dental amalgam for the restoration of posterior teeth. This trend is primarily due to esthetics, but it is also driven by the continuous litany of unproven health claims concerning mercury and its role in environmental waste issues. Composites have improved significantly from the first-generation, large-particle macrofilled materials to the latest nanomer-based restoratives. Nanoparticle composites, over time, retain their surface luster to the same degree as the adjacent enamel. These new materials show gloss retention without compromising their physical properties. As advanced as modern composite restoratives may be, their performance can only be realized by the proper use of an adhesive agent. The adhesive agents introduced a decade ago have been have shown to be highly effective through long-term clinical trials. These adhesives, requiring etching, priming, and resin-bonding steps, will successfully bond with composites that polymerize with light as well as chemical initiation. Current self-etching and "all-in-one" formulations have been shown to perform adequately in laboratory testing. However, their long-term clinical performance has yet to be established. In deciding to use these simplified bonding agents, the clinician must weigh the benefit of convenience with a potential sacrifice of long-term performance.

The global popularity of glass ionomer and resin-modified ionomer cements has increased. Glass ionomer materials have excellent pulpal biocompatibility, bond strength, and resistance to microleakage. Recently, a new glass ionomer–based pit and fissure sealant was introduced. With a water-based chemistry and long-term fluoride release, this sealant might be an ideal material for difficult placements.

There will be continual improvement of dental materials and devices. As these new technologies are introduced to the marketplace, it is crucial that their performance be validated in controlled clinical trials and not just certified by in vitro laboratory testing. The long-term clinical success of a restoration continues to depend on an adequate knowledge of the restorative materials' properties as well as a skilled clinical technique.

Alan A. Boghosian, DDS

Clinical Evaluation of an "All-in-One" Bonding System to Non-carious Cervical Lesions—Results at One Year

Burrow MF, Tyas MJ (Univ of Melbourne, Australia)
Aust Dent J 248:180-182, 2003   1–1

Background.—The practice of bonding to dentin with resin-based materials in recent years has increased, as improvements have been made in reliability, bond strength, and simplification of placement techniques. However, these systems remain technique-sensitive for several reasons, such as the need for multiple steps and variations in the bonding substrate, especially dentin. Recently, several manufacturers have introduced resin-based adhesives that combine the etching, priming, and bonding steps into a single application. These all-in-one systems are simpler to use and less technique-sensitive because they eliminate the washing and drying steps. However, it has also been reported that all-in-one systems do not adhere as well to dentin that has a thick smear layer produced by an instrument such as a coarse diamond stone. Adhesion problems may also occur on sclerotic dentin found on the surface of noncarious cervical lesions. However, few clinical trials of these all-in-one bonding systems have been reported. The 1-year results of a clinical trial of an all-in-one bonding system with a resin composite placed in nonundercut noncarious cervical lesions were assessed.

Methods.—The trial included 51 nonundercut, noncarious cervical lesions restored with an all-in-one bonding system and a resin composite in 15 patients with a mean age of 57.5 years. The restorations were evaluated at 6 months and at 1 year for their presence or absence and for marginal staining in comparison with standardized color photographs.

Results.—At 1 year, of 51 restorations, 42 (82%) were intact and available for evaluation. A slight degree of marginal staining was observed around 3 restorations, but this staining was determined to have no clinical significance.

Conclusions.—The all-in-one bonding system with the resin composite assessed in this study is a promising material for the restoration of noncarious cervical lesions.

▶ This article reports the clinical effectiveness of a self-etching bonding agent in noncarious cervical lesions. Fifty-one Palfique Estilite composite resin restorations were examined at 1 year and evaluated using color photographs. At 1 year, 46 of the original 51 restorations were examined with 100% retention. Although I question whether 1-year studies should be published routinely, this article provides one of a very few clinical studies on self-etching bonding agents. My advice is to wait until clinical trials prove the effectiveness of self-etching adhesives. To date, there are not enough clinical data to support their use. Why experiment on your patients with unproven bonding agents?

J. O. Burgess, DDS, MS

Effect of Self-Etching Primer Application Method on Enamel Bond Strength

Miyazaki M, Hinoura K, Honjo G, et al (Nihon Univ, Tokyo)
Am J Dent 15:412-416, 2002   1–2

Background.—Self-etching primer systems have been developed to simplify and shorten bonding procedures. Self-etching 2-step bonding agents simultaneously demineralize and prime the tooth surface with acidic monomers followed by bonding agent penetration into tooth substrate. Concern has been expressed regarding the durability of enamel bonding with self-etching primer systems, as they do not use phosphoric acid for etching enamel. The hypothesis was that the bond to enamel with self-etching primers could be increased with agitation during their application.

Methods.—Five commercial self-etching primer systems—Imperva Fluoro Bond, Mac Bond II, Clearfil Liner Bond II Σ, Clearfil SE Bond, and Unifil Bond—were used in this investigation. Bovine mandibular incisors were mounted in self-curing resin, and the facial enamel surfaces were ground wet on 600-grit SiC paper. Self-etching primers were applied either with no agitation (inactive) or with agitation by brush (active), and resin-based composites were condensed into the mold on the enamel surface and light cured. Fifteen specimens per test group were stored in 37°C water for 24 hours, or followed by 3000 or 10,000 thermal cycles and subjected to shear tests at a crosshead speed of 1 mm/min.

Results.—Active application provided greater bond strengths than inactive application. Significant differences were noted in bond strength among the Fluoro Bond, Mac Bond II, and Unifil Bond systems in active versus inactive application.

Conclusions.—Active application of self-etching primer improves bond strength of some self-etching materials.

▶ The newest bonding agents are the sixth-generation or self-etching bonding agents, which eliminate the etch-and-rinse step. This article measured the shear bond strength to bovine enamel when the self-etching bonding agents (Imperva Fluoro Bond, Mac Bond II, Clearfil Liner Bond II Σ, Clearfil SE Bond and UniFil Bond) were applied with and without agitation. Bond strength was measured at 24 hours and after 3000 and 10,000 thermocycles. Agitation increased the enamel shear bond strength for all materials except Clearfil SE Bond when the adhesive was applied following the manufacturers' directions. As a general rule, apply self-etching bonding agents to enamel with agitation.

J. O. Burgess, DDS, MS

The Effect of Current-Generation Bonding Systems on Microleakage of Resin Composite Restorations

Yazici AR, Baseran M, Dayangaç B (Hacettepe Univ, Ankara, Turkey)
Quintessence Int 33:763-769, 2002   1–3

Background.—The marginal seal of a restoration has a direct effect on the success and longevity of that restoration. Good marginal adaptation to the tooth structure reduces marginal discoloration, secondary caries, postoperative sensitivity, and pulpal irritation related to microleakage. Microleakage of resin composites has been a significant concern for clinicians, particularly with respect to restorations having margins located in dentin. Adequate bonding of resin composite to enamel is achieved by acid etching, a clinically proven technique; however, dentin bonding is more complicated because of its composition and histologic structure. The microleakage of current-generation dentin bonding systems in Class II resin composite restorations was determined.

Methods.—The study was conducted on 70 noncarious extracted human premolar teeth. Class II (occlusodistal or occlusomedial) cavity preparations with a gingival margin 2 mm apical to the cementoenamel junction were prepared, and the prepared teeth were randomly divided into 5 groups and treated with different-generation bonding systems. These systems included the Optibond FL, Gluma One Bond, Clearfil SE Bond, acid etching plus Clearfil SE Bond, and Prompt L-Pop. All of the cavities were restored with a posterior resin composite and thermocycled 200 cycles at 5°C to 55°C. The teeth were immersed in 0.5% basic fuchsin dye for 24 hours, sectioned longitudinally, and evaluated for dye penetration.

Results.—No statistically significant differences were observed in the degree of microleakage in the occlusal walls. For the gingival walls, statistically significant differences were observed only between the Clearfil SE Bond and the Prompt L-Pop groups and between the Clearfil SE Bond with acid etching and Prompt L-Pop groups. The greatest amount of microleakage was found in the Prompt L-Pop specimens.

Conclusions.—Most of the 5 dentin bonding systems included in this test were able to eliminate microleakage completely in the occlusal walls, yet some systems showed statistically significant differences in the amount of leakage in the gingival walls.

▶ This article examined the microleakage of fourth-, fifth- and sixth-generation bonding agents. As I define classes of bonding agents (which differs from the authors), Optibond FL is a fourth-generation (etch, prime and bond) system using 3 bottles. Gluma One is a fifth-generation system using 2 steps (etch and bond) requiring 2 bottles. Clearfil SE Bond and Prompt L-Pop are self-etching systems that do not use a separate etch and rinse step. Most researchers believe that the bond and seal to intact enamel is poor with self-etching bonding agents. This article is significant in that it reports no improvement in the leakage of Clearfil SE Bond when the enamel is etched with phosphoric acid prior to placing the SE Bond. SE Bond is an interesting bonding agent and seems to be the best of the self-etching bonding agents. A number of abstracts published in the *Journal of Dental Research* last year report that SE Bond bonds to intact and ground enamel equally well.

J. O. Burgess, DDS, MS

Microleakage of Adhesive Resin Systems in the Primary and Permanent Dentitions

Schmitt DC, Lee J (Univ of the Pacific, Calif; San Clemente, Calif)
Pediatr Dent 24:587-593, 2002   1–4

Introduction.—A crucial characteristic of dental restorative materials is their marginal integrity along the tooth restorative interface. The in vitro microleakage of fourth-generation filled and unfilled dentin bonding systems was compared with fifth-generation filled and unfilled adhesive resin bonding systems and examined in both primary and permanent teeth.

Methods.—Eighty extracted or exfoliated human noncarious teeth (40 primary and 40 permanent) were placed in 1 of 8 groups. Groups 1, 3, 5, and 7 were primary teeth; groups 2, 4, 6, and 8 were permanent teeth. Groups 1 and 2 were bonded with Optibond FL (Kerr), groups 3 and 4 were bonded with Scotchbond Multipurpose (3M).

All teeth received a Class V cavity preparation and the cavosurface margins were positioned entirely in enamel. They were restored with TPH Spectrum Shade A1 (Dentsply Caulk). All teeth were thermocycled, stained with basic fuchsin, sectioned, and examined under the microscope. Measurements were documented in absolute millimeters and relative grades as determined by 2 evaluators.

Results.—There were no significant differences in microleakage between the fourth- and fifth-generation adhesive resin systems ($P = .1447$), whether filled or unfilled or applied on primary or permanent teeth ($P = .6308$). There were significant differences in the amount of microleakage at the gingival and occlusal surfaces in all groups ($P = .0001$). The 1-bottle, fifth-generation adhesive resin systems allowed easier application with the same effectiveness as the 2-bottle, fourth-generation systems.

Conclusion.—There was no significant difference in microleakage between the fourth- and fifth-generation dentin bonding systems, whether filled or unfilled or applied to primary or permanent teeth. There were significant differences for all groups in the amount of microleakage at the gingival and occlusal surfaces. One-bottle, fifth-generation adhesive resin systems allow easier application with the same effectiveness as the 2-bottle, fourth-generation systems.

▶ Adhesive systems have become simpler and easier to use. However, their indications for use have become more limited. As an example, many single fifth-generation and self-etching sixth-generation systems provide little or no bond strength when chemical or dark set, duel-cured restoratives are used. This is encountered with core buildup procedures, where the core will fall off when the tooth is prepared. Numerous clinical trials have shown that multi-component systems outperform fifth- and sixth-generation systems. But several in vitro studies, including the results of this study, demonstrate that bond strength to dentin is comparable to earlier systems. The results of laboratory investigations can only provide the comparative performance of materials tested. The true behavior of a restorative material can only be determined by controlled clinical trials.

A. A. Boghosian, DDS

Dentin Permeability: Self-Etching and One-Bottle Dentin Bonding Systems

Grégoire G, Joniot S, Guignes P, et al (Univ of Toulouse III, France)
J Prosthet Dent 90:42-49, 2003   1–5

Background.—A variety of dentin bonding systems have been developed by manufacturers as dental practitioners have increased their understanding of the chemical, biological, and physical complexities of dentin, collagen, and the smear layer. Bonding systems are available with or without a prior acid etch. Clinicians must be aware of the most effective systems and which will provide the best seal. The infiltration of physiologic saline solution across dentin disks after application of self-etching or 1-bottle total-etch bonding systems was measured.

Methods.—One-mm-thick dentin disks were cut from 36 extracted noncarious human third molars. Segments parallel to the occlusal surface in the incisal portion of the pulp cavity were tested. The 36 disks were divided into 6 groups, each of which tested with 1 of the following 6 dentin bonding systems: (1) Optibond Solo Plus, (2) Excite, (3) Prime & Bond NT, (4) Single Bond, (5) Clearfil SE Bond, and (6) Prompt L-Pop. The first 4 bonding agents were total-etch adhesives while systems (5) and (6) were self-etching systems. Hydraulic conductance measurements were made by recording the volume of saline passing through the 1-mm disks. Both sides of each dentin disk were etched with 36% phosphoric acid for 30 seconds and measurements made every 30 seconds for 15 minutes. The initial measurement was used as the reference value for each specimen. The measurements were repeated after formation of a smear layer and again after the bonding agent was applied.

Results.—The 4 systems with conventional phosphoric acid etching—Optibond Solo Plus, Single Bond, Excite, and Prime & Bond NT—provided the greatest mean reduction (40%) of saline through the dentin. The 2 self-etching systems reduced saline passage by 36% (Prompt L-Pop) and 16% (Clearfil SE Bond). With the exception of Single Bond and the Prime & Bond NT groups, standard deviations were as high as 50% of the mean.

Conclusions.—The 4 bonding systems using conventional etching provided a greater decrease in dentin permeability than the 2 self-etching systems tested. Permeability decrease was significantly less for the Prompt L-Pop system compared with all other systems tested.

▶ This study measured and compared the fluid movement through dentin when the dentin was coated with 4 total-etch 2-step bonding agents and 2 self-etching bonding agents. Prompt L-Pop had the least reduction and may not be useful for hypersensitive root surfaces.

J. O. Burgess, DDS, MS

Four-Year Water Degradation of Total-Etch Adhesives Bonded to Dentin
De Munck J, Van Meerbeek B, Yoshida Y, et al (Catholic Univ of Leuven, Belgium; Okayama Univ, Japan; Hokkaido Univ, Sapporo, Japan; et al)
J Dent Res 82:136-140, 2003   1–6

Background.—Most total-etch adhesives on the market today perform well in bond strength tests, at least when tested shortly after application and under controlled in vitro conditions. However, the oral cavity presents a daunting restorative challenge, with temperature extremes, chewing loads, and chemical challenges from acids and enzymes. Marginal deterioration of composite restorations occurs and significantly shortens restoration lifetime. Exposure to water is one of the factors known to degrade tooth-composite bonds. During the total-etch procedure, phosphoric acid-etching almost completely removes hydroxyapatite surrounding collagen, allowing resin monomers to infiltrate, wet, and interact with hydroxyapatite-depleted collagen. Unfortunately, incomplete hybridization, which leaves collagen unprotected and vulnerable to hydrolytic degeneration, frequently occurs.

Methods.—The study tested 2 hypotheses: (1) no degradation of microtensile bond strength to dentin will be observed between 2-step and 3-step total-etch adhesives and (2) a composite-enamel bond will protect the adjacent composite-dentin bond against degradation. Quantitative and qualitative failure analyses were performed by correlating field-emission scanning electron microscopy (Fe-SEM) and transmission electron microscopy (TEM).

Results.—No significant reduction was noted in the microtensile bond strength of any adhesive after indirect exposure to water. In contrast, direct exposure resulted in a significant reduction in the microtensile bond strength of both 2-step adhesives tested.

Conclusions.—Resin bonded to enamel seals and protects the resin-dentin bond against degradation, while 4-year direct exposure to water adversely affects bonds created with 2-step total-etch adhesive systems.

▶ This article expands past work by others showing that the bond of composite resins to tooth declines with water storage time. Using two 2-step (Optibond Solo and Single Bond) and two 3-step (Optibond Dual Cure and Scotchbond MP) total-etch adhesives, specimens were bonded and stored in water for 4 years, and then microtensile testing was completed. Direct exposure to water decreased the bond strength of the 2-step but not the 3-step adhesives. Internal sections of the tooth, those dentin surfaces not exposed directly to water since they were protected by an enamel bond and seal, did not have a decline. As this study demonstrates, long-term bonding to enamel with bonding agents is successful. However, bonding to dentin as in a restoration with a gingival margin ending in dentin is not stable with newer bonding agents. Older total-etch bonding agents provide better long-term bonds to dentin. As with many newer products, simplified bonding agents, such as the fifth-generation, 2-step systems used here are not advances. Newer does not always mean better. In our efforts to use the newest materials, we may be producing less-durable restorations.

J. O. Burgess, DDS, MS

Effect of Changing Application Times on Adhesive Systems Bond Strengths

Nour El-Din AK, Abd El-Mohsen MM (Baylor College of Dentistry, Texas)
Am J Dent 15:321-324, 2002   1–7

Background.—The efficacy of an adhesive system to dentin surfaces is determined by its bonding ability and sealing capacity. Intertubular and intratubular resin penetration are thus very important to achieving effective dentin bonding. Infiltration of resin is controlled by several parameters, the most important ones being the permeability of the dentin substrate, the diffusibility of the resin monomer, and the techniques of application. One technique that may optimize resin monomer infiltration and, thus, create more stable and stronger bonds is lengthening the application time. The effects of increasing the priming time and the adhesive curing time on the shear bond strength of the new dentin bonding systems were determined.

Methods.—This study evaluated 2 multistep total-etch dentin bonding systems (Scotchbond Multi-Purpose Plus [SBMP+] and Optibond FL [OB FL]) and one 1-bottle total-etch dental bonding system (Single Bond). One hundred flat dentin specimens were prepared for extracted human molars. Superficial dentin was exposed and the specimens were randomly assigned to the 3 bonding systems, with at least 5 specimens used for each test condition. For the multistep systems, 40 specimens were divided into 4 groups with priming times of 10, 20, 30, and 40 seconds, and each group was further subdivided into 2 subgroups with adhesive resin precuring times of 20 and 40 seconds. The Single Bond specimens were divided into 4 subgroups with a waiting time of 10, 20, 30, and 40 seconds before drying and curing of its 1-bottle adhesive. A universal testing machine was used to test shear bond strength at a crosshead speed of 0.5 mm/min. The results were analyzed using analysis of variance and Duncan's multiple-range tests.

Results.—For the multistep bonding systems, increasing the priming time up to 30 or 40 seconds resulted in a significant increase in the mean shear bond strength values. No significant increase was noted in the mean shear bond strength values as a result of lengthening the adhesive resin precuring time, with the exception of the 30- and 40-second priming times. For the Single Bond system, increasing the 1-bottle adhesive waiting time before drying and curing to 30 seconds provided a statistically significant increase in shear bond strength.

Conclusions.—An increase in the time between primer application and drying (the priming time) can provide a significant increase in the shear bond strength values, which may be clinically significant. The values obtained in this study were above the bond strength of 20 MPa that was thought to be the minimum strength necessary to resist polymerization shrinkage.

▶ This article examines the hypothesis that one 2-step (Single Bond) and two 3-step (Scotchbond MP and Optibond FL) total-etch bonding agents would have higher bond strengths with longer application times of the primer or with longer adhesive curing times. Once again, the bond strength of the "simplified" newer bonding agent was less than the older 3-step bonding agents. Increased application times increased bond strength when curing time was increased. Having control over the priming and curing steps is a significant advantage with total-etch 3-step bonding agents. Although it was not stated in this article, I would assume that the curing light guide was placed against the bonding surface. I wonder if the bond strength would have decreased more if the light had been placed 5 or 6 mm away from the bonding surface. This would be the clinical case when curing the adhesive on the gingival margin.

J. O. Burgess, DDS, MS

Hybridization Efficiency of the Adhesive/Dentin Interface With Wet Bonding
Wang Y, Spencer P (Univ of Missouri-Kansas City)
J Dent Res 82:141-145, 2003   1–8

Background.—The strength of the adhesive-dentin bond is dependent on the quality of the hybrid layer. Ideally, the adhesive monomers will surround the collagen fibers exposed after removal of the mineral by acid etching. However, recent studies have shown that this objective is frequently not achieved, and it is unclear how well the resin monomers seal the dentin collagen fibrils under wet bonding conditions. The quality and molecular structure of adhesive/dentin (a/d) interfaces formed with wet bonding were compared with those of adhesive-infiltrated demineralized dentin (AIDD) produced under controlled conditions with optimum hybridization.

Methods.—The study was conducted on 6 extracted unerupted human third human molars stored at 4°C in 0.9% weight per volume of NaCl containing 0.002% sodium azide. One fraction was obtained from each tooth and demineralized, dehydrated, and infiltrated with Single Bond adhesive under optimum conditions. The remaining adjacent fraction was treated with Single Bond by wet bonding. The AIDD and a/d interface sections were stained with Goldner's trichrome, and corresponding sections were analyzed with micro-Raman spectroscopy.

Results.—Under wet bonding, the a/d is not an impervious collagen/polymer network but rather a porous web composed predominantly of collagen and 2-hydroxyethyl methacrylate (HEMA), with lesser amounts of the BisGMA component. The collagen fibers at the base of the demineralized dentin were not fully enveloped by either the HEMA or the BisGMA.

Conclusions.—The histomorphologic and spectroscopic findings suggest that the a/d interface under wet bonding is a porous collagen web that is primarily infiltrated by HEMA and that BisGMA, the critical dimethacrylate component that is the greatest contributing factor to the crosslinked polymeric adhesive, infiltrates only a fraction of the total wet, demineralized, intertubular dentin layer.

▶ This article provides significant insight to the problems with bonding systems. Clinicians experience frustration with bonding systems when patients return with complaints of postoperative sensitivity, especially with posterior composite resin restorations. This study measured and quantified the amount of primer and adhesive that penetrated and surrounded demineralized dentin. Using 1 bonding agent (Single Bond), the authors produced a 6-µm-thick demineralized layer of dentin, applied the Single Bond, and polymerized the adhesive. They were able to measure with good precision the amount of penetration of the bonding agent into the demineralized dentin and the amount that surrounded the collagen. Their results clearly demonstrate that the bottom of the hybrid layer is porous, only partially encasing the exposed collagen fibers. This probably produces a layer that leaks with time and allows the bond to degrade. Single Bond (and most commonly used fifth-generation bonding agents) is composed of HEMA and Bis-GMA. The HEMA component of the bonding agent penetrated further than the Bis-GMA component. At the base of the demineralized dentin, neither HEMA nor the Bis-GMA totally encased the collagen fibers. This is an excellent article that should be reviewed by anyone interested in bonding mechanisms.

J. O. Burgess, DDS, MS

Effect of Multiple Application of a Dentin Adhesive on Contraction Gap Width of a Resin-Based Composite

Koike T, Hasegawa T, Itoh K, et al (Showa Univ, Tokyo)
Am J Dent 15:159-163, 2002   1–9

Introduction.—The most important role of the dentin bonding system is maintaining the dentin bonding system between the unpolymerized resin-based composite paste and the dentin cavity wall until completion of the polymerization of the resin-based composite. The efficacy of the multiple application of a total-etch dentin adhesive was examined by determining (1) the contraction gap width of a light-activated resin-based composite in a cylindrical dentin cavity and (2) the early tensile bond strength to a flat dentin surface with the Single Bond Dental Adhesive System.

Methods.—The contraction gap width was measured in a cylindrical dentin cavity (3×1.5 mm) treated with either a single coat or double coat of the Single Bond adhesive and restored with Silux Plus or Z-100. For the control, the cavity was treated with an experimental dentin bonding system composed of ethylenediamine tetraacetic acid (EDTA), 35% GM, and Clearfil Photo Bond. Early tensile bond strengths of Silux Plus or Z-100 were ascertained on the flat dentin surface treated with the 3 bonding procedures as in the contraction gap experiment within 10 minutes after final cure.

Results.—The contraction gap of Silux Plus and Z-100 was prevented by the double coats of the Single Bond adhesive. The contraction gap of Z-100 was not prevented by the single coat of the Single Bond and the experimental system. When the film thickness of the Single Bond system was below 2 μm, the gap was not averted. The tensile bond strengths of Silux Plus and Z-100 to flat dentin mediated with the 3 bonding procedures were not significantly different ($P > .05$).

Conclusion.—Bonding efficacy of the total-etch, blot dry, and multiple bonding application system was definitely better than the experimental bonding system because contraction gap formation of the Z-100 was completely prevented. Acid etching on the dentin cavity wall creates a collagen-rich layer on the superficial substrate dentin. Nanoleakage is possibly seen when monomer infiltration or water replacement is not adequate. Such a leakage on the bottom of the hybrid layer may produce serious secondary caries, which are commonly seen in the clinical cases of the adhesive bridge.

▶ "If the liquid adhesive does not wet the surface of the adherend. . .then the adhesion between the liquid and the adherend will be negligible or nonexistent." This statement was taken from chapter 2 of the seventh edition of *Skinner's Science of Dental Materials*, authored by the late Ralph Phillips and published in 1973. A decade after that quote, the first dentin adhesive was introduced on the market. It was 2 decades later that consistently effective adhesives were made available for bonding procedures. While the chemical composition has changed over the years, the principles of adhesion as quoted in 1973 have not. This study finds that the resistance to microleakage improves with the placement of a second coat of adhesive. Single-component adhesives, such as the one investigated in this study, as well as some self-etching adhesives do not always provide an adequately coated or sufficiently thick enough layer to permit adequate sealing or bonding to composite. This issue does not exist with the multicomponent systems. Furthermore, multicomponent adhesives have greater versatility than simplified systems, with far fewer indication restrictions. While simplicity is always welcome, efficacy should not be compromised.

A. A. Boghosian, DDS

Bond Strength to Primary Tooth Dentin Following Disinfection With a Chlorhexidine Solution: An In Vitro Study

de Sousa Vieira R, da Silva IA Jr (Santa Catarina Federal Univ, Florianópolis, Brazil)

Pediatr Dent 25:49-52, 2003   1–10

Background.—Enamel adhesion using acid etching is a well-established technique in restorative dentistry. However, the search continues for adhesive systems that bond efficiently with dentin. Some bonding agents bond effectively, but bacteria left under restorations may be a source of secondary decay. Antibacterial solutions have been studied as an alternative procedure for reduction and elimination of bacteria from cavity preparations. The effect on shear bond strength of chlorhexidine used as a cavity disinfectant on primary tooth dentin was determined.

Methods.—The study included 30 teeth divided into 3 groups. In group 1, the dentin was acid etched with a 37% phosphoric acid for 15 seconds and then washed and dried. In group 2, a commercial chlorhexidine solution (Cav Clean) was applied for 40 seconds, washed, and dried after acid etching for 15 seconds. In group 3, dentin was treated with a 37% phosphoric acid gel containing 2% digluconate of chlorhexidine (Cond AC) for 15 seconds. Single Bond adhesive was applied to all specimens, and composite cylinders were built. A universal testing machine was used to shear the specimens at a crosshead speed of 0.5 mm/min, and results were calculated in MPa. The failure mode was also recorded.

Results.—Analysis of variance indicated the mean shear bond strength of group 2 (17.99 MPa) was significantly less than that of group 1 (19.88 MPa) and group 3 (19.57 MPa). After debonding, cohesive failure of the material was observed in 63% of specimens, adhesive failure in 24%, and cohesive failure of dentin in 10%.

Conclusions.—The dentin adhesive Single Bond is adversely affected by a cavity disinfectant with 2% chlorhexidine, with significantly less shear bond strength than the etch gel with chlorhexidine and the acid etch alone.

▶ This article tested the shear bond strength of Single Bond, a 2-step total-etch bonding system, to dentin in primary teeth when the teeth were disinfected with chlorhexidine. In this study, the disinfectant was applied in the etchant and as a separate step following etching. When the chlorhexidine was applied as a separate step, it decreased bond strength. The question is why was this testing done and why was it accepted for publication? It is well established that phosphoric acid is an effective antimicrobial agent. So why test other antimicrobial agents and increase the application time for the bonding procedure? Once bacteria are dead, they are dead, and another step to kill them is unnecessary, time consuming, and expensive.

J. O. Burgess, DDS, MS

Effects of HEMA/Solvent Combinations on Bond Strength to Dentin

Carvalho RM, Mendonca JS, Santiago SL, et al (Univ of São Paulo, Brazil; Univ of Hong Kong; Med College of Georgia, Augusta)
J Dent Res 82:591-601, 2003   1–11

Background.—Air drying demineralized dentin matrix may collapse the collagen matrix up to 65 vol%. This shrinkage causes a reduction in the interfibrillar spaces that serve as diffusion channels for resin infiltration, which compromises hybrid layer formation and bonding of adhesive systems to dentin. One approach to preventing collagen collapse is to rewet the dentin surface with water before bonding. Another approach is to use a bonding agent that contains water or other strong H-bonding solvents that are capable of breaking interpeptide collagen hydrogen bonds formed when collagen collapses as in dried dentin. Other adhesives use ethanol or acetone as solvents, rather than water. When these water-free adhesives are applied to demineralized, dried, collapsed dentin, the re-expansion will be dependent on the ability of solvents or monomers to associate with collagen and break interpeptide hydrogen bonds. The hypothesis that dentin bond strengths are dependent on the ability of experimental 2-hydroxy-ethyl-methacrylate (HEMA)/solvent primers to re-expand the collagen matrix was tested.

Methods.—Dentin surfaces were acid-etched with 37% phosphoric acid for 20 seconds, air-dried for 30 seconds, primed with either 35%/65% (v/v) HEMA/water, HEMA/methanol, HEMA/ethanol, or HEMA/propanol for 60 seconds, and bonded with 4-methacryloyloxyethyl trimellitate anhydride-tri-*n*-butyl borane (4-META-TBBO) adhesive. The samples were stored in water for 1 day and then prepared for microtensile bond strength testing. Transmission electron microscopy was used to measure the width of interfibrillar spaces in the hybrid layers.

Results.—The HEMA/ethanol primer produced the highest bond strength, and the HEMA/propanol primer produced the lowest bond strength. A direct correlation was noted between the bond strengths and the width of the interfibrillar spaces.

Conclusions.—The solubility parameters of HEMA/solvent mixtures have a significant effect on bond strengths to dentin. The challenge to manufacturers is to develop products that include solvents with the ability to maintain the structure of the demineralized dentin matrix in an expanded configuration during and after resin infiltration.

▶ The amount of dentin wetness that will produce the best bond strength has been examined in multiple articles. This well-written article examines the microtensile bond strength to dentin when the solvent in the bonding agent was changed from ethanol, to methanol, to water, and to propanol. Since drying causes collagen collapse and a significant reduction in bond strength after phosphoric acid etching and rinsing, techniques have developed to prevent overdrying demineralized dentin. This article demonstrates that while water-based materials are helpful, they will not eliminate the problems associated with overdrying. Best is to use the high-volume suction to remove excess moisture after rinsing and avoid overdrying dentin.

J. O. Burgess, DDS, MS

Aging Affects Two Modes of Nanoleakage Expression in Bonded Dentin
Tay FR, Hashimoto M, Pashley DH, et al (Univ of Hong Kong; Hokkaido Univ, Japan; Med College of Georgia, Augusta; et al)
J Dent Res 82:537-541, 2003   1–12

Background.—Hydrolytic degradation of resin-dentin interfaces is a factor in the reduction of bond strengths created by dentin adhesives. This degradation is aggravated by the incorporation of hydrophilic and ionic resin monomers into contemporary adhesives because hydrophilicity and hydrolytic stability of resin monomers are generally antagonistic properties. Hydrolytic degradation cannot occur in the absence of water uptake in bonded interfaces. The hypothesis that water sorption and hydrolytic degradation are morphologically manifest by the uptake of ammoniacal silver nitrate, which traces hydrophilic areas and water-filled channels within matrices was tested. It is thought that water sorption is nonuniform and can be traced by the use of silver nitrate.

Methods.—The study included 10 extracted human third molars that were bonded with an experimental filled adhesive and aged in artificial saliva or nonaqueous mineral oil (control specimens). Specimens immersed in 50% wt/vol ammoniacal silver nitrate for up to 12 months were examined for changes in silver nitrate uptake.

Results.—In the teeth aged in artificial saliva, reticular silver deposits initially identified within the bulk of hybrid layers were gradually reduced over time but later replaced by similar deposits located along the hybrid layer-adhesive interface. With aging, the silver uptake in the water-binding domain of the adhesive layers increased, an effect that resulted in water tree formation.

Conclusions.—Leakage can contribute to a decrease in bond strength at resin-dentin interfaces. The water-filled channels that form in the hybrid layer may function as sites of hydrolytic degradation of the resin-dentin bond.

▶ This is one of the first articles to describe the mechanism of declining bond strengths in dentin bonding. Using an experimental bonding agent, the authors bonded to dentin, aged half the specimens, and then examined them with transmission electron microscopy. The results demonstrate that bonds to dentin degrade over time by the formation of water channels. Since Wang and Spenser (Abstract 1–8) have demonstrated that the hybrid layer is porous, the formation and expansion of "water channels" and "water trees" are reasonable to describe the formation of water within the hybrid layer. Exposing collagen to water produces breakdown in the hybrid layer, resulting in lower dentin bond strength with time. The channels are produced through several mechanisms, but poor agitation of the bonding agent, poor curing of the adhesive, and the adhesive composition all play a role in the breakdown. This is an important finding and furthers the science of our knowledge of dentin bonding.

J. O. Burgess, DDS, MS

Contraction Stress of Flowable Composite Materials and Their Efficacy as Stress-Relieving Layers

Braga RR, Hilton TJ, Ferracane JL (Depto. de Materials Dentarios da FOUSP, São Paulo, Brazil; Oregon Health and Science Univ, Portland)
J Am Dent Assoc 134:721-728, 2003   1–13

Introduction.—The stress created by polymerization contraction of resin-based composite material is the first threat to a restoration's marginal integrity. Flowable composites were evaluated to determine whether they produce lower polymerization contraction stress, compared to nonflowable composites. Also examined was whether the use of a precured layer of flowable composite material can significantly decrease the contraction stress produced by a subsequent increment of nonflowable composite material.

Methods.—Four flowable and 6 nonflowable composite materials were evaluated for contraction stress in a tensiometer. A 1.4-mL–thick layer of flowable composite or unfilled resin was applied and precured in the test apparatus to evaluate the stress relief provided by a low-modulus material during light curing of a subsequent layer of highly filled composite. The flexible moduli of the precured materials were ascertained via a 3-point bending test.

Results.—The range of stress values was 6.04 to 9.10 MPa. No significant differences were seen in stress between flowable and nonflowable composites. The microfilled composites created lower contraction stress, compared to hybrids. The flexural modulus of the flowable composites varied between 4.1 and 8.2 GPa. The stress was 42% lower when a precured layer of nonflowable composite material was used. Stress reduction was significant for only 1 of the flowable materials (Filtek Flow).

Conclusion.—The flowable composites created stress levels similar to those of nonflowable materials. Most of the flowable materials did not provide significant stress reduction when used under a nonflowable composite. The use of a flowable resin-based composite for restorative material is not likely to decrease the effects of polymerization stress. Stress reduction depended on the elastic modulus of the lining material when a thin layer was used under a nonflowable composite.

▶ The next abstract (Abstract 1–14) examined the issue of fracture toughness of flowable composite restoratives. This is a highly important consideration when a flowable material is used as a posterior restorative. Flowable composites are also used as liners, presumably acting as a mitigator of marginal interface stress resulting from polymerization shrinkage of the restorative.

This study concludes that flowable composites placed as a liner do not appreciably reduce the contraction stress produced from the polymerization of the overlaying composite restorative. In the opinion of the authors, the major benefit derived by the use of a flowable composite or filled adhesive is ease in obtaining the complete coverage of the tooth structure. When placing a viscous posterior restorative material in a deep Class II cavity, it is often difficult to avoid air entrapment at the proximal box line angles. The use of a flowable material before the placement of a high-viscosity restorative can greatly assist in achieving an adequate cavity seal.

A. A. Boghosian, DDS

Fracture Toughness of Nine Flowable Resin Composites
Bonilla ED, Yashar M, Caputo AA (Univ of California at Los Angeles)
J Prosthet Dent 89:261-267, 2003   1–14

Introduction.—Flowable composites are used in many different clinical applications. The ability of these materials to resist crack propagation is not well described. The resistance to crack propagation, as measured by the fracture toughness, was compared in 9 flowable composites.

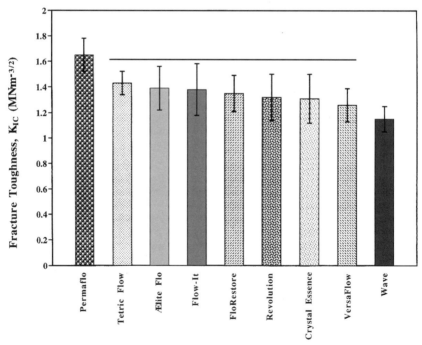

FIGURE 5.—Mean fracture toughness values for 9 flowable composites tested. *Vertical bars* represent ± 1 standard deviation. The *horizontal bar* connects groups of materials that were not statistically significantly different ($P < .05$). (Reprinted by permission of the publisher from Bonilla ED, Yashar M, Caputo AA: Fracture toughness of nine flowable resin composites. *J Prosthet Dent* 89:261-267, 2003. Copyright 2003 by Elsevier.)

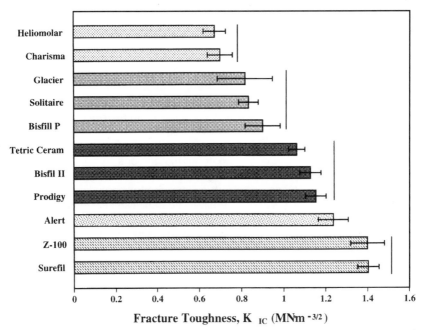

FIGURE 7.—Fracture toughness values for several packable composite restorative resins. *Horizontal lines* represent ± standard deviation. Groups of materials not statistically different (*P* < .05) are connected by *vertical bars.* Data adapted from Bonilla ED, Mardirossian G, Caputo AA: Fracture toughness of posterior resin composites. *Quintessence Int* 32:206-210, 2001. (Reprinted by permission of the publisher from Bonilla ED, Yashar M, Caputo AA: Fracture toughness of nine flowable resin composites. *J Prosthet Dent* 89:261-267, 2003. Copyright 2003 by Elsevier.)

Methods.—The 9 composites were: AeliteFlo, Crystal Essence, Flow-It, FloRestore, Permaflo, Revolution, Tetric Flow, VersaFlow, and Wave. Ten specimens of each composite were created with a brass mold used with a 3-mm preformed notch. The final dimensions of each specimen were 2 × 4.2 × 20 mm. Each specimen was light polymerized to manufacturer specifications and stored in air for 24 hours. The fracture toughness value, K_{IC} (MNm$^{-3/2}$), for every specimen was determined via a 3-point bending mode and a single-edge notched beam at a crosshead speed of 0.125 mm/min until fracture.

Results.—The flowable composites had a spectrum of fracture toughness with mean significant differences that ranged from 1.15 ± 0.10 MNm$^{-3/2}$ for Wave to 1.65 ± 0.13 MNm$^{-3/2}$ for Permaflo (*P* < .05) (Fig 5). The remaining materials made up 1 group with intermediate K_{IC} values that were similar (*P* > .05) to each other yet were significantly different from Wave and Permaflo. Comparisons of fracture toughness with the filler content by volume of each composite showed no correlation. The K_{IC} values of Permaflo and Tetric Flow were higher, compared to the hybrid and packable posterior composites (Fig 7).

Conclusion.—There were no significant differences among 7 of the 9 evaluated composites in their resistance to fracture. Permaflo had the greatest resistance to crack propagation. There was no association between the filler content by volume and the fracture toughness of these flowable composites.

▶ All dental restorative materials must satisfy 2 fundamental requirements. They must possess adequate physical properties and have suitable handling characteristics for them to be properly placed. Flowable composite materials were developed to restore microcavity preparations and be used as cavity liners since traditional hybrid composites are difficult to use in these applications. Similarly, packable composites were developed to assist in obtaining better interproximal contacts with posterior restorations.

This study shows that fracture toughness does not increase with higher filler concentrations. Based on this study, one might conclude that flowable composites can be successfully used in all posterior applications. However, the resistance to wear of flowable composites is significantly poorer than for macrofilled composites. Therefore, their use should be limited to only very conservative restorations in the posterior.

A. A. Boghosian, DDS

Marginal and Internal Adaption of Class II Restorations After Immediate or Delayed Composite Placement
Dietschi D, Monasevic M, Krejci I, et al (Univ of Geneva; Academic Ctr for Dentistry Amsterdam)
J Dent 30:259-269, 2002   1–15

Introduction.—Composite polymerization shrinkage has been decreased in modern composite formulations, yet it continues to be challenging, especially when proximal limits extend below the cementum-enamel junction. The influence of the delay in adhesive application and composite buildup on restoration adaptation was examined in Class II restorations.

Methods.—The root length of freshly extracted human third molars was adjusted to fit into a test chamber of a mechanical loading device. After proper positioning, the specimens were fixed with light-curing composite on a metallic holder. The root base was embedded with self-curing acrylic resin to complete tooth stabilization. Box-shaped Class II cavities with parallel walls and beveled enamel margins were prepared and randomly assigned to 1 of 4 experimental groups corresponding to the 2 adhesive systems and the delay in composite placement.

All cavities were filled by means of a horizontal layering technique immediately after adhesive placement (IP) or after a 24-hour delay (DP). A filled 3-component adhesive (Optibond, Fla; OB) and a single-bottle, unfilled one (Prime & Bond 2:1; PB) were evaluated. Marginal adaptation was examined before and after each phase of mechanical loading (250,000 cycles at 50 N, 250,000 cycles at 75 N, and 500,000 cycles at 100 N).

Internal adaptation was assessed after test completion. Gold-plated resin replicas were examined in the scanning electron microscope, and restorative quality was assessed in the percentages of continuity (C) at the margins and within the internal interface, after sample section.

Results.—Adaptation to beveled enamel was satisfactory in all groups. After loading, the adaptation to gingival dentin degraded more in PB-IP (C = 55.1%) versus PB-DP (C = 86.9%) or OB-DP (C = 89%). More internal defects were seen in PB samples (IP: C = 79.2% and DP: C = 86.3%) versus OB samples (IP: C = 97.4% and DP: C = 98.3%).

Conclusion.—The filled adhesive (OB) allowed a better adaptation, compared with the 1-bottle brand (PB), hypothetically by forming a stress-absorbing layer, thus limiting development of adhesive failures. Postponing occlusal loading (using the indirect approach) also improved restoration adaptation.

▶ Polymerization shrinkage is inherent to any tooth-colored restorative material. A major role of the bonding agent is to compensate for the shrinkage of the composite. The use of a liner or base material between the adhesive and the composite may also provide stress relief from polymerization shrinkage. The application of a liner that serves as an "elastic" material to prevent adhesive failures in Class V restorations has been well documented in the literature. These materials include glass ionomer cement, filled adhesives, and flowable composites.

One significant conclusion from this study suggests that improved internal adaptation to dentin resulted when using a multicomponent adhesive versus a single-bottle system. Achieving a successful result with an adhesive can only be realized if it completely wets out and coats the adherend. Considering this notion, the benefits of providing an "elastic layer" within the restoration might be secondary to attaining a uniformly bonded surface.

A. A. Boghosian, DDS

Dimensional Stability of Dental Restorative Materials and Cements Over Four Years
Hermesch CB, Wall BS, McEntire JF (Univ of Texas, San Antonio)
Gen Dent 51:518-523, 2003   1–16

Background.—Unlike the polymerization shrinkage that occurs in some restorative materials, dimensional expansion has not been well studied. It has been noted in several studies that hygroscopic expansion can compensate for polymerization shrinkage, thereby reducing the size of marginal gaps. This reduction may be favorable to some degree if the expansion is not too great, but the tooth or material may fracture when the hygroscopic expansion exceeds polymerization shrinkage. Hygroscopic expansion can occur for up to 18 months and may last longer. The linear dimensional change of dental restorative materials and cements stored in water for 4 years immediately after curing was determined.

Methods.—The study included 19 commercially available products, representing 7 classes of dental materials. These classes included amalgam, composite resin, resin cement, glass ionomer cement, zinc phosphate cement, compomer, resin-modified glass ionomer cement, and hybrid monomer. Six cylindrical specimens were fabricated for each of the 19 materials, in accordance with the manufacturers' recommendations.

Results.—After 4 years, 5 of the 19 materials manifested net shrinkage, and the remaining 14 materials demonstrated net expansion. This expansion exceeded 3.5% in 1 product, which corresponded to 10% volumetric expansion.

Conclusions.—Many factors must be considered in the selection of dental restorative materials, including the long-term dimensional stability of a material. Some materials introduced recently can expand with time, and it is important that manufacturers, when introducing a new material, provide data on its dimensional stability.

▶ Most esthetic dental restorative materials, especially composite resins, shrink during polymerization. If the material absorbed enough water to balance the shrinkage perfectly, little long-term stress would remain on the restored tooth, but as the literature shows, the shrinkage of composite is greater than the water swelling that occurs after the composite restoration is placed. This article recorded the swelling produced from 19 different materials during 4 years. Excessive swelling can be harmful and can fracture teeth or cemented ceramic crowns. These data should be essential in your decision-making process and should be supplied for every dental cement. Cements with excessive expansion should not be used, especially with ceramic restoration or to cement posts. Some slight expansion with restorative materials is desirable to help seal the restorative margin.

J. O. Burgess, DDS, MS

Effect of Smear Layer on Root Demineralization Adjacent to Resin-Modified Glass Ionomer
AL-Helal AS, Armstrong SR, Xie XJ, et al (Univ of Iowa, Iowa City)
J Dent Res 82:146-150, 2003   1–17

Introduction.—The cariostatic influence of resin-modified glass ionomer (RMGI) on secondary root caries is well known. This beneficial effect may depend on the method of cavity surface treatment. Caries resistance and inhibition zone formation seem to be linked to the amount of fluoride released from glass ionomers and subsequent fluoride uptake by adjacent cavosurfaces.

Two-dimensional mapping by electron probe microanalysis has shown that teeth restored with conventional and resin-modified glass ionomers take up greater amounts of fluoride, with penetration deeper into dentin versus enamel. The potential role of the smear layer on the development and inhibition of secondary root caries adjacent to RMGI was examined.

Methods.—Four cavity surface treatments before placement of RMGI were examined. They were nontreatment, polyacrylic acid, phosphoric acid, and Scotchbond Multi-Purpose adhesive for control. The specimens were aged for 2 weeks in synthetic saliva and thermocycled and underwent an artificial caries challenge (pH 4.4).

Results.—Polarized light microscopy and microradiography revealed significantly less demineralization with the phosphoric acid cavity surface treatment (P = .05 or less). Dentin fluoride profiles ascertained by electron probe microanalysis supported both the polarized light microscopy and microradiography findings.

Conclusion.—Removal of the smear layer with phosphoric acid contributes significantly enhanced resistance to secondary root caries formation adjacent to RMGI restorations.

▶ RMGI restoratives may very well be the most underutilized, clinically proven materials available to the restorative dentist. Their adhesive strength to dentin and enamel is comparable to bonded composite restorations as demonstrated in long-term clinical trial investigations. The therapeutic benefits of fluoride release and uptake inherent to RMGI materials offers a significant advantage when resorting a caries-prone patient. This artificial root-surface caries investigation concludes that the removal of the smear layer enhances the caries resistance of dentin adjacent to RMGI restorations.

Cavity surface pretreatment agents are offered by many manufacturers of RMGI products. Several laboratory investigations have concluded that pretreatment conditioning of dentin may not significantly improve dentin adhesion. However, pretreatment of enamel did significantly increase bond strengths. When considering the results of this investigation and the potential benefits of enhanced surface adhesion, the routine use of pretreatment conditioners is recommended when placing RMGI restorations.

A. A. Boghosian, DDS

A 3-Year Clinical Evaluation of Glass-Ionomer Cements Used as Fissure Sealants

Pereira AC, Pardi V, Mialhe FL, et al (UNICAMP, Piracicaba-SP, Brazil)
Am J Dent 16:23-27, 2003   1–18

Introduction.—Changes in caries prevalence in Brazil and around the world in the past 2 decades are primarily because of water fluoridation and fluoridated dentifrices. The use of sealants, changes in treatment philosophy by dentists, educational procedures for health in dentistry, and changes in diet pattern are also responsible for the reduction in caries prevalence. Resistance and adherence to dental structures have improved with the development of resin-modified (glass-ionomer) cements. The retention and caries-preventive effectiveness of 2 ionomeric materials (conventional and resin-modified) were assessed.

Methods.—A total of 208 schoolchildren aged 6 to 8 years were randomly assigned to either an experimental or control group (100 and 108 children, respectively). All children had permanent first molars that were sound and unsealed. Two hundred conventional glass-ionomer (Ketac Bond) and 200 resin-modified glass-ionomer (Vitremer) sealants were applied in the experimental group (400 teeth). There were 432 first molars in the control group. Clinical evaluations were performed at 6, 12, 24, and 36 months after sealant application.

Results.—The total retention rates for Ketac Bond were 26%, 12%, 3%, and 4% at 6, 12, 24, and 36 months, respectively; for Vitremer, the rates were 61%, 31%, 14%, and 13%, respectively. The between-group differences were significant. The experimental group had an incidence of caries that was 93%, 78%, 49%, and 56% lower than controls ($P < .01$) for the 4 evaluation time points, respectively.

Conclusion.—The retention rates for ionomeric materials were low, but the materials had a significant cariostatic effect. The presence of active incipient caries was statistically correlated with caries incidence in the first molars after 36 months, in relation to either experimental group or controls.

▶ The only effective immunization against occlusal caries, available to the dental profession, is through the application of pit and fissure sealants. Numerous longitudinal clinical trials have demonstrated the effectiveness of resin-based pit and fissure sealants that are properly placed. Any deviation from correct acid etching, rinsing, isolation, and appropriate polymerization can significantly reduce the anticipated outcome. The study investigates the use of glass-ionomer materials for sealants. Fewer steps are required for placement compared with resin-based sealants. The water component of ionomers may make them more tolerant to a contaminated placement field. The retention rates of sealants observed in this study are consistent with the reduced physical properties of ionomer materials. However, despite the rather low retention rates, their cariostatic effectiveness remained high. A new conventional glass-ionomer pit and fissure sealant was recently introduced this year. Based on the results of this clinical study, an additional effective option can be considered for use over traditional resin-based sealants.

A. A. Boghosian, DDS

How Storage and Mixing Effect a Resin-Modified Glass Ionomer
Winkler MM, Walker R (Louisiana State Univ, New Orleans)
Gen Dent 51:52-53, 2003   1–19

Introduction.—Many clinicians may be using triturators older than 20 years to mix encapsulated resin-modified glass ionomer (RMGI) restorative materials. Older triturators were designed for amalgam capsules, which are very different from RMGI capsules. The impact of storage time and mixing speed of an older (>20 years), common brand triturator (Vari Mix II) on the working time of RMGI restorative material was examined.

Methods.—Two batches of RMGI were used: 1 fresh (at least 18 months before expiration date) and 1 older (within 1 month of the expiration date). Only the high and low speeds on the triturator were used to illustrate the full spectrum of effects produced by variations in mixing speed. The lowest speed was used to ascertain whether it caused a significantly faster setting time versus the recommended time. After testing at these speeds, the triturator was altered to achieve the manufacturer's recommended speed (4000 rpm) for the RMGI, since this speed was under the lowest calibrated mixing speed. Both batches of RMGI were triturated at 3 speeds: lowest (L1, 4600 rpm), highest (H3, 6250 rpm), and recommended (4000 rpm). The working time was considered to be the time in seconds from the start of the mix until the load started to increase. Ten capsules were mixed for each storage time/mixing speed, and mean working times were determined.

Results.—The mean working times of the fresh and old capsules were not significantly different at the manufacturer's recommended speed of 4000 rpm. At L1 speed, the lowest speed attained by an average older triturator, and at H3 speed, a significant difference was seen between fresh and old capsules. The working times were significantly shorter at both L1 and H3 speeds versus 4000 rpm for the old capsules. For the fresh capsules, the working times at 4000 rpm and at 4600 rpm were not significantly different; the working time at H3 was significantly shorter than the other 2 speeds.

Conclusion.—At the manufacturer's recommended speed of 4000 rpm, there were no significant differences in working times between fresh and old RMGI capsules. At higher mixing speeds, the working time for the old capsules was significantly less than for fresh capsules. It is important to use the correct mixing speed to safeguard consistent working times for RMGI materials, particularly when they are close to their expiration date.

▶ Unlike ready-to-place materials such as light polymerized composite, the physical properties of dental materials that require mixing can be significantly affected by improper manipulation. Formats such as cartridge-dispensed impression materials removed the need for trained skills when mixing and dispensing. Streak-free mixes can be routinely achieved through static and dynamic mixing formats. Also, infringement on sufficient work time can be greatly reduced with auto-mixed impression materials. Despite the benefits of encapsulated, auto-mixed glass ionomer cement, the results of this study show that certain parameters must be followed to realize expected working times and achieve ultimate physical properties. One very important factor is to avoid the use of expired materials and to read the directions for use enclosed with the product.

A. A. Boghosian, DDS

Fracture Resistance of Teeth Restored With Two Different Post-and-Core Designs Cemented With Two Different Cements: An In Vitro Study. Part I

Mezzomo E, Massa F, Líbera SD (Universidade Luterana do Brasil (ULBRA), Canoas)

Quintessence Int 34:301-306, 2003   1–20

Background.—Integral parts of dental reconstruction of a coronal structure are the posts and cores that provide the retention and stability for the artificial crown. Fracture resistance in teeth restored with cast posts and cores was evaluated.

Method.—Forty clean maxillary premolars were selected and the crowns horizontally sectioned. The 40 specimens were randomly divided into 4 groups and treated as follows: group 1, restored with cast posts and cores cemented with zinc-phosphate cement with cervical ferrule; group 2, restored with cast posts and cores cemented with resin cement with cervical ferrule; group 3, restored with cast posts and cores cemented with zinc-phosphate cement without cervical ferrule; and group 4, restored with cast posts and cores cemented with resin cement without cervical ferrule (Fig 1).

Results.—The 20 specimens with ferrule (groups 1 and 2) showed greater resistance than the nonferruled specimens in groups 3 and 4. There was no difference according to which cement was used.

Discussion.—Maximal conservation of dentin, as shown in a review of the literature, is the main factor in choosing a restoration procedure for endodontically treated teeth. Fracture resistance of teeth is improved when they are restored with materials that have a low elasticity modulus compared with hard materials. Cervical ferrule and resin cement were found to be the best performers in restored teeth.

▶ Preservation of tooth structure, both vital and nonvital, is one of the most important factors contributing to increasing the longevity of the restoration and remaining tooth structure. Smaller posterior composite restorations will have better wear resistance than larger ones. Teeth restored with amalgam will be less prone to fracture if the isthmus width can be held smaller. With

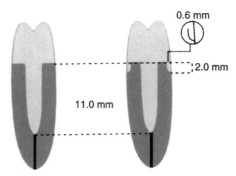

FIGURE 1.—Diagram of the 2 restoration designs tested. (Courtesy of Mezzomo E, Massa F, Líbera SD: Fracture resistance of teeth restored with two different post-and-core designs cemented with two different cements: An in vitro study. Part I. *Quintessence Int* 34:301-306, 2003.)

indirect restorations, this study concludes that endodontically treated teeth requiring post and cores will have greater resistance to fracture when a ferrule design is used.

The results of this study also indicate that using an adhesive resin cement provides better resistance to fracture than does zinc-phosphate cement. Every attempt should be made to retain as much tooth structure as possible, especially at the gingival margin. Additionally, if an endodontically treated tooth can be built up to support a full coverage restoration without the use of a post, further resistance to fracture can be realized.

A. A. Boghosian, DDS

Resin-Ceramic Bonding: A Review of the Literature
Blatz MB, Sadan A, Kern M (Louisiana State Univ, New Orleans; Christian Albrechts Univ Kiel, Germany)
J Prosthet Dent 89:268-274, 2003   1–21

Background.—An increasing number of all-ceramic materials and systems are available for clinical use. Adhesive bonding techniques used with these all-ceramic systems provide a wide range of restorative dentistry treatments with excellent esthetic results. The brittleness of some ceramic materials, specific treatment modalities, and certain clinical situations require resin bonding of the complete ceramic restoration to the supporting tooth structures for long-term clinical success. Ideally, specific treatment modalities and their long-term durability are best tested in controlled clinical trials. However, in vitro investigations are vital to the identification of superior materials before their clinical evaluation, particularly, in comparative studies of bonding agents and cements. The literature on the resin bond to dental ceramics was reviewed.

Methods.—A search was conducted of the PubMed database to identify in vitro studies involving the resin bond to ceramic materials. The search was restricted to peer-reviewed English-language articles published between 1966 and 2001.

Results.—The resin bond to silica-based ceramics has been well-researched and documented, but few in vitro studies of the resin bond to high-strength ceramic materials have been published. The preferred methods for surface treatment are acid etching with hydrofluoric acid (HF) solutions and subsequent application of a silane coupling agent. Adhesive cementation may not be required for final insertion of high-strength all-ceramic restorations with proper mechanical retention. However, resin bonding and adequate ceramic-surface conditioning are necessary in some clinical situations. The preferred treatments for glass-infiltrated aluminum-oxide ceramics are either airborne particle abrasion with Al_2O_3 and use of a phosphate-modified resin cement or tribochemical surface treatment in combination with conventional Bis-GMA resin cement.

Conclusions.—Resin bonding to high-strength ceramic materials is less predictable, and significantly different bonding methods are required for high-strength ceramics than with silica-based ceramics. Additional in vitro studies and controlled clinical trials of resin bonding to high-strength ceramics are needed.

▶ This very thorough review of ceramic bonding provides an excellent background for bonding all ceramic restorations. Not only are problems reviewed when bonding to high-strength core materials but also practical solutions are provided. All ceramic systems with high-strength zirconia cores are now viable replacements for single crowns and perhaps multiple-unit fixed partial dentures due to the improved flexural strength of the core. This article provides a thorough and concise discussion of all ceramic systems and provides enough background to enable the individual clinician to select the ceramic material most appropriate for the clinical situation. This article is a must-read!

J. O. Burgess, DDS, MS

Clinical Evaluation of Solitaire-2 Restorations Placed in United Kingdom General Dental Practices: 1-Year Report
Burke FJT, Crisp RJ, Bell TJ, et al (Univ of Birmingham, England; Douglas, Isle of Man, UK; York, UK; et al)
Quintessence Int 34:594-599, 2003   1–22

Background.—The increasing esthetic focus among patients has increased the demand for tooth-colored restorative materials for posterior teeth. Resin composite is a commonly used tooth-colored restorative material, but resin composite restorations are technique sensitive. For example, difficulties in achieving satisfactory interproximal contact have been reported with 1 study reporting 2.5 times as many defective contacts with composite Class II restorations as amalgam. Resin composite cannot be pushed against the matrix band to help establish a tight proximal contact, especially since composite shrinks during polymerization. In addition, since clinicians often use amalgam placement techniques for placement of resin composite restorations, manufacturers have developed packable composites in recent years to allow clinicians to condense composite. The efficacy of 1 packable composite, Solitaire-2, used with 2 adhesives, GLUMA Solid Bond and GLUMA One Bond, in Class I and II cavity restorations in permanent teeth was assessed.

Methods.—The study was conducted among the practices of 5 members of the Product Research and Evaluation by Practitioners (PREP) Panel, a group of dental practitioners in the United Kingdom. Each of the 5 panel members placed 20 Solitaire-2 restorations in patients with no history of adverse reaction to the restorative materials used, no occlusal parafunction or pathologic tooth wear, and no medical or dental history that could have complicated the placement of restorations or influenced the performance of the restorations. All of the patients selected had a history of regular visits to their dental practitioner. The restorations were reviewed at 1 year by the

PREP panel member who placed the restoration and by a trained and calibrated evaluator using well-established criteria for evaluation.

Results.—Of the 100 restorations placed, 88 restorations (33 Class I and 55 Class II) in 49 patients were reviewed at 1 year. One Class II restoration was replaced at 10 months, after detection of a fracture across the distal box. The remaining restorations (99%) were intact, and no secondary caries was detected.

Conclusions.—In 99% of cases evaluated in this report, the Solitaire-2 restorations, placed in conjunction with the GLUMA Solid Bond adhesive and the GLUMA One Bond system, were performing satisfactorily at 1 year of follow-up.

► This article reports the clinical performance of Solitaire-2 composite resin in Class I and Class II restorations in a general practice setting. At 1-year recall, 88 of the 100 restorations were evaluated. Although this study is designed to evaluate the composite resin restorative material in a private practice setting, only 40 restorations were placed in Class II restorations in molars. This article was interesting in that it evaluates the composite resin in a private practice setting, not the controlled environment of a dental school. However, both settings are important. A controlled clinical trial reports the best performance possible with the material and controls many variables that might limit success. The private practice setting, in many cases, examines the abuse tolerance of the restorative material. Both settings are essential for the ultimate clinical success of the material, and, therefore, both should be conducted. This report, while favorable, evaluates the composite resin for too short a period to truly determine the long-term success of the composite resin.

J. O. Burgess, DDS, MS

The Effect of Six Polishing Systems on the Surface Roughness of Two Packable Resin-Based Composites
Reis AF, Giannini M, Lovadino JR, et al (Campinas State Univ, Piracicaba/SP, Brazil)
Am J Dent 15:193-197, 2002   1–23

Introduction.—Proper finishing and polishing of posterior composite restorations are crucial steps that enhance both esthetics and longevity of restored teeth. Surface roughness, related to improper finishing and polishing, can produce excessive surface staining, increased wear rates, and increased plaque accumulation, which compromise the clinical performance of the restoration. The effect of 6 different finishing and polishing agents on the surface roughness of 2 packable resin-based composites was compared, and their polished surfaces were examined with a scanning electron microscope.

Methods.—Solitaire and Alert composite samples were prepared and polished with Poli I and Poli II aluminum oxide pastes, Ultralap diamond paste, Enhance finishing points, Politip rubber polishers, fine and extra fine diamond burs, and 30-blade tungsten carbide burs according to the directions of the manufacturer. The polished surfaces were examined with a profilometer and a scanning electron microscope.

Results.—Solitaire composite resin had the smoothest surfaces when polished with the Poli I and II aluminum oxide pastes, Ultralap diamond paste, Politip finishing points, and 30-blade tungsten carbide burs. The smoothest surfaces for the Alert composite samples were observed with the 30-blade tungsten carbide burs.

Conclusion.—Alert had a significantly greater surface roughness, compared with Solitaire, for most of the agents assessed. The smoothest surfaces for Solitaire were achieved with polishing pastes, 30-blade carbide burs, and Politip. Carbide burs produced the best finish for Alert.

▶ There are 3 phases involved with the completion of a composite restoration after its placement. The first step involves contouring the restoration to establish proper occlusion of anterior form. Rotary instruments such as diamonds and carbides are used for contouring. The second step, finishing, removes contouring marks and develops secondary and tertiary anatomy in posterior restorations. Thirty-fluted carbides, ultrafine diamonds, and abrasive impregnated rubber points can be effectively used. The final step, glossing, brings the surface luster of the restoration equal to that of the adjacent enamel. As demonstrated in this study, carbide burs used to finish the appropriate composite produced a very smooth surface. Contouring, finishing, and glossing of contemporary small particle hybrid and nano-filled composites can be performed with multifluted carbide burs followed by appropriate polishing pastes. Not only will this technique yield an enamel-like appearance, the resultant surface will also be free from surface defects that can lead to fracture.

A. A. Boghosian, DDS

Depth of Cure and Microleakage With High-Intensity and Ramped Resin-Based Composite Curing Lights
Jain P, Pershing A (Southern Illinois Univ School of Dental Medicine, Alton)
J Am Dent Assoc 134:1215-1223, 2003   1–24

Background.—The increasing number of resin-based composite restorations being placed by dentists has spurred a search for new methods and curing lights that will decrease curing time and reduce marginal gaps caused by polymerization shrinkage. Recently, curing lights have been developed with higher intensities and shorter curing cycles to shorten curing time for an increment of composite resin. Ramped- and stepped-intensity curing lights have been marketed. These curing units have curing cycles that begin at lower power and increase to higher levels as the curing cycle proceeds. Soft-start polymerization may create less stress at the resin-based composite-enamel/dentin joint and reduce marginal gaps. Whether high-intensity curing lights used in high-intensity or ramped-intensity modes affect microleakage of resin-based composite restorations and whether different types of resin-based composites cured in these modes meet the standard established by the National Standards Institute/American Dental Association for depth of cure were determined.

Methods.—Five high-intensity lights, including 3 plasma arc lights and 2 quartz-tungsten-halogen lights, were compared in their regular and ramped-intensity modes with a quartz-tungsten-halogen 40-second light. The main outcome measures were microleakage 1 month after bonding and curing depth for different resin-based composite types. Curing depth was measured using a scratch test.

Results.—Light curing with the Optilux 501 for 10 seconds and the ADT PowerPAC for 10 seconds provided higher microleakage values than light curing with other lights. The microhybrid resin-based composite was the only material that met the ANSI/ADA Specification no. 27 (1993):7.7 for depth of cure after light curing with all of the lights tested. The greatest depth of cure was obtained with microhybrid resin-based composite, whereas flowable resin-based composite had the least depth of cure.

Conclusions.—Curing with high-intensity lights will result in different curing depths when different categories of resin-based composites are used. Light curing with some high-intensity lights compared with halogen lights may result in higher microleakage values. Caution is recommended when light curing flowable resin-based composite with high-intensity light.

▶ This is another article based on an in vitro study that adds to the debate on fast versus slow composite resin curing. The authors compared ramped, conventional curing and fast (plasma arc curing light) and measured the leakage of Class V resin restorations as well as depth of cure on several composites. Curing composites depend on the curing light and the composite resin used. Curing composite resin depends on the spectral output of the curing light, the power density of the unit, and the time of curing. The amount and type of photoinitiation in the composite, its translucency, shade, and type resin also determine the effectiveness of polymerization. The results of this study are of limited value and demonstrate that the energy density should be calculated and applied when determining the amount of curing time applied to each specimen. To apply the same amount of energy to each composite, it is necessary to calculate the product of curing time and power. This should be standardized for each light. Then and only then can you show differences for each composite. This calculation was not made, and therefore the results, although interesting, are not scientific.

J. O. Burgess, DDS, MS

Light-Emitting Diode Curing: Influence on Selected Properties of Resin Composites

Asmussen E, Peutzfeldt A (Univ of Copenhagen)
Quintessence Int 34:71-75, 2002   1–25

Background.—Halogen curing units have been used for more than 2 decades for polymerization of resin composites. However, other types of light-curing units have been marketed recently. Among these new types of units is the plasma arc curing (PAC) unit. PAC units have high power density, and the manufacturers of these units claim that polymerization may be accomplished with significantly shorter curing times than with lower-powered halogen curing units. However, some studies have questioned the efficacy of PAC units. The light-emitting diode (LED) curing unit is another recent polymerization device. The minimal heat generated by these units is one of the main advantages of the LED unit. In addition, a cooling fan is not needed, and LEDs consume so little energy that they can be powered by rechargeable batteries. The efficacy of 2 recently introduced LED polymerization units was compared with that of a conventional halogen curing unit, and the selected properties of resin composites polymerized with these curing units were determined.

Methods.—Three different brands of resin composite were used to investigate flexural strength and modulus in 3-point bending tests, depth of polymerization as determined by removal of uncured material after irradiation, polymerization contraction as evaluated with the bonded-disk method, and degree of conversion as measured by Fourier transform infrared spectroscopy.

Results.—The properties of resin composites polymerized with LED curing units were found to be equal to or inferior to those properties provided by curing with halogen light. However, both the flexural strength and the depth of polymerization obtained from LED curing met the requirements determined by the International Standards Organization (ISO).

Conclusions.—The LED units used for polymerization of resin composites resulted in composites that were equivalent or moderately inferior to those cured with a conventional halogen unit, although the flexural strength and depth obtained with LED polymerization fulfilled ISO requirements. The degree of conversion is a significant determinant of the properties of resin composites, and lower conversion rates of the resin composite were obtained with LED light units than with halogen lights.

▶ LED curing units are here to stay. Although the initial units had low power density (200-300 mW/cm²), second-generation LED curing lights have significantly greater output and broader spectral distribution. Some of the newest LED curing units will cure all photopolymerizable materials. Unfortunately, this article used first-generation LED-curing lights and compared them to a quartz tungsten halogen-curing light; therefore, the results were not as favorable as with the newest second-generation LED-curing lights. The article provides good background on LED-curing lights and anyone considering purchasing one should review this article.

J. O. Burgess, DDS, MS

2 Esthetic Dentistry

Introduction

In the past 30 years, interest in the area of esthetic dentistry has revolutionized dentistry. Clinical activity in dentistry has greatly increased because of esthetic dentistry. It is anticipated that numerous esthetic-oriented techniques will increase in use, including all types of veneers, tooth-colored crowns and intracoronal restorations, bleaching, orthodontics, and facial surgery.

This year, the literature has returned to the basic fundamentals of esthetic dentistry. Many of the studies emphasized self-etching bonding agents and principles of bonding. In the articles offered this year, the focus is on the presented research related to adhesion.

Frederick M. McIntyre, DDS, MS

Technical

Marginal Discrepancies and Leakage of All-Ceramic Crowns: Influence of Luting Agents and Aging Conditions

Gu X-H, Kern M (Zhejiang Univ, Hangzhou, People's Republic of China; Christian-Albrechts Univ, Kiel, Germany)
Int J Prosthodont 16:109-116, 2003
2-1

Background.—Long-term performance of all-ceramic crowns may be affected by marginal discrepancies, leakage, and fracture resistance. Luting agents are an important contributor to marginal discrepancies in crown restorations; particularly in the posterior region, a less complex luting procedure may help to avoid adverse effects related to local oral conditions. The effects of 3 types of luting agents on marginal discrepancy and leakage of all-ceramic crowns were investigated in an in vitro study.

Methods.—Forty-eight all-ceramic crowns were prepared and luted onto extracted human molars. In groups of 16, the crowns were luted with a zinc phosphate cement, Harvard Cement; a compomer cement, Dyract; or an adhesive composite resin luting system, Panavia F. Sixteen metal-ceramic crowns luted with Harvard Cement served as control units. The specimens were artificially aged with 3500 thermocycles, with or without 600,000 loading cycles in a chewing simulator. Marginal discrepancies were assessed using an impression-replica technique with scanning electron microscopy, and leakage was measured by the dye penetration method.

Results.—The control metal-ceramic crowns had significantly larger discrepancies at the porcelain shoulder margins. Otherwise, marginal discrepancies were similar between groups and were not significantly affected by fatigue testing. However, marginal leakage differed significantly between the different luting agent groups, being lowest with Panavia F and intermediate with Dyract. The use of Harvard Cement was associated with severe leakage into the pulp chambers via the dentinal tubules. Leakage was similar with or without simulated chewing.

Discussion.—In all-ceramic crowns, the use of an adhesive composite resin luting system is associated with the least amount of leakage, compared with a compomer cement and a zinc phosphate cement. Marginal discrepancies are similar across the 3 luting agents.

Conclusions.—Panavia F performs well in minimizing leakage of all-ceramic crowns and provides clinically acceptable marginal discrepancies.

▶ When all-ceramic restorations were first introduced, marginal discrepancy was a major concern. Fabrication of all-ceramic restorations relied on platinum foil matrixes or refractory die materials. Both of these techniques required extraordinary efforts to produce clinically acceptable margins. Today, pressable ceramics and CAD/CAM technology have greatly improved the accuracy of the all-ceramic margin. However, there is still concern that stress-related fatigue due to mastication can produce microleakage, which would lead to clinical failure. This article reported results of a study evaluating marginal discrepancies and leakage of all-ceramic crowns cemented with different luting agents.

F. M. McIntyre, DDS, MS

In Vitro Evaluation of Long-term Bonding of Procera AllCeram Alumina Restorations With a Modified Resin Luting Agent

Blatz MB, Sadan A, Arch GH Jr, et al (Louisiana State Univ, New Orleans; Univ of Michigan, Ann Arbor)
J Prosthet Dent 89:381-387, 2003   2–2

Background.—Laminate veneers and resin-bonded fixed partial dentures were recently included in the range of clinical indications for CAD/CAM-fabricated densely sintered, high-purity aluminum-oxide ceramic restorations (Procera AllCeram, Nobel Biocare, Goteborg, Sweden). Laminates such as these rely on a strong and long-term durable resin bond. Air particle abrasion and a phosphate-modified luting agent have the potential to provide this type of bond to aluminum oxide ceramics, but the efficacy of this agent on the Procera AllCeram intaglio surface has not been determined.

The microroughness inherent in this surface may affect bond strengths because micromechanical interlocking is a primary factor in the adhesion of resins to ceramic materials. The purpose of this study was to evaluate the bond strength of a phosphate-modified resin luting agent with and without silanization to an air particle–abraded Procera AllCeram intaglio surface compared with a conventional resin-bonding system before and after artificial aging.

Methods.—Sixty square specimens of Procera AllCeram with the Procera intaglio surface were air particle–abraded with aluminum oxide. Composite cylinders were fabricated with Z-250 composite and bonded to the ceramic specimens with either Panavia 21 TC (Kuraray, Osaka, Japan) or Rely X ARC (control) and their corresponding bonding/silane coupling agents. Panavia was also used without silanization. Subgroups of 10 specimens were stored in distilled water for either 3 or 180 days. Shear bond strength was then tested with a universal testing machine (Mpa) until fracture. The 180-day specimens underwent thermocycling at 2000 cycles every 30 days, for a total of 12,000 cycles. Failure modes were examined with a light microscope.

Results.—Significant differences were noted between the short-term and long-term groups. Bond strength with Rely X ARC and its silane coupling agent decreased significantly after artificial aging. Panavia 21, after silanization, showed significantly different early and late bond strengths but attained its highest bond strength after artificial aging. There was not a significant difference in bond strength of Panavia without silanization at the early and late time points (Fig 4). Failure modes were mainly adhesive at the ceramic surface for all groups.

Conclusion.—Panavia 21 in combination with its corresponding bonding/silane coupling agent can provide an acceptable resin bond to the air particle–abraded intaglio surface of Procera AllCeram restorations after

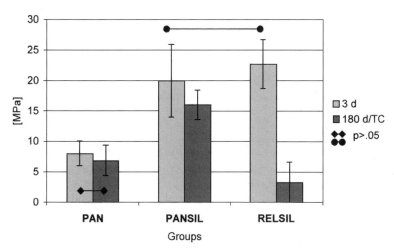

FIGURE 4.—Mean early (3 day) and late (180 day/thermocycling) bond strength values and standard deviations *(Mpa)*. *Horizontal bars* indicate no statistical difference (α = .05). (Reprinted by permission of the publisher from Blatz MB, Sadan A, Arch GH Jr, et al: In vitro evaluation of long-term bonding of Procera AllCeram alumina restorations with a modified resin luting agent. *J Prosthet Dent* 89:381-387, 2003. Copyright 2003 by Elsevier.)

artificial aging. The most dramatic decrease in bond strength occurred with the conventional resin luting agent.

▶ Sintered aluminum oxide ceramic materials such as Procera present luting difficulty because the surface of the material cannot easily be bonded. Several techniques are advocated to improve the surface for bonding. Air abrasion and silanization have been advocated to prepare the surface for bonding with a luting composite such as Panavia 21. This study evaluates bond strengths achieved using Panavia 21 or Rely X ARC to bond Procera that has been air abraded or air abraded and silanated.

F. M. McIntyre, DDS, MS

Water Treeing—A Potential Mechanism for Degradation of Dentin Adhesives
Tay FR, Pashley DH (Univ of Hong Kong; Med College of Georgia, Augusta)
Am J Dent 16:6-12, 2003   2–3

Background.—Advances in dentin bonding research have resulted in the refinement of 2 divertive bonding strategies: the total-etch technique and the self-etch technique. There is now considerable evidence that deterioration of the structural integrity of resin-dentin bonds created with either technique occurs over time. This breakdown has been attributed to slow water hydrolysis, which may occur either in the resin or protein component of the bonded interfaces. Water available from the adhesives used in either technique may be trapped within resin-dentin interfaces.

It would be desirable to remove water completely after bonding, but the presence of 2-hydroxyethyl methacrylate (HEMA), acidic monomers, and dissolved calcium and phosphate ions may lower the vapor pressure of water, which makes it difficult to remove water before polymerization. HEMA-containing adhesives used on wet dentin may also create domains of microporous poly(HEMA) hydrogels, which permit the movement of water, solvated ions, and polar molecules. Water treeing is a well-recognized degradation phenomenon in the dielectric insulation cable industry. Water treeing is responsible for the water-induced deterioration of polymer insulation of electrical cables after aging. This study tested the hypothesis that water channels are present along the adhesive-dentin interface that can be detected with transmission electron microscopy examination of tracer penetration.

Methods.—Several different commercially available total-etch and self-etch adhesives as well as an experimental self-etch adhesive were bonded to dentin and enamel (Table). Bonded-resin tooth slabs were then immersed in 50 wt% conventional silver nitrate or 50 wt% basic, ammoniacal silver nitrate for 24 hours. The slabs were then exposed to a photodeveloping solution and prepared for examination with transmission electron microscopy.

Results.—All of the adhesives displayed nanoleakage within hybrid layers with both types of silver nitrate. Water trees in the form of interconnecting, dendritic silver deposits were observed along the surface of the hybrid layers

TABLE.—Composition of the 2-Step, Single Bottle, Total-Etch, Self-Priming Adhesives and the Single-Step, Self-Etch Adhesives Used in the Study

Category	Adhesive	Composition
Two-step, single bottle, total-etch adhesives	Single Bond	Water, ethanol, Bis-GMA, HEMA, UDMA, Bisphenol A glycerolate, dimethacrylate, polyalkenoic acid copolymer, photoinitiator, stabilizer
	Excite	Water, ethanol, HEMA, Bis-GMA, glycerine dimethacrylate, phosphoric acid acrylate, highly dispersed silica, photoinitiator, stabilizer, pigments
	PQ1	8% ethanol, HEMA, proprietary monomers, proprietary natural resins, 40% barium borosilicate glass fillers, photoinitiator, stabilizer
Single-step, self-etch adhesives	Prompt L-Pop	Water, methacrylated phosphoric acid esters, fluoride complex, photoinitiator (BAPO), stabilizer, parabenes
	Reactmer Bond	Reactmer Bond A: Water, acetone, F-PRG fillers, FASG fillers, initiators (TMBA, *p*-TSNa)
		Reactmer Bond B: 4-AET, 4-AETA, HEMA, UDMA, photoinitiator
	RZ II	Base liquid: Water, acetone, 4-META, triacrylate, monomethacrylate, photoinitiator, stabilizer
		RZ brush: Initiator (*p*-TSNa), amine

Abbreviations: *4-AET*, 4-Acryloxyethyltrimellitic acid; *4-AETA*, 4-acryloxyethyltrimellitic anhydride; *4-META*, 4-methacryloxyethyltrimellitic anhydride; *BAPO*, bis-acyl phosphine oxide; *Bis-GMA*, bisphenol A diglycidyl ether dimethacrylate; *F-PRG*, full-reaction type pre-reacted glass ionomer filler; *FASG*, fluoroaluminosilicate glass; *HEMA*, 2-hydroxyethyl methacrylate; *p-TSNa*, p-toluenesulfinic acid sodium salt; *TMBA*, trimethyl barbituric acid; *UDMA*, urethane dimethacrylate.

(Courtesy of Tay FR, Pashley DH: Water treeing—A potential mechanism for degradation of dentin adhesives. *Am J Dent* 16:6-12, 2003.)

that extended perpendicularly into the adhesive layers. With ammoniacal silver nitrate, additional isolated, unconnected silver grains were noted within the adhesive.

Conclusion.—This study demonstrated interconnecting water trees and isolated silver grains in resin adhesive layers that may be attributed to the entrapment of water. The consequences of these defects are minor if they remain static; however, they could be of clinical significance if further studies show that these defects are self-propagating or permit the further ingress of water.

▶ Clinical observation has documented breakdown and microleakage between tooth and composite along vertical walls of preparation. Flexure of the interface between the tooth and the composite has been the explanation routinely given. This article introduces another possible explanation for marginal breakdown. It is a common phenomenon seen in the cable industry in which there is cable degradation to water contamination. The term given is water treeing. Tay and Pashley tested the adhesive-dentin interface to detect whether this phenomenon might be present at the composite interface.

F. M. McIntyre, DDS, MS

Efficacy of Self-Etching Primer on Sealing Margins of Class II Restorations

Fabianelli A, Kugel G, Ferrari M (Univ of Siena, Italy; Tufts Univ, Boston)
Am J Dent 16:37-41, 2003   2–4

Background.—There is a steadily increasing demand among patients for tooth-colored restorations rather than amalgam restorations. One of the major problems with resin restorations is microleakage, which may result from the polymerization shrinkage of resin material, which creates a gap between cavity wall and the restoration. It is apparent the microleakage cannot be prevented routinely, even with the development of adhesives that can produce adhesion to dentin comparable to the adhesion to enamel than can be achieved. However, dentin adhesives have been developed with hydrophilic groups and high wettability, and these new adhesives can penetrate a chemically conditioned dentin to create a mechanical interlocking based on the formation of a hybrid layer and resin tags penetrating into opened dentin tubules. Self-etching primers have been proposed to simplify handling properties, reduce working time, and avoid the collapse of collagen fibrils. The sealing ability of different types of restorative-adhesive combinations was evaluated, and etch patterns were correlated with leakage scores.

Methods.—The study used 56 posterior molars, which were divided randomly into 4 groups of 14 specimens each. A standardized adhesive Class II preparation with the cervical margin placed 1 mm below the cement-enamel junction, and an occlusal reduction of 2 mm was performed. No bevels were used. Four combinations of bonding system/restorative material were tested. Group 1 consisted of Excite (EX) combined with Tetric Ceram (TC) as control. Group 2 consisted of Prompt L-Pop applied for 15 seconds in combination with TC. The third group consisted of Etch and Prime 3.0 in combination with Definite restorative material, and group 4 consisted of Prompt L-Pop applied for 30 seconds in combination with TC. The resin composite was applied, and 10 specimens from each group were processed for leakage test.

Results.—EX showed less dye penetration at occlusal margins than the other 3 groups. However, there were no statistically significant differences among the groups at the dentin margin. Scanning electron microscopy showed a rougher and more uniform enamel etch pattern when phosphoric acid (EX) was applied than was obtained with self-etching adhesive systems. All groups showed resin tags and adhesive lateral branches at the dentin site.

Conclusion.—The sealing ability of self-etching priming bonding systems at the enamel margins is less effective than the sealing ability of phosphoric acid bonding systems.

▶ When All-Bond was introduced to the profession, it became the benchmark by which other bonding agents were compared. It was the first effective universal dentinal bond agent the profession had. It was a generation IV product that had multiple steps for application; however, it could be used as a light-cure or self-cure bonding agent, which allowed its use with several different materials. Generation V dentinal bonding agents were introduced to eliminate multiple steps of application but were still based on acid-etch wet bond techniques. Limitation became evident with self-cured composite materials. Activators have been introduced to overcome the problem, but the results are still not as good as those of generation IV products. Recently, self-etch bonding agents have been introduced to further eliminate application steps. Controversy has been associated with self-etch bond strengths to enamel. Reports of successful enamel bonding have been mixed. This article compares acid-etch technique with self-etch agents for enamel bonding.

F. M. McIntyre, DDS, MS

Influence of Resin Composite Polymerization Techniques on Microleakage and Microhardness
Amaral CM, Bedran de Castro AKB, Pimenta LAF, et al (Univ of Campinas, São Paulo, Brazil)
Quintessence Int 33:685-689, 2002   2–5

Introduction.—Resin composite restorations are the most esthetic direct placement restorations currently available. Resin composite is being used with increasing frequency due to its mechanical properties and patients' desire for esthetics. Yet, these materials have limitations, including polymerization shrinkage, deflection of cusps, production of internal stress, and postoperative sensitivity. The influence of conventional and soft-start polymerization technique on the microleakage and microhardness of Class II resin composite restorations placed in bulk or by an incremental technique were examined in vitro in bovine teeth.

Methods.—One hundred twenty Class II cavities were prepared in bovine teeth; they were randomly placed in 4 groups: bulk placement and conventional polymerization (Conv 1); buccolingual increments and conventional polymerization (Conv 3); bulk placement and soft-start polymerization (Soft 1); buccolingual increments and soft-start polymerization (Soft 3). All cavities were restored by means of the Z100/Single Bond system. After thermocycling, the specimens were immersed in 2% methylene blue solution, then assessed for microleakage. Half of the samples were embedded in

---

TABLE 1.—Relative Frequency (Percentage) of Microleakage Scores for Each Group

Group	\multicolumn{5}{c}{Score}				
	0	1	2	3	4
Conv 1	54.44	28.89	10.00	0.00	6.67
Conv 3	70.11	29.89	0.00	0.00	0.00
Soft 1	42.53	49.43	7.78	0.00	3.33
Soft 3	63.22	33.33	3.33	0.00	0.00

Note: Fisher exact test; $P = .00071$ for all comparisons.
Abbreviations: Conv, Conventional polymerization; *Soft,* soft-start polymerization.
(Courtesy of Amaral CM, Bedran de Castro AKB, Pimenta LAF, et al: Influence of resin composite polymerization techniques on microleakage and microhardness. *Quintessence Int* 33:685-689, 2002.)

TABLE 2.—Knoop Hardness Number for Each Group and for Each Depth of the Restoration

| | Depth (µm) | | | | | |
| | 100 | | 2500 | | 5000 | |
Group	Mean	SD	Mean	SD	Mean	SD
Conv 1	139.20	26.28	143.10	28.14	150.04	34.20
Conv 3	140.24	26.24	147.19	24.38	144.25	22.65
Soft 1	137.26	20.09	143.02	22.94	143.14	20.73
Soft 3	143.94	16.90	139.61	14.78	144.80	19.42

Coefficient of variation = 9.82%. Means not significantly different (vertically or horizontally) (analysis of variance; $P > .05$).
Abbreviations: Conv, Conventional polymerization; *Soft,* soft-start polymerization.
(Courtesy of Amaral CM, Bedran de Castro AKB, Pimenta LAF, et al: Influence of resin composite polymerization techniques on microleakage and microhardness. *Quintessence Int* 33:685-689, 2002.)

polyester resin, then polished. The Knoop microhardness of the restorations was determined.

Results.—No dye penetration was observed in 54.44% of Conv 1, 70.11% of Conv 3, 42.53% of Soft 1, and 63.22% of Soft 3 specimens. Significant differences in microleakage were observed between groups (Table 1). No significant differences in microhardness were seen in any group at any depth (Table 2).

Conclusion.—Less microleakage occurred with the incremental placement technique. The soft-start system produced sufficient polymerization, yet could not improve marginal sealing.

▶ I read articles such as this with great interest because of my interest in light-curing techniques. The curing light is one of the most important instruments we use in our dental office today, yet one of the least understood. How much time is enough? What intensity is needed? Is halogen better than light-emitting diode? Bulk fil versus incremental fil? Our studies have shown that 20 seconds of cure may be optimal with the proper intensity. Shorter cure times appear to be better than longer cure times with high intensity. Forty seconds may not have been the correct time to obtain different results. Also bulk cure works better with transenamel illumination for short durations. There is still a lot to be investigated before we will have the correct answers.

F. M. McIntyre, DDS, MS

Fracture Resistance of Endodontically Treated Teeth Restored With Composite Posts
Newman MP, Yaman P, Dennison J, et al (Univ of Michigan, Ann Arbor)
J Prosthet Dent 89:360-367, 2003   2–6

Introduction.—The success of esthetic restorative techniques has prompted increased patient demands for these techniques, especially for anterior teeth. This has significantly increased the use of all-ceramic crowns, along with endodontic post and core materials that do not affect the esthetic results. There are few data concerning the physical properties of the post systems. The effect of 3 fiber-reinforced composite post systems on the fracture resistance and mode of failure of endodontically treated teeth was examined.

Methods.—Ninety maxillary central incisors were divided into 9 groups of 10 teeth each: 8 experimental (ParaPost) and 1 control. Eighty teeth were assigned to 2 experimental groups: narrow and flared canal groups (Fig 1 and Table 1). In the narrow canal group, post spaces were designed with the corresponding reamer to restore the teeth with FibreKor, Luscent anchors, and Ribbond posts of 1.5 mm, 1.6 mm, and 2.0 mm in diameter, respectively. Thin-walled canals were simulated in the flared canals group. Teeth in this group were restored with the same posts and were cemented into tapered 2-mm–wide canals devised with a tapered diamond bur. Prefabricated posts (FibreKor and Luscent anchors) for narrow and flared canals were cemented with an autopolymerized resin cement and a flowable composite, respectively.

Customized Ribbond posts were luted with a light-polymerized composite for both canal types. An additional set of 20 Ribbond posts with coronal sections of variable size and shape, named "Ribbond nonstandardized," were also prepared and assessed. Specimens were loaded to failure (kilograms) using a universal testing machine at a crosshead speed of 0.05 cm/min until failure.

Results.—There were no significant differences between flared and narrow canals in mean load to failure between the post systems, with the exception of the Ribbond posts ($P < .01$). The mean load in the narrow canal group ranged from 4.55 kg for the Ribbond standard to 12.9 kg for the Luscent anchors. The low mean load in the flared canal group was 9.04 kg for FibreKor; the high mean load was the same for both Luscent anchors and Ribbond standard (12.87 kg and 12.87, respectively). Overall, the ParaPost control group had the highest load value (18.33 kg; $P < .05$) (Fig 2).

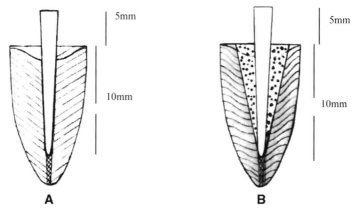

FIGURE 1.—A, Representation of post dimensions of standard group. **B,** Flared canal group. (Courtesy of Newman MP, Yaman P, Dennison J, et al: Fracture resistance of endodontically treated teeth restored with composite posts. *J Prosthet Dent* 89:360-367, 2003.)

TABLE 1.—Description of Experimental Groups

Group (n = 10)	Post System	Specimen Group Preparation and Luting Agents
Narrow canals		
1,1	FibreKor 1.5 mm Glass fiber	Diameter of post space 1.5 mm Luting agents: Cement-it and 3M Scotchbond Multi-Purpose
1,2	Dentatus Luscent anchors 1.6 mm Glass fiber	Diameter of post space 1.6 mm Luting agents: Cement-it and 3M Scotchbond Multi-Purpose
1,3	Ribbond standard 1.6 mm Woven polyethylene fiber	Diameter of post space 1.6 mm Two pieces of 2 mm × 28 mm Ribbond folded in half and placed across each other inserted into the canal Luting agents: Flow-it and 3M Scotchbond Multi-Purpose
Flared canals		
2,1	FibreKor 1.5 mm Glass fiber	Diameter of post space 2.0 mm Luting agents: Flow-it Self and 3M Scotchbond Multi-Purpose
2,2	Dentatus Luscent anchors 1.6 mm Glass fiber	Diameter of post space 2.0 mm Luting agents: Flow-it Self and 3M Scotchbond Multi-Purpose
2,3	Ribbond standard 2.0 mm Woven polyethylene fiber	Diameter of post space 2.0 mm Three pieces of 2 mm × 28 mm Ribbond folded in half and placed across each other inserted into the canal Luting agents: Flow-it and 3M Scotchbond Multi-Purpose
Control		
1,4	Parapost XH 1.5 mm Stainless steel	Diameter of post space 1.5 mm Luting agents: Cement-it and 3M Scotchbond Multi-Purpose
Narrow		
1,5	Ribbond Nonstandardized 1.6 mm Woven polyethylene fiber	Diameter of post space 1.6 mm Two pieces of 2 mm × 28 mm Ribbond folded in half and placed across each other inserted into the canal Luting agents: Flow-it and 3M Scotchbond Multi-Purpose
Flared		
2,5	Ribbond Nonstandardized 2.0 mm Woven polyethylene fiber	Diameter of post space 2.0 mm Two pieces of 2 mm × 28 mm Ribbond folded in half and placed across each other inserted into the canal Luting agents: Flow-it and 3M Scotchbond Multi-Purpose

(Courtesy of Newman MP, Yaman P, Dennison J, et al: Fracture resistance of endodontically treated teeth restored with composite posts. *J Prosthet Dent* 89:360-367, 2003.)

Ribbond nonstandardized had a mean load to failure of 24.91 kg and 31.95 kg for the narrow and flared canal groups, respectively. The results for these groups were excluded from analysis due to their uncontrolled core sizes and high standard deviations. No root fractures were observed in any of the experimental groups.

Conclusion.—Although all fiber-reinforced composite posts achieved lower load values than metal posts, their performance may be favorable since none of the esthetic post failures resulted in root failure. These new-

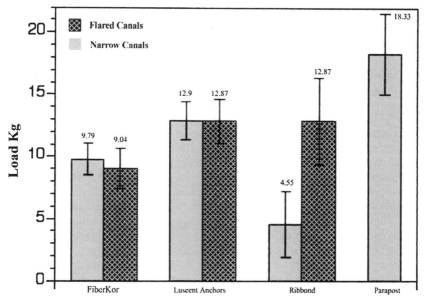

FIGURE 2.—Mean load values and standard error bars of experimental groups by canal type. (Courtesy of Newman MP, Yaman P, Dennison J, et al: Fracture resistance of endodontically treated teeth restored with composite posts. *J Prosthet Dent* 89:360-367, 2003.)

generation post systems are promising and need to be followed up with long-term, controlled clinical trials.

▶ The restorative philosophy for endodontically treated teeth has changed significantly over the years. The cast post core is no longer advocated as the standard for restoration of endodontically treated teeth. Conservation of dentin is the key concept today. Direct placement of post core restorations conserves tooth structure because there is no need to prepare a path of withdrawal for the post. The material choices have changed. More emphasis is being placed on using materials that are biocompatible with the physical properties of enamel and dentin. Fiber posts appear to be gaining popularity because their properties relate well to tooth structure. These authors studied the fracture resistance of endodontically teeth treated with composite posts.

F. M. McIntyre, DDS, MS

Effect of Etching and Airborne Particle Abrasion on the Microstructure of Different Dental Ceramics

Borges GA, Sophr AM, de Goes MF, et al (Univ of Uberaba, Brazil; Pontificial Catholic Univ of Rio Grande do Sul, Brazil; Univ of Campinas, Piracicaba, Brazil; et al)

J Prosthet Dent 89:479-488, 2003   2–7

Introduction.—Dental ceramics are highly esthetic restorative materials which have the advantages of translucence, fluorescence, chemical stability, biocompatibility, high compressive strength, and a coefficient of thermal expansion similar to that of tooth structure. Ceramics are frail under strain. This weakness can be attributed to the presence and propagation of microflaws present on the surface of the material.

This makes ceramic susceptible to fracture during the luting procedure and under occlusal force. The surface topography of 6 different ceramics after hydrofluoric acid etching or airborne aluminum oxide particle abrasion treatments was examined.

Methods.—Five copings of each of the following were fabricated on a die stone master cast: IPS Empress, IPS Empress 2 (0.8 mm thick), Cergogold (0.7 mm thick), In-Ceram Alumina, In-Ceram Zirconia, and Procera (0.8 mm thick). Each coping was longitudinally sectioned into 4 equal parts using a diamond disk. The resulting sections were randomly sorted into 3 groups, depending on subsequent surface treatments, as follows: group 1, specimens without additional surface treatments, as received from the laboratory (control); group 2, specimens treated by use of airborne particle abrasion with 50-μm aluminum oxide; and group 3, specimens treated with 10% hydrofluoric acid etching (20 seconds for IPS Empress 2; 60 seconds for IPS Empress and Cergogold; and 2 minutes for In-Ceram Alumina, In-Ceram Zirconia, and Procera).

Results.—Airborne particle abrasion changed the morphological surface of IPS Empress, IPS Empress 2, and Cergogold ceramics. The surface topography of these ceramics demonstrated shallow irregularities not obvious in controls. For Procera, the 50-μm aluminum oxide airborne particle abrasion caused a flattened surface. Airborne particle abrasion of In-Ceram Alumina and In-Ceram Zirconia did not alter the morphological characteristics; the same shallow pits detected in controls remained.

For IPS Empress 2, 10% hydrofluoric acid caused elongated crystals scattered with shallow irregularities. For IPS Empress and Cergogold, the morphological characteristic was honeycomb-like on the ceramic surface. The surface treatment of In-Ceram Alumina, In-Ceram Zirconia, and Procera did not alter their superficial structure.

Conclusion.—Hydrofluoric acid etching and airborne particle abrasion with 50-μm aluminum oxide increased the irregularities on the surfaces of IPS Empress, IPS Empress 2, and Cergogold. Similar treatment of In-Ceram Alumina, In-Ceram Zirconia, and Procera did not alter their morphological microstructure.

▶ Advances in dental ceramics have been dramatic over the past 15 years. The introduction of the porcelain veneer in the early 1980s created the revolution in ceramic materials that is occurring today. Tom Greggs introduced one of the first porcelains developed for porcelain veneers in the early 1980s. Ivoclar followed with their lucite-reinforced porcelain Fortune. Empress was developed by Ivoclar in the late 1980s, and became the catalyst for the development of many of the new ceramics today. Today we have porcelain restorations that can be computer-aided design/computer-aided manufacturing generated and porcelains that can be used to fabricate fixed partial dentures. These new porcelains have required new luting systems and techniques. This article evaluates etching and abrasion on the microstructure of different ceramics.

F. M. McIntyre, DDS, MS

LED and Halogen Lights: Effect of Ceramic Thickness and Shade on Curing Luting Resin

Barghi N, McAlister EH (Univ of Texas, San Antonio)
Compend Contin Educ Dent 24:497-506, 2003   2–8

Background.—Halogen-source lights provide excellent polymerization of photoactivating composite resins but require routine monitoring and maintenance to ensure adequate light output. Blue light–emitting diode (LED) curing lights are now commercially available. These lights have achieved good hardness, compressive strength, and depth of cure in studies that used photoactivated composite resins. The potential effects of ceramic thickness and color on the microhardness of resin cements cured with the use of LED versus halogen curing lights were assessed.

Methods.—Porcelain specimens were made using 2 shades: the low-chroma, high-value shade A1 and the high-chroma, low-value shade C4 in thicknesses of 1 and 2 mm. A 0.5-mm–thick layer of composite luting resin was placed under each specimen, then cured for 30 or 60 seconds with an LED or halogen curing light. Control specimens were cured under a layer of clear Mylar. Surface hardness testing was then performed at a load of 15 N.

Results.—With cure times of 30 or 60 seconds, the surface hardness of the LED-cured specimens was similar to that of the control specimens. The

---

TABLE 2.—Materials and Methods (Experimental Groups and Subgroups)

	40-A1				40-C4		
20-1 mm		20-2 mm		20-1 mm		20-2 mm	
10-LED	10-Halogen	10-LED	10-Halogen	10-LED	10-Halogen	10-LED	10-Halogen
5 at 5 at	5 at 5 at	5 at 5 at	5 at 5 at	5 at 5 at	5 at 5 at	5 at 5 at	5 at 5 at
30 60	30 60	30 60	30 60	30 60	30 60	30 60	30 60
sec sec	sec sec	sec sec	sec sec	sec sec	sec sec	sec sec	sec sec

Abbreviations: A1, Shade A1 porcelain; *C4*, shade C4 porcelain; *LED*, light-emitting diode lamp; *halogen*, tungsten halogen lamp; *sec*, seconds.
(Reprinted with permission from *The Compendium of Continuing Education in Dentistry* from Barghi N, McAlister EH: LED and halogen lights: Effect of ceramic thickness and shade on curing luting resin. *Compend Contin Educ Dent* 24:497-506, 2003.)

2-mm specimens of C4 porcelain showed lower surface hardness with the halogen light with curings of 30 or 60 seconds. The LED curing light offered more consistent surface hardness results, although a cumulative comparison of the 2 lights showed similar results (Table 2).

Conclusion.—An LED curing light achieves consistently good surface hardness of composite luting resin specimens under porcelain of differing thicknesses and shades. In contrast, porcelain thickness and shade may have a greater effect on the cure achieved by a halogen light.

▶ Halogen light has long been the standard for the polymerization of composite materials. LED light sources are the most recent development in light-cure polymerization of composite materials. The Esthetic Dentistry Education Center at the University of Buffalo School of Dental Medicine has been studying LED light sources versus halogen light sources over the past 2 years. The studies by the esthetic dentistry residents and 2 prosthodontic residents have found similar results, as reported in this article. LED light sources are proving to be an excellent alternative to halogen light.

F. M. McIntyre, DDS, MS

Influence of NaOCl Deproteinization on Shear Bond Strength in Function of Dentin Depth

Toledano M, Perdigão J, Osorio E, et al (Univ of Granada, Spain; Univ of Minnesota, Minneapolis)
Am J Dent 15:252-255, 2002   2–9

Background.—Acid etching of dentin is used to improve adhesion in a variety of restorative and preventive dental procedures. This etching leaves the collagen fibrils without mechanical support with the exception of that caused by the water contained within the nanospaces between adjacent collagen fibers. The role of collagen fibrils in dentin adhesion has been questioned, and some authors have reported that dentin collagen does not contribute to dentin adhesion and may even interfere with the bonding mechanisms because of the fragile structure of the collagen fibers after etching. This study evaluated the effect of collagen removal with application of 5% sodium hypochlorite (NaOCl) on the shear bond strength of an acetone-based adhesive on superficial versus deep dentin.

Methods.—Superficial and deep dentin in 40 noncarious human third molars was exposed by sectioning of the occlusal surface immediately under the enamel-dentin junction or close to the pulp chamber. After polishing of the dentin disks, they were assigned to 36% orthophosphoric acid either for 15 seconds or for 15 seconds followed by 5% NaOCl for 2 minutes. The dentin adhesive was applied according to the manufacturer's instructions, followed by TPH resin-based composite. The specimens were stored in water for 24 hours at 37°C and thermocycled x500, and shear bond strengths were determined. Analysis of variance and Student's *t*-test were used for statistical analysis of data.

Results.—Superficial dentin resulted in statistically higher mean shear bond strength than deep dentin for acid-etched specimens. However, statistically similar mean shear bond strengths were obtained from deep and superficial dentin after NaOCl application. The mean shear bond strength on superficial dentin was not affected by collagen removal; however, shear bond strength on deep dentin was increased with the removal of collagen.

Conclusion.—The application of NaOCl after etching increases shear bond strength on deep dentin but does not affect the shear bond strength on superficial dentin when an acetone-based adhesive is used.

▶ Dr Paul Belvedere has advocated the use of NaOCl for years to clean the dentin interface. This article has shown that debridement of the dentin with NaOCl can increase shear bond strengths within deep dentin. Deep dentin usually yields lower bond strength than superficial dentin because of its physical properties. NaOCl deproteinizes the deeper dentinal tissues to yield shear bond strengths similar to superficial dentin. Clinically, we can increase our shear bond strengths to dentin within deeper restorations, which increases the longevity of our restorative dentistry.

F. M. McIntyre, DDS, MS

Clinical

Clinical Evaluation of Teeth Restored With Quartz Fiber–Reinforced Epoxy Resin Posts

Malferrari S, Monaco C, Scotti R (Univ of Bologna, Italy)
Int J Prosthodont 16:39-44, 2003   2–10

Introduction.—Several post-and-core restorations have been introduced by both researchers and manufacturers to provide reliable systems for reconstruction of endodontically treated teeth. The survival rate of 180 endodontically treated teeth (132 patients) (Table 1) restored with the use of quartz-fiber posts and composite resin material was examined over a 30-month evaluation period.

Methods.—The posts of Æstheti-Plus quartz-fiber posts were luted with the All-Bond 2 adhesive system and C&B Resin Cement according to the manufacturer's recommendations. The core was created with the use of Core-Flo or Bis-Core. All-ceramic crowns or metal-ceramic crowns were applied as final restorations. Parameters used to evaluate clinical failure were

TABLE 1.—Distribution of Treated Teeth According to Type

Jaw	Central Incisors	Lateral Incisors	Canines	Premolars	Molars
Maxilla	43	17	28	24	8
Mandible	9	11	16	8	16
Both	52	28	44	32	24

(Courtesy of Malferrari S, Monaco C, Scotti R: Clinical evaluation of teeth restored with quartz fiber–reinforced epoxy resin posts. *Int J Prosthodont* 16:39-44, 2003.)

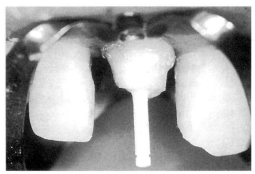

FIGURE 1.—Æstheti-Plus quartz-fiber post cemented in a maxillary right central incisor. (Courtesy of Malferrari S, Monaco C, Scotti R: Clinical evaluation of teeth restored with quartz fiber–reinforced epoxy resin posts. *Int J Prosthodont* 16:39-44, 2003.)

as follows: displacement, detachment, or fracture of posts; core or root fracture; and crown or prosthesis decementation. Patients were re-assessed at 6, 12, 24, and 30 months.

> *Technique.*—After root preparation is performed, the fiber post is reduced to the proper length, which is at least equal to the length of the clinical crown, while respecting the apical gulla percha seal of 4 mm. The root canal was treated with 32% phosphoric acid for 15 seconds, rinsed with deionized water, and gently dried. Equally mixed primes A and B (Bisco) are applied in the canal and on the post surface and gently dried. The 2 components of the self-curing C&B Resin Cement (Bisco) are mixed and applied at the edge of the root and on the post, which is immediately placed in the prepared canal (Figs 1 and 2).

> *Results.*—There were 3 failures in 30 months (1.7% failure rate). All occurred during the temporary phases during removal of the resin temporary restoration. One cohesive failure involving a margin of the composite core

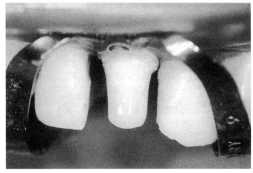

FIGURE 2.—Completed core buildup. (Courtesy of Malferrari S, Monaco C, Scotti R: Clinical evaluation of teeth restored with quartz fiber–reinforced epoxy resin posts. *Int J Prosthodont* 16:39-44, 2003.)

occurred 2 weeks after placement, and 2 adhesive fractures were observed after 2 months. These fractures were located between the cement and the dentin walls of the canals. The restoration was successfully replaced in all 3 failed cases.

Conclusion.—Good clinical results were observed in the rehabilitation of endodontically treated teeth with the use of quartz-fiber posts during a 30-month evaluation period. There was no incidence of crown or prosthesis decementation, and there were no post, core, or root fractures.

▶ The philosophy for restoring teeth endodontically has changed dramatically from the classic approach of the 1970s. It is no longer believed that posts strengthen endodontically treated teeth. Posts are used today to provide a foundation for restoring an endodontically treated tooth when insufficient tooth structure remains to retain the core restoration. The conservation of dentin and the development of a ferrule of tooth structure provide strength to the endodontically treated tooth. Several materials are now used as posts in endodontically treated teeth. This article reports a clinical evaluation of teeth restored with a quartz fiber–reinforced epoxy resin post.

F. M. McIntyre, DDS, MS

3 Prosthodontics

Introduction

Prosthodontics is the single largest area of income to general dentists. The older population with increased life expectancy, discretionary funds to spend, and a desire to look and feel better has stimulated growth. All-ceramic crowns, computer-aided design/computer-aided manufacturing, and all-ceramic fixed partial dentures are increasing in their use. Removable complete and partial dentures are still a major part of dentistry today. Developments of new tooth forms, better denture bases, and refinements in framework metals continue to offer excellent service for our patients.

Included in this year's chapter are articles related to diagnosis, the technical aspects of prosthetic restoration procedures, and interesting clinical studies related to occlusion. Occlusion is presently a highly controversial subject in the practice of prosthodontic procedures today.

Frederick M. McIntyre, DDS, MS

Diagnosis

Initial In Vitro Evaluation of DIAGNOdent for Detecting Secondary Carious Lesions Associated With Resin Composite Restorations
Boston DW (Temple Univ, Philadelphia)
Quintessence Int 34:109-116, 2003   3–1

Introduction.—Secondary caries often necessitate replacement of resin composite restorations. There is evidence that the diagnosis of secondary caries is often inaccurate. Laser fluorescence has been created as an adjunct to smooth surface and pit-fissure caries lesion identification; the DIAGNOdent (DD) system is commercially available for this purpose. The potential of DD readings to identify secondary enamel and dentin carious lesions linked with resin composite restorations were examined in a set of preserved extracted adult teeth.

Methods.—Thirty test sites adjacent to resin composite restorations in 15 extracted teeth were assessed visually and with DD readings for enamel and dentin caries. Findings were compared to gold standard diagnosis ascertained by sectioning through each site and subsequent microscopic observation. Sensitivity, specificity, accuracy, and likelihood ratios at optimum threshold values for enamel and dentin caries were calculated. Visual and

TABLE 1.—DIAGNOdent Readings by Reading Site and Diagnosis Class

DIAGNOdent Reading Site/ Diagnosis Class	Minimum Reading	Maximum Reading	Mean	SD
Tooth/restoration margin				
Enamel positive*	20	62	36.67	19.49
Enamel negative†	0	58	17.42	15.66
Dentin positive‡	9	62	34.00	20.97
Dentin negative§	0	37	13.89	10.83
Tooth, 1 mm from margin				
Enamel positive*	1	23	11.50	8.46
Enamel negative†	0	34	7.25	8.77
Dentin positive‡	1	34	13.18	9.74
Dentin negative§	0	22	5.16	6.72
Restoration, 1 mm from margin				
Enamel positive*	5	29	17.00	19.49
Enamel negative†	0	37	11.38	10.30
Dentin positive‡	3	29	15.91	9.39
Dentin negative§	0	37	10.53	10.54
Cross-sectioned surface				
Enamel positive*	8	51	30.83	15.52
Enamel negative†	0	16	3.71	4.18
Dentin positive‡	25	99	66.45	33.18
Dentin negative§	2	24	7.32	5.38
Center of healthy smooth surface of tooth	3	9	5.87	1.78
Center of resin composite restoration surface	5	22	12.07	5.11

*n = 6.
†n = 24.
‡n = 11.
§n = 19.
Abbreviation: SD, Standard deviation.
(Courtesy of Boston DW: Initial in vitro evaluation of DIAGNOdent for detecting secondary carious lesions associated with resin composite restorations. *Quintessence Int* 34:109-116, 2003.)

DD diagnostic methods were compared via receiver operator characteristic (ROC) analysis.

Results.—Histologic examination showed that the incidence of enamel caries was 20% and of dental caries was 36.67% (Table 1). All composite restorations in the extracted teeth fluoresced (range, 5-22) (Figs 1 and 2). For enamel caries identification with DD, the optimum threshold of 22 or greater generated a sensitivity of 0.67 and a specificity of 0.79. For dentin caries identification with DD, the optimum threshold of 22 or greater produced a sensitivity and specificity of 0.73 and 0.84, respectively (Table 2).

The receiver operating characteristic analysis revealed that DD readings contain diagnostic information. The DD readings for dentin caries diagnosis provided better diagnostic results compared to visual readings for the 30 test sites; these results did not vary significantly (Table 3).

Conclusion.—The DD readings may be useful in identifying secondary carious lesions associated with resin composite restorations. Instrument design factors and technique need to be optimized to improve performance beyond that obtained from visual detection alone.

▶ For years, dentists have relied on radiographs and tactile examination to determine if caries are present within tooth structure. Some clinicians have advocated that changes in color within the enamel can help identify carious le-

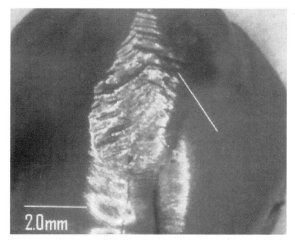

FIGURE 1.—The visual appearance of 1 diagnostic site located on the facial margin of a facial-distal-lingual resin composite restoration in a maxillary right canine can be seen. The location of the diagnostic site is marked by the *white line* traversing the tooth/restoration margin. Internal discoloration of the adjacent tooth structure was noted on examination and the site was rated as "enamel caries definitely present" and "dentin caries definitely present" visually. The DIAGNOdent (DD) reading taken at the tooth/restoration margin was 61. At 1 mm from the margin onto the tooth structure, the DD reading was 11, and at 1 mm from the margin onto the restoration, the DD reading was 8. (Courtesy of Boston DW: Initial in vitro evaluation of DIAGNOdent for detecting secondary carious lesions associated with resin composite restorations. *Quintessence Int* 34:109-116, 2003.)

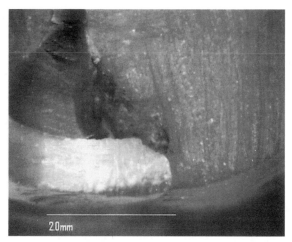

FIGURE 2.—The microscopic appearance of the site from Figure 1 after sectioning and application of caries dye can be seen. On microscopic examination, the adjacent enamel was rated as chalky and crumbling upon explorer probing, and the adjacent dentin was rated as soft, stained, and stainable with caries dye. In this view, some carious dentin adjacent to the resin composite restoration is missing due to explorer probing for softness. Gold standard rating for both enamel and dentin caries was rated positive for this site. DIAGNOdent readings taken directly on the exposed enamel and dentin adjacent to the resin composite restoration prior to probing or application of caries dye were 44 for enamel and 70 for dentin. (Courtesy of Boston DW: Initial in vitro evaluation of DIAGNOdent for detecting secondary carious lesions associated with resin composite restorations. *Quintessence Int* 34:109-116, 2003.)

TABLE 2.—Test Results by Type and Location of Diagnosis Technique

Type/Location of Diagnostic Technique	Best Threshold Value (≥)	Sensitivity	Specificity	Accuracy	Likelihood Ratio	AUC	P
Enamel caries diagnosis (scale 0-99)							
DD at restoration margin	26	.67	.79	.77	3.20	.8542	.0081*
DD 1 mm onto tooth structure	23	.17	.96	.80	4.00	.6910	.1516*
DD 1 mm onto restoration	29	.17	.96	.80	4.00	.6875	.1607*
Dentin caries diagnosis (scale 0-99)							
DD at restoration margin	22	.73	.84	.80	4.61	.8254	.0034*
DD 1 mm onto tooth structure	23	.18	1.00	.70	∞	.7871	.0094*
DD 1 mm onto res-toration	23	.45	.89	.73	4.32	.6842	.0968*
Visual diagnosis for dentin caries (scale 1-5)	5	.45	.68	.60	2.16	.6029	.0787†
Visual diagnosis for enamel caries (scale 1-5)	5	.83	.71	.73	3.20	.8056	.6475†

*Probability of the null hypothesis that area under the curve (AUC) is not different from the AUC of no information (0.5).
†Probability of the null hypothesis that there is no difference between AUC for visual diagnosis at AUC for DIAGNOdent (DD) diagnosis.
(Courtesy of Boston DW: Initial in vitro evaluation of DIAGNOdent for detecting secondary carious lesions associated with resin composite restorations. *Quintessence Int* 34:109-116, 2003.)

sions. Transillumination has been used to detect interproximal caries. Within the last 10 years, caries detectors have been marketed to stain caries within the tooth. When I was at the KAVO factory in 1999, I was introduced to the DD unit for the first time. Since that time, I have had the opportunity to evaluate it on several occasions. It appears to be a promising instrument for use in your dental office.

F. M. McIntyre, DDS, MS

TABLE 3.—Test Results for Combinations of Visual and DIAGNOdent Information

Positive Dentin Caries Diagnosis Defined by:	Sensitivity	Specificity	Accuracy
Visual means alone	.4545	.6842	.6000
DD values alone	.7273	.8421	.8000
Visual or DD values must be positive for dentin caries	.8182	.6842	.7333
Visual and DD values must be positive for dentin caries	.3636	1.0000	.7667

Abbreviation: DD, DIAGNOdent.
(Courtesy of Boston DW: Initial in vitro evaluation of DIAGNOdent for detecting secondary carious lesions associated with resin composite restorations. *Quintessence Int* 34:109-116, 2003.)

Planning Restorative Treatment for Patients With Severe Class II Malocclusions

Ambard A, Mueninghoff L (Univ of Alabama at Birmingham)
J Prosthet Dent 88:200-207, 2002   3–2

Introduction.—Ideally, severe Angle skeletal Class II malocclusions should be identified at an early age and corrected orthodontically. Described was a clinical protocol in which fixed prosthodontic procedures are used to restore patients with severe Class II skeletal malocclusions.

Class II Malocclusions.—Under the protocol for the occlusal rehabilitation of patients with severe Angle skeletal Class II malocclusions, an occlusal device is used for 2 reasons: (1) to locate the most appropriate maxillary-mandibular relationship for function and range of motion at an established vertical dimension of occlusion and (2) to accurately transfer this relationship to an articulator for fabrication of provisional and definitive restorations. The advantages of using an evidence-based protocol are that no irreversible procedures are initiated until the patient is comfortable and the treatment results are visualized clearly. After a harmonious physiologic relationship is established, treatment can become technical.

Conclusion.—Frequent use of an occlusal device to locate the most harmonious deprogramed position of the mandible has also proven beneficial in full-mouth reconstruction and in patients with muscular incoordination.

▶ Class II malocclusions are the most difficult restorative challenges we have. Anterior guidance can be difficult to achieve, especially if there is a change in the vertical dimension of occlusion (VDO). As the VDO is increased, the arc of closure changes and the relationship of the maxillary and mandibular incisors will change. This article reviews the characteristics associated with a Class II malocclusion and reports on one treatment protocol that can be used to treat Class II malocclusions. I would caution you about using 1 technique to treat all Class II malocclusions. Increasing VDO is not always advantageous for the patient.

F. M. McIntyre, DDS, MS

Mandibular Adaptive Reposturing: The Etiology of a Common and Multifaceted Autodestructive Syndrome

Giffin KM (Brandon, Miss)
Gen Dent 51:62-67, 2003   3–3

Introduction.—As with other joints, positional stability and integrity of the TMJ are maintained through muscle forces. These forces attempt to hold the TMJ condyles and articular disks in an optimal spatial relationship and in close apposition to joint interfaces within the glenoid fossa, which minimizes dislocation of articular surfaces. It resists heavy force loading without joint damage or discomfort. Optimal condylar position is referred to as centric relation (CR) and the condylar position dictated by maximum dental intercuspation is described as centric occlusion. Frequently, maximum intercuspation (MI) is referred to as interocclusal position or maximum interocclusal position. It is directed through sensory feedback from periodontal proprioceptors and is a neuromuscularly favored and protective mandibular position for the dentition; it literally drives the stomatognathic system. The etiology of the autodestructive syndrome was discussed.

Etiology and Treatment.—When MI and CR are not in harmony, the mandible takes on adaptive reposturing to try to achieve as much MI as mechanically possible. This can cause an autodestructive syndrome that damages various stomatognathic components. Diurnal and nocturnal clenching and/or bruxism, along with other parafunctional activities mediated at various neurologic levels, can complicate this problem.

Effective management of the autodestructive syndrome necessitates establishment of harmony between CR and MI. Mandibular adaptive reposturing (MAR) can be managed with orthognathic surgery and refined with orthodontics, equilibration, and/or reconstructive dentistry as needed. Various joint prostheses can by used that may remedy or lessen a joint problem and eradicate MAR in patients with a severely degenerated TMJ not responsive to more conservative approaches.

Conclusion.—Because MI drives the stomatognathic system, homeostasis necessitates balance between CR and MI. If this does not occur, MAR will take place automatically to maximize intercuspation, with the potential for the development of stomatognathic pathology.

▶ Too often, dentistry is focused on tooth-tooth restorative dentistry, ignoring the other elements of the stomatognathic system. The restorative dentist treats the symptoms of the disease, not the cause. To treat the cause, the dentist must ask the question "Why?", and to answer the question there must be an understanding of functional and anatomical harmony within the system. The dentist must be able to recognize the signs of instability within the stomatognathic system in order to treat the underlying cause. This article discusses the etiology related to the autodestructive breakdown of the stomatognathic system.

F. M. McIntyre, DDS, MS

Pulmonary Risk of Intraoral Surface Conditioning Using Crystalline Silica
Mayer B, Raithel H, Weltle D, et al (Univ of Cologne, Germany; Univ of Erlang-en-Nuernberg, Germany)
Int J Prosthodont 16:157-160, 2003   3–4

Introduction.—Repair of broken or abraded ceramic or resin facings of fixed prostheses is frequently needed in prosthetic dentistry. To avoid the time-consuming and expensive replacement of fixed dentures, new intraoral techniques based on tribochemical (chemical binding caused by kinetic energy) use of SiO_x have been created and provide excellent results in cases of cracked facing.

The retention between repair resin and metal or ceramic surfaces can be enhanced significantly with the use of Rocatec particles, which are Al_2O_3 granules covered with crystalline silica that are tribochemically broken on the repair surfaces.

There is concern about the pulmonary risk with these 5-μm particles, which are commonly regarded as respirable dust that can be deposited in the lung parenchyma. The pulmonary risk caused by possible respirable dust of Al_2O_3 and SiO_x resulting from chairside tribochemical sandblasting procedures in a dental office was examined.

Methods.—Dust (Al_2O_3 particles [mean size, 30 μm] covered with SiO_x) was gathered with the use of a trap near the working field. Quantitative morphological determination and identification were performed with scanning electron microscopy and energy dispersive x-ray analysis. Forty blasting processes (working pressure, 2.3 bars; flow rate, 6 to 6.5 g Rocatec or Cojet powder/min; total time, 20 minutes) were aimed at a dummy to obtain maximum pollution of the workplace. The respirable dust fraction was determined by personal air samplers with an 8-μm cellulose-nitrate filter and a volume flow rate of 2 L/min. Masses of the respirable dust fraction were ascertained. Respirable free crystalline silica was identified by infrared spectroscopy.

Results.—Measurements of total respirable dust (particle size over 5 μm) showed a mean workplace air pollution of 0.26 mg/m³ for sandblasting processes without suction. Use of dental suction produced a significantly reduced mean concentration for respirable dust of 0.21 mg/m³. With and without dental suction, the workplace air pollution of respirable crystalline silica was always under 0.02 mg/m³. Independent of dental suction, the pollution of the sandblasting clinician did not vary significantly ($P = .42$) from that of the assistant.

Conclusion.—Concern about the risk of oral tribochemical methods and possible impairment of the health of patients and dental staff is groundless. Under extreme conditions, even without protective measures, the concentrations of respirable dust particles in the air are well beneath the current threshold value of 1.5 mg/m³. The concentration of the harmful free crystalline silica in the air is also well beneath the current threshold value of 0.15 mg/m³. Under normal conditions, intraoral surface conditioning using crystalline silica is not dangerous to the health of dental patients or staff.

▶ Intraoral repairs of fractured porcelain can be enhanced with the use of microetching. Microetching increases the bonding area for a micromechanical bond between the porcelain and composite repair. Studies have shown that it provides a better surface for repair than a surface prepared with a fine diamond. I have used microetching for several years now to repair porcelain. I have always had concerns about the inhalation of the powder. I use a rubber dam whenever possible for the protection of the patient. When a rubber dam cannot be used, I have used a 4 × 4 gauze which I wet with H_2O and place in the mouth as a trap for the powder. These authors studied the pulmonary risks associated with microetching.

F. M. McIntyre, DDS, MS

Technical

The Retention of Complete Crowns Prepared With Three Different Tapers and Luted With Four Different Cements

Zidan O, Ferguson GC (Univ of Minnesota, Minneapolis; Waterville, Me)
J Prosthet Dent 89:565-571, 2003   3–5

Background.—In the 1950s and 1960s, the traditional standards for crown retention were established on the basis of analysis of the geometric configurations of the area—taper, height, and surface area. Of these, the taper has been the most investigated and most discussed feature. Luting is the primary function of a traditional nonadhesive luting cement, such as zinc phosphate. With these cements, retention is dependent mainly on the geometry of the preparation.

Zinc phosphate has traditionally been the cement of choice, and its clinical success is well documented. However, newer classes of cements—such as conventional glass ionomers, resin-modified glass ionomers, and resins—are formulated with adhesive properties. The role of these adhesive properties in the retentive strength of crowns with different degrees of taper is unclear. This study evaluated the retention of full crowns prepared with 3 different tapers and cemented with 2 conventional and 2 adhesive resin systems.

Methods.—A total of 120 sound human molars were randomly assigned to 1 of 12 groups representing the 4 cements: zinc phosphate, conventional glass ionomer, and 2 adhesive resin cements. Three tapers of 6°, 12°, and 24° were used with each cement, with the 6° taper considered the control within each cement group. Crowns were cast with a high noble alloy. Retention was measured by separation of the metal crowns from the prepared teeth under tension on a universal testing machine. Analysis of variance was used to test the main effects on the retentive strength of full crowns, namely, cements, tapers, and failure modes.

Results.—There was a significant difference in the main effect cement and taper. The mean retentive strength values of both the zinc phosphate and the conventional glass ionomer were significantly lower than the mean retentive strength values of the 2 adhesive resin cements. The difference between the retention of crowns with the 6° taper from retention with the 12° taper was not significant; however, there was a significant different in retention between the 6° taper and the 24° taper and between the 12° and 24° tapers. The types of failure were adhesive in the cement in 65% of cases, cohesive in the tooth in 31% of cases, and assembly failure in 4% of cases. The type of failure was dependent on the degree of taper and type of cement.

Conclusion.—The use of resin luting agents provided retention values that were twice the value of zinc phosphate or conventional glass ionomer cement.

▶ For years, zinc phosphate cement was the only reliable cement for permanently cementing restorations. Reliable as it was, it was the weakest link in the restoration of the tooth. In order to compensate for the cement interface, preparation design required attention to resistance and retention design. Taper of the preparation walls was limited to 4° to 8°. Today, the restorative dentist has several luting agents for cementation of restorations. The dentist must understand the advantages and disadvantages of the various luting agents. This article compared the effects of cement and taper using zinc phosphate, C & B Metabond, and Panavia.

F. M. McIntyre, DDS, MS

Preparation Design and Margin Distortion in Porcelain-Fused-to-Metal Restorations

Shillingburg HT Jr, Hobo S, Fisher DW (Univ of California, Los Angeles)
J Prosthet Dent 89:527-532, 2003   3–6

Background.—The design of the preparation used for porcelain-fused-to-metal crowns, so widely used today, must incorporate stabilization factors to address any possible interaction between the 2 materials when porcelain is added to the metal coping. The metal-plus-porcelain copings may not fit as well as before, with the labial margin most often the area of greatest distortion. Various configurations have been used to blend strength and esthetics in this part. An evaluation was performed on 4 labial finish lines to see what effect their configurations had on the stability of labial margins of porcelain-fused-to-metal crowns during the porcelain firing stages.

Methods.—The 4 finish lines assessed were the chamfer, the heavy chamfer with bevel, the shoulder with bevel, and the shoulder. A standardized coping design was employed to avoid differences in contour, collar size, or thickness of the veneering area that could influence the fit. The coping wax patterns were produced by using a split mold that was warmed, lubricated, assembled, and secured with a U-clamp that was precision fitted. After the castings were done and treated, they were put through the firing stage, with each casting being treated identically and measurements taken at each step. Once the baked thickness of 0.3 mm was achieved, the body and incisal porcelain were applied, and all copings were glazed. Final measurements were taken.

Results.—The means were determined for the labial opening measurements. The 4 finish lines had wider labial opening measurements through the first addition of body porcelain. The shoulder with bevel was the only finish line that did not continue to widen through the second body porcelain bake. Only slight changes were found with glazing. Significant differences were noted between the shoulder with bevel and both of the chamfer configurations; the shoulder and both chamfers had marginally significant differences. The 2 chamfer lines showed no significant differences, nor did the 2 shoulder lines. A significant difference was seen between the 2 shoulders and the 2 chamfers when body porcelain was added and at all succeeding steps, excluding the bevels.

Discussion.—In these porcelain-fused-to-metal restorations, the shoulder and shoulder with bevel finish lines exhibited significantly less distortion in the labial margins than the chamfer and chamfer with bevel finish lines. The openings of the chamfer (47.1 µm) and the heavy chamfer with bevel (29.3 µm) were large enough to be of clinical significance.

▶ This article is a classic revisited concerning preparation design and marginal distortion. Although all-ceramic crowns are used more often in dentistry than ever before, the porcelain-fused-to-metal restoration is still the dominant restoration placed. Distortion of the metal margin underlying the porcelain interface is a common problem. Too often, porcelain-fused-to-metal crowns are prepared with inadequate reduction and improper margin design to resist marginal distortion. Reviewing this article will benefit you and your patients.

F. M. McIntyre, DDS, MS

Bonding of Silicone Prosthetic Elastomers to Three Different Denture Resins

Polyzois GL, Frangou MJ (Univ of Athens, Greece; Athens, Greece)
Int J Prosthodont 15:535-538, 2002   3–7

Introduction.—Composite or implant-retained facial prostheses use a denture resin substructure or retentive matrix. The denture resin component needs to be securely bonded to the silicone material of the prosthesis. The reliability of the silicone-denture resin interface is crucial to the success and serviceability of the prosthesis because of the forces applied to the bone during placement and removal of the prosthesis and during mold-opening and deflasking procedures. The interfacial bond strength between various types of silicone facial elastomers and denture resins was examined.

Methods.—Cosmesil and Ideal were the facial materials that were evaluated, and the denture resins were SR 3/60, SR 3/60 Quick, and Triad (Table 1). The "overlap-joint" model was used to assess the bond strength (Fig 1). Within 1 week of polymerization, 10 samples for each silicone/resin group were placed in tension until failure.

TABLE 1.—Materials Used in the Study

Material	Type of Chemistry	Polymerization Method
Denture resin		
SR 3/60, Ivoclar	Heat-curing acrylic resin	8 h at 70°C (dry heat)
SR 3/60 Quick, Ivoclar	Autopolymerizing acrylic resin	20 min at room temperature
Triad VLC, Dentsply	Urethanedimethacrylate resin	10 min visible light curing
Silicone elastomer		
Cosmesil, Principality Medical	Condensation reaction	24-h room-temperature vulcanizing
Ideal, Orthomax	Addition reaction	24-h room-temperature vulcanizing

(Courtesy of Polyzois GL, Frangou MJ: Bonding of silicone prosthetic elastomers to three different denture resins. *Int J Prosthodont* 15:535-538, 2002.)

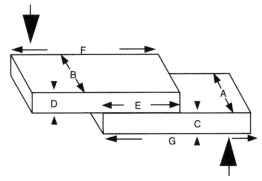

FIGURE 1.—Overlap-joint specimens and their dimensions. A = B = 13 mm; C = D = 3 mm; E = 23 mm; F = G = 48 mm. (Courtesy of Polyzois GL, Frangou MJ: Bonding of silicone prosthetic elastomers to three different denture resins. *Int J Prosthodont* 15:535-538, 2002.)

Results.—All samples failed adhesively to the extent that the silicone elastomer separated from the denture resin, suggesting that the tensile strength of the silicone was greater than the bond strength to the resin. There were significant differences in bond strength due to the denture resin variable ($P = .019$), the silicone elastomer variable ($P < .001$), and their interaction ($P < .001$). The primary effect of the silicone elastomer was the most important factor. This was followed by the denture resin, determining the bone strength. Three combinations of Cosmesil silicone with the denture resins (groups A, C, E) revealed significantly stronger ($P < .05$) bond strengths compared with the respective combinations with Ideal silicone (groups B, D, F) (Table 2).

Conclusion.—Cosmesil condensation-type silicone always revealed higher bond strength with the 3 different types of denture resins compared with Ideal addition silicone, keeping other variables linked with the silicone-resin bond fixed.

▶ There have been cases where there has been severe ridge resorption in which I have used a soft liner to increase comfort for the patient. My experiences with the materials has been the same as for many others. The material begins to break down and debond at the edges. I have tried many different sur-

TABLE 2.—Bond Strength of Silicone Facial Elastomers to Denture Resins (n = 10)

Denture resin	Group	Cosmesil Mean	SD	Group	Ideal Mean	SD
SR 3/60	A	0.19[a]	0.044	B	0.03[b]	0.007
SR 3/60 Quick	C	0.23[a]	0.044	D	0.03[b]	0.005
Triad VLC	E	0.18[a]	0.046	F	0.04[c]	0.009

Note: Figures are in megapascals. Means with the same superscribed letter were not statistically different at the $\alpha = 0.05$ level.
Abbreviation: SD, Standard deviation.
(Courtesy of Polyzois GL, Frangou MJ: Bonding of silicone prosthetic elastomers to three different denture resins. *Int J Prosthodont* 15:535-538, 2002.)

face preparations and marginal designs. Some have worked better than others, but I have never been able to obtain a satisfactory result for more than 6 months. This article reports the results obtained by using different techniques to increase the bond between elastomers and denture resins.

F. M. McIntyre, DDS, MS

The Effect of Design Modifications on the Torsional and Compressive Rigidity of U-Shaped Palatal Major Connectors
Green LK, Hondrum SO (US Army Dental Activity, Fort Benning, Ga; US Army Dental Materials Lab, Fort Gordon, Ga)
J Prosthet Dent 89:400-407, 2003   3–8

Introduction.—The major connector of a removable partial denture (RPD) acts to unite the various components of the prosthesis into a single unit and distributes the forces placed on the RPD to all supporting structures. Diminishing the rigidity of a mandibular major connector decreases the ability of the RPD to resist horizontal stresses. The failure to provide sufficient rigidity can result in patient discomfort and possible damage to oral structures. The effects of changing the width, thickness, and shape on the rigidity of U-shaped maxillary major connectors were examined.

Methods.—Twenty maxillary frameworks consisting of 5 frameworks each of 4 different U-shaped removable partial denture designs were fabricated with the use of a nickle-chrome alloy. The designs included an 8-mm–wide U-shaped strap with a 6-mm posterior strap (A-P strap), a 13-mm–wide U-shaped strap (Wide), and 8-mm–wide U-shaped strap that widened to 13 mm at midline (Notch), and an 8-mm–wide U-shaped strap twice the thickness of the other straps (Thick). A fifth group of 5 frameworks was created by removing the posterior strap from the A-P strap frameworks (A strap).

Two testing points were marked on every framework that corresponded to the first premolar and second molar positions. After mounting the frameworks in a universal testing machine, vertical (torsional) and horizontal (compressive) loads were applied using a 10-kilonewton load cell at a crosshead speed of 2 mm/min until a deflection of 1 mm occurred. A force-deflection curve was produced for each test, and slope of curves (newtons per millimeter) was compared with analysis of variance and the Scheffé F test ($\alpha = 0.05$).

Results.—The Thick group was significantly more rigid ($P < .05$) than the other frameworks when torsional loads were applied to both the premolar (22.42 newtons/mm) and molar (10.88 newtons/mm) areas, and when a compressive load was applied to the premolar (232.85 newtons/mm) area. The A-P strap group was significantly more rigid ($P \geq .05$), compared to other designs when a compressive load was applied to the molar (69.56 newtons/mm) area (Figs 3 and 4). The Thick and the A-P strap groups were significantly more rigid ($P < .05$), compared to the Notch and A strap groups.

Torsion

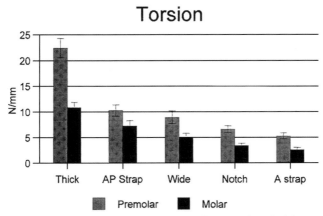

FIGURE 3.—Mean force-deflection value (newtons per millimeter) and standard deviation for frameworks when tested with torsional load. (Courtesy of Green LK, Hondrum SO: The effect of design modifications on the torsional and compressive rigidity of U-shaped palatal major connectors. *J Prosthet Dent* 89:400-407, 2003.)

Conclusion.—Doubling the thickness of the anterior strap of a U-shaped maxillary major connector enhanced the rigidity of the framework to the torsional loads. A posterior strap added to the U-shaped connector was more effective in maintaining work rigidity to compressive forces as the length of the arch increased.

▶ The major connector for a maxillary removable partial denture has been studied extensively in the literature. It provides the rigidity to protect the abutment teeth and is primary to the retention of the partial denture. To create rigidity requires, in many cases, maximum coverage of the palate. For patients, there can be problems related to tongue, space, and position. It can also dis-

Compression

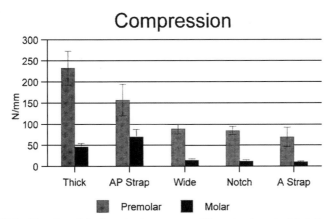

FIGURE 4.—Mean force-deflection value (newtons per millimeter) and standard deviation for frameworks when tested with compressive load. (Courtesy of Green LK, Hondrum SO: The effect of design modifications on the torsional and compressive rigidity of U-shaped palatal major connectors. *J Prosthet Dent* 89:400-407, 2003.)

rupt taste. The U-shaped palatal major connector has been used by dentists for years to try to alleviate patients' complaints. This article revisits the effect of design modification on the rigidity of the U-shaped palatal major connector.

F. M. McIntyre, DDS, MS

Clinical

Cervical Dentin Hypersensitivity: Part III: Resolution Following Occlusal Equilibration

Coleman TA, Grippo JO, Kinderknecht KE (Shaftsbury, Vt; Western New England, Springfield, Mass; West Virginia Univ, Morgantown)
Quintessence Int 34:427-434, 2003   3–9

Background.—Stress-induced hard tissue lesions, termed "abfractive lesions," are related to cervical dentin hypersensitivity (CDH) in that they are usually found on the cervical facial surfaces of premolars and molars. This relationship may indicate that CDH develops in response to excessive functional or parafunctional occlusal stress. The changes that occur in CDH in response to occlusal equilibration were investigated retrospectively.

Methods.—A random selection of 250 active-care patients underwent analysis for links between CDH and its resolution with occlusal equilibration. A treatment group of 82 patients and a delayed treatment group of 19 patients were formed, wherein occlusal equilibration was done after CDH was verified by means of the air indexing method (Table 1). A third group of 149 patients had no detectable and verified CDH over the 17 years of the study.

Results.—Of the 2 treatment groups, 43.6% had CDH of 1 tooth and 22.8% of 2 teeth; 1 patient had CDH of 13 teeth. Overall, 246 teeth were verified to have CDH over the 17 years studied. All of the 246 teeth with

TABLE 1.—Summary of Comparisons of Groups A, B, and C (1979 to 1996)

| | Groups | | | | | | | | |
| | A | | | B | | | C | | |
	Female	Male	Both	Female	Male	Both	Female	Male	Both
No. of patients	42	40	82	13	6	19	77	72	149
Age at beginning of dental care									
Mean	37	41	39	32	45	36	39	42	40
Median	48	46	47	38	46	41	35	41	38
Standard deviation	11	12	12	10	13	20	19	15	17
Mean no. of teeth	26	27	26	26	26	26	25	24	24
Mean years in treatment	9	10	10	13	17	14	9	9	9
No. of patients with active parafunction (%)	23	18	41 (50.0%)	7	2	9 (47.4%)	12	11	23 (15.4%)

Note: A includes patients with verified cervical dentin hypersensitivity (CDH) equilibrated within 30 days; B, patients with verified CDH equilibrated at 30 days or greater; C, patients with no verified CDH.

(Courtesy of Coleman TA, Grippo JO, Kinderknecht KE: Cervical dentin hypersensitivity: Part III. Resolution following occlusal equilibration. *Quintessence Int* 34:427-434, 2003.)

TABLE 2.—Equilibration Data and Equilibrated Cervical Dentin Hypersensitivity Associated With Recent Dental Treatment for Groups A and B

	Groups					
	A (n = 82)			B (n = 19)		
	Female	Male	Both	Female	Male	Both
Total equilibration visits for positive air indexed teeth*			220			30
Mean visits to resolve CDH			2			2
Total patients relieved of CDH by occlusal equilibration			82			19
Patients with recurrent CDH following equilibration (%)			12 (15)			1 (5)
Total equilibration visits for secondary positive air indexed teeth*			19			3
Average no. of visits to resolve secondary occurrence of CDH			2			3
Percentage of patients requiring 4 or more visits of occlusal equilibration to resolve CDH			12			10
No. of incidents of CDH†	66	55	121	15	6	21
No. of incidents of CDH related to dental treatment (%)†	19 (29)	18 (33)	37 (31)	9 (60)	1 (17)	10 (48)
Operative	8	9	17	4	0	4
Crown	5	4	9	5	1	6
Fixed bridge	6	3	9	0	0	0
Extractions (more than 7 days postop)	0	1	1	0	0	0
Partial denture	0	1	1	0	0	0

Note: A includes patients with verified cervical dentin hypersensitivity (*CDH*) equilibrated within 30 days; B, patients with verified CDH equilibrated at 30 days or greater; C, patients with no verified CDH.
*One treatment visit may relate to equilibration of several teeth diagnosed with verified CDH.
†Some patients had multiple CDH teeth.
(Courtesy of Coleman TA, Grippo JO, Kinderknecht KE: Cervical dentin hypersensitivity: Part III. Resolution following occlusal equilibration. *Quintessence Int* 34:427-434, 2003.)

CDH had occlusal equilibration and resulting resolution of the CDH (Table 2). Generally, 2 visits were required for resolution. Fifteen percent of the treatment group and 5% of the delayed treatment group had recurrent CDH, which also resolved in an average of 2 visits by occlusal equilibration. For 31% of the treatment group and 48% of the delayed treatment group,

TABLE 3A.—Distribution of Occlusal Equilibrations for Groups A and B

	Groups			
	A		B	
Treatment Time	Mean No. of Days	Total Incidents	Mean No. of Days	Total Incidents
Between diagnosis and first treatment	7	121	92	21
Between first and second treatment	17	57	19	7
Between second and third treatment	15	26	14	3
Between third and fourth treatment	8	15	12	2

Note: A indicates patients with verified cervical dentin hypersensitivity equilibrated within 30 days; B, patients with verified cervical dentin hypersensitivity equilibrated at 30 days or greater.
(Courtesy of Coleman TA, Grippo JO, Kinderknecht KE: Cervical dentin hypersensitivity: Part III. Resolution following occlusal equilibration. *Quintessence Int* 34:427-434, 2003.)

TABLE 3B.—Location of Occlusal Equilibrations for Groups A and B

| | | Group A | | | | Group B | | |
Adjustment	First	Second	Third	Fourth+	First	Second	Third	Fourth+
Working	65	31	10	3	8	2	0	0
Nonworking	10	1	0	0	3	2	1	1
Centric	5	1	1	1	1	0	0	0
Protrusive	4	1	0	0	3	0	0	0
Working and nonworking	28	19	11	8	6	3	2	1
Centric and protrusive	2	0	0	0	0	0	0	0
Working and centric	5	2	2	1	0	0	0	0
Working/nonworking/centric	2	2	2	2	0	0	0	0
Total	121	57	26	15	21	7	3	2

Note: A indicates patients with verified cervical dentin hypersensitivity equilibrated within 30 days; B, patients with verified cervical dentin hypersensitivity equilibrated at 30 days or greater.

(Courtesy of Coleman TA, Grippo JO, Kinderknecht KE: Cervical dentin hypersensitivity: Part III. Resolution following occlusal equilibration. *Quintessence Int* 34:427-434, 2003.)

the CDH diagnosis was related to hyperfunctional contacts from recent dental treatment. Those in the treatment group had initial occlusal equilibration at an average of 7 days after diagnosis and for those in the delayed group, the average was 92 days (Tables 3A and 3B). Most of the adjustments required involved working cusp inclines, which corresponded to the overwhelming buccal locations of CDH.

Discussion.—A direct relationship was found between CDH and occlusal disharmony. Undertaking careful occlusal analysis and equilibration will likely eliminate CDH.

▶ There is controversy in the literature related to factors contributing to CDH. The controversy centers on whether occlusion is a factor. Some investigators believe that cervical lesions are created by abrasive or erosive processes only. Others relate cervical lesions to occlusal trauma and use the term "abfraction lesion." Some recent studies have concluded that CDH is probably multifactorial. The present study confirms that verified and quantified CDH can be directly related to occlusal disharmony.

F. M. McIntyre, DDS, MS

Tooth Preparations Designed for Posterior Resin-Bonded Fixed Partial Dentures: A Clinical Report

Chow TW, Chung RWC, Chu FCS, et al (Univ of Hong Kong, China)
J Prosthet Dent 88:561-564, 2002   3–10

Introduction.—Many designs for posterior resin-bonded fixed partial dentures (RBFPD) have been developed, yet there is no standardized RBFPD design. A logical tooth preparation approach for posterior abutments to receive resin-bonded retainers was discussed. The groove, plate, and strut approach necessitates minimal tooth substance removal and avoids many shortcomings linked with the early RBFPD design.

Preoperative Assessment/Path of Insertion.—A comprehensive clinical assessment of periodontal health, endodontal status, coronal structure, and occlusal relationship must be performed. Study casts need to be surveyed to ascertain the most appropriate path of insertion. By inserting the prosthesis from a slightly lingual direction for the mandibular arch or palatal for the maxillary arch, dislodgement of the prosthesis in an occlusal direction can be reduced by the use of rigid retainers.

Framework Design and Tooth Preparation.—The grooves on proximal and palatal/lingual surfaces of abutment teeth have 2 main functions: to define the path of insertion and to provide retention and resistance form to the retainer against the dislodging forces acting on the pontic. Grooves on the proximal surfaces can efficiently resist rotation of the pontic along the axis created by the occlusal rests.

The palatal/lingual framework (plate) or the retainer is important for retention of the RBFPD. It is helpful to have a large area of enamel to aid in bonding the plate to the abutment tooth. A minimum 180° encirclement of the tooth has been suggested. Its vertical extension is determined by the path of insertion and the location and degree of the abutment undercut. The proximal extension is limited by esthetics and the proximal contact.

Material rigidity is an important feature of cast restorations. Without adequate thickness, deformation or bending of the plate of a circumferential retainer can occur during laboratory fabrication. The occlusal strut gives rigidity to the resin-bonded retainer in a similar way as an occlusally placed groove preparation of the conventional crown. In addition to producing rigidity and enhanced support to the RBFPD through its geometrical configuration, the strut joining the mesial and distal aspects of the plate results in a 360° encirclement of the palatal/lingual cusp. This encirclement gives resistance to palatal/lingual dislodgement of the retainer. If an existing occlusal restoration is present, an occlusal cavity can be created and included in the RBFPD by removing the restoration to ensure retentive features.

Conclusion.—The groove, plate, and strut design is a conservative and esthetic approach to RBFPD preparation design which allows straightforward fabrication of the prosthesis.

▶ In the early 1970s, the Maryland bridge became a popular treatment alternative to a conventional bridge for replacement of a single tooth. It was designed to conserve the enamel on the abutment teeth. Only base metals could be used at that time in order to properly etch the metal. Many of the early bridges began to fail because of the conservative nature of the prep design and the relatively weak resin luting systems we had available at the time. Anteriorly, there was the problem of graying abutment teeth due to the base metal wings. Today, many of the problems have been solved with better preparation design, stronger resin luting systems, and gold base metals. This article discusses tooth preparation design for posterior RBFPDs.

F. M. McIntyre, DDS, MS

Rehabilitating a Patient With Bruxism-Associated Tooth Tissue Loss: A Literature Review and Case Report

Yip KH-K (Univ of Hong Kong, China)

Gen Dent 51:70-74, 2003   3–11

Introduction.—Tooth loss from bruxism is associated with various dental problems, including tooth sensitivity, excess reduction of clinical crown height, and possible changes of occlusal relationship. Several treatment modalities are available that emphasize prevention and rehabilitation with adhesive techniques. The management of excess tooth tissue loss in a patient with a history of bruxism was described.

Case Report.—Woman, 43, with a history of tooth grinding of many years was seen for her appearance and sensitive gums. She had no history of using erosive agents. She had severe wear of her anterior teeth, multiple missing posterior teeth, a retained root, 2 teeth with nonvital pulps, and marginal gingival inflammation. Articulated study casts revealed a deep anterior overbite and unstable posterior tooth contacts. Treatment objectives were to avoid further tooth tissue loss and to improve both the function and appearance of the dentition.

Initial advice and treatment included oral hygiene instruction and scaling, endodontic treatment, extraction of retained roots, and creation of a maxillary acrylic occlusal splint at a reestablished occlusal vertical dimension. Initial restorative treatment involved anterior and posterior resin composite tooth buildup with the use of vacuum-formed matrices fabricated from diagnostic wax-ups. Adjustments were repeated until the patient was comfortable.

After resin composite buildup and a 4-week assessment period, porcelain veneers were placed on the mandibular anterior teeth and ceramo-metal crowns were positioned on the maxillary anterior teeth to establish anterior guidance. The patient's anterior guide was examined 4 weeks later. Posterior restorations, including gold onlays and crowns and 3 ceramo-metal fixed partial dentures, were placed segmentally during the next 2 months. A new maxillary acrylic occlusal splint was created; soft splint is not an option with bruxism. The patient reported less tooth grinding and clenching.

Conclusion.—Full-mouth oral rehabilitation for this patient involved creating multiple porcelain veneers, adhesive gold onlays, ceramo-metal crowns, and fixed partial dentures. The prognosis is favorable for this patient with the use of an occlusal splint and compliance with good oral hygiene.

▶ Developments in esthetic dentistry have created a demand by individuals with worn dentitions to have their teeth restored. Wear can be related to attrition, abrasion, and erosion. Bruxism creates worn dentitions through the process of attrition. Whether bruxism is CNS driven or occlusally originated is controversial. In this article, the author discusses the rehabilitation of a patient with bruxism-associated tooth wear. He assumes that all patients need a change in vertical dimension in occlusion (VDO), which is not necessarily always the case. He also discusses the use of a splint to test VDO, which is also a controversial issue. When treating patients with worn dentitions, it is important to obtain additional diagnostic records—such as cephalometrics, centric relation, evaluation of the functional envelope, and anterior tooth position—because in many cases, there is no loss in VDO, but a change in occlusal plane orientation which needs to be corrected.

F. M. McIntyre, DDS, MS

4 Periodontics

Introduction

Several useful systematic reviews were published this past year, including assessments on guided tissue regeneration, periodontal root coverage techniques, and toothbrush efficacy. These types of reviews provide clinicians with the highest level of scientific assessment when considering an evidence-based approach to therapy. I have chosen to include a few of the more definitive reviews in the hope of helping you get a sense of what the best evidence really is in certain areas. New insights have also been gained in the past year regarding genetic markers for periodontal disease and the pitfalls of the very popular idea that periodontal disease may be a significant factor in heart disease. In the area of esthetic periodontal/implant surgeries, there have been reports to help clinicians gain some discernment in soft tissue grafting and the soft tissue dimensions around maxillary anterior single-tooth implants. This year also saw some large strides made in tissue engineering using adenoviral vectors and bone morphogenetic proteins, as well as some more clinically applicable documentation of the value of an antiseptic-containing dentifrice in slowing periodontal disease progression over 5 years. Hopefully, these selections will prove useful to your clinical practice and help you visualize the future of periodontal therapy.

Andrew Dentino, DDS, PhD

Genetics and Periodontal Disease

The Interleukin-1 Polymorphism, Smoking, and the Risk of Periodontal Disease in the Population-Based SHIP Study
Meisel P, Siegemund A, Grimm R, et al (Ernst Moritz Arndt Univ, Greifswald, Germany)
J Dent Res 82:189-193, 2003   4–1

Introduction.—Several trials have demonstrated a role for interleukin (IL)-1 gene cluster polymorphisms in the risk assessment for periodontal diseases. The role of IL-1 polymorphism as a risk factor for periodontal diseases was examined in The Study of Health in Pomerania, a randomized, population-based, cross-sectional investigation.

Methods.—Of 210,000 inhabitants in the German part of Pomerania, 3148 research subjects were randomly selected and examined for a broad range of diseases and environmental/behavioral risk factors. A total of 1085 research subjects aged 40 to 60 years were genotyped for the IL-1 genotype composite polymorphism in relation to periodontal variables.

Results.—An increased risk of periodontal disease was identified for IL-1 genotype-positive smokers. The odds ratio adjusted for age, sex, education, and plaque was 2.50 (95% CI, 0.73-1.62; P = .676). No such increase was seen for IL-1 positive nonsmokers (odds ratio, 1.09).

Conclusion.—Synergistic actions of smoking and IL-1 associated genetic factors may explain the relationship of identified risk factors.

▶ In the past, the usefulness of being able to test for the IL-1 genotype has been seriously questioned, as most clinicians wouldn't treat patients any differently if they knew that they were IL-1 positive. However, these data by Meisel et al suggest that testing for IL-1 positivity in young smokers with gingivitis or early periodontitis could theoretically provide a significant public health benefit because more aggressive maintenance could then be instituted.

A. Dentino, DDS, PhD

Association of the − 1087 *IL 10* Gene Polymorphism With Severe Chronic Periodontitis in Swedish Caucasians
Berglundh T, Donati M, Hahn-Zoric M, et al (Göteborg Univ, Sweden)
J Clin Periodontol 30:249-254, 2003   4–2

Purpose.—Severe forms of periodontitis may be related to alterations of genes affecting cytokine function. Polymorphisms of the gene for interleukin-10 (*IL-10* gene)—which suppresses proinflammatory cytokines and enhances proliferation of conventional and autoreactive B cells—have been linked to disease, including autoimmune disorders. A specific polymorphism of the *IL-10* gene was evaluated for possible association with severe chronic periodontitis.

Methods.—The case-control study included 60 Swedish adults (mean age, 54.5 years) with severe, generalized chronic periodontitis. All patients had greater than 50% bone loss at all teeth. The control subjects were 39 periodontally healthy persons of similar age. Genotyping for a polymorphism in the promoter region of the *IL-10* gene—associated with a G to A transition at the − 1087 position—was performed by polymerase chain reaction with restriction endonuclease mapping.

Findings.—The homozygous GG genotype was detected in 40.0% of patients with chronic periodontitis versus 20.5% of control subjects. Among nonsmokers in these 2 groups, the rates were 61.3% versus 20.6%. In contrast, the homozygous AA genotype was detected in 9.7% of nonsmokers in the case group, compared with 35.3% of nonsmoking control subjects. More than 90% of nonsmokers with chronic periodontitis had at least 1 G allele.

Conclusion.—In this Northern European population, the −1087 polymorphism of the *IL-10* gene is associated with severe chronic periodontitis. This association is particularly apparent among nonsmokers, with an associated odds ratio of 6.1. Some effect of *IL-10* on autoreactive B cells may play an important role in the pathogenesis of periodontal disease.

▶ This retrospective case-control cross-sectional study examined the possible association of an *IL-10* single nucleotide polymorphism at position 1087 between severe, chronic periodontitis and healthy control subjects in a Swedish Caucasian population. In nonsmokers, there was an odds ratio of 6.1, strongly suggesting an association between this single DNA base pair alteration and severe chronic periodontitis. These observations are consistent with findings by Al-Rasheed and coworkers,[1] who documented accelerated periodontal bone loss in *IL-10*–deficient mice compared to wild-type mice, which further supports the importance of *IL-10* as a protective regulator of inflammation.

This work adds another genetic marker to the growing list which includes the IL-1, Fc receptor, and vitamin D receptor genes, to name a few. These genetic variations all play different roles in periodontitis susceptibility. The development of clinical tests for these and other genetic markers of periodontitis susceptibility should eventually provide a significant public health benefit as dentistry moves from a primarily surgical profession to more of a health surveillance profession.

A. Dentino, DDS, PhD

Reference

1. Al-Rasheed A, Scheerens H, Rennick DM, et al: Accelerated alveolar bone loss in mice lacking interleukin-10. *J Dent Res* 82:632-635, 2003.

Periodontics and Systemic Diseases

Bias Induced by Self-Reported Smoking on Periodontitis–Systemic Disease Associations

Spiekerman CF, Hujoel PP, DeRouen TA (Univ of Washington, Seattle)
J Dent Res 82:345-349, 2003
4–3

Introduction.—Standard regression methods rely on the assumption that the independent variables used are without appreciable error. The use of an imperfect measure, such as self-reported smoking, to adjust for tobacco exposure will hamper full adjustment for the effects of smoking. The "leftover" confounding due to the inadequate adjustment may affect estimates of association for any of the variables in the model. The impact is similar to leaving out an important confounding variable. Presented are the results of standard statistical analyses that show false-positive associations between measures of periodontal disease and outcomes ascertained completely by serum cotinine levels, even after adjustment for tobacco exposure based on self-reported smoking data.

Methods.—Data from the Third National Health and Nutrition Examination Survey, performed in 2 stages from 1988 to 1991 and 1991 to 1994, were used to examine associations between attachment loss and serum cotinine levels after adjustment by self-reported number of cigarettes smoked. Cotinine, a metabolite of nicotine, should not be associated with attachment loss if self-reported smoking captures the effect of tobacco on attachment levels.

Results.—Adjustment for self-reported cigarette smoking did not completely remove the association between attachment loss and serum cotinine level (r = 0.075, n = 1507, P = .003). Simulation studies suggested similar outcomes for time-to-event data.

Conclusion.—These findings show the difficulty in distinguishing the effects of periodontitis from those of smoking with regard to smoking-associated outcomes. Further trials should address outcomes of analyses on separate cohorts of individuals who smoke and those who have never smoked.

▶ Tobacco exposure is a very important risk factor for periodontitis and is strongly implicated in, if not the strongest risk factor for, many systemic diseases currently linked with periodontitis. Studies carried out to date demonstrating an association between periodontitis and many other tobacco-related illnesses have used self-reported cigarette smoking to estimate tobacco exposure. In a clever study design, the authors demonstrate the hazards of relying on self-reported smoking habits and convincingly demonstrate that such a measure is not sufficient to completely remove the confounding effects of smoking. They go on to suggest that future studies should report separate analyses for smokers and never smokers.

A. Dentino, DDS, PhD

Soft Tissue Concerns

Dimensions of Peri-implant Mucosa: An Evaluation of Maxillary Anterior Single Implants in Humans

Kan JYK, Rungcharassaeng K, Umezu K, et al (Loma Linda Univ, Calif; Univ of Washington, Seattle)
J Periodontol 74:557-562, 2003   4–4

Purpose.—Most previous assessments of the biological dimensions of osseointegrated dental implants have been histologic studies in animals. There are no data on the contribution of soft tissue support from adjacent teeth on the interproximal dimension of the peri-implant mucosa associated with anterior single-tooth replacements. The dimensions of the peri-implant mucosa around 2-stage anterior maxillary single implants were assessed after 1 year of service, including the effects of the peri-implant biotype.

Methods.—The study included 45 patients with 45 maxillary anterior single-implant crowns, with a mean functional period of 32.5 months. Bone sounding was performed to assess the dimensions of the peri-implant mucosa, including not only the implant restoration but also the adjacent natural teeth. Bone-sounding sites were the mesial (MI), midfacial (F), and distal (DI)

TABLE 1.—Bone-Sounding Measurements of Anterior Implant Single Crowns Comparing Thick and Thin Biotypes

	Bone-Sounding Depth (Mean ± SD, mm)		
Site	Thick Biotype ($n = 28$)	Thin Biotype ($n = 17$)	P Value
MT	4.46 ± 0.78	3.76 ± 0.53	0.002*
MI	6.54 ± 1.05	5.56 ± 1.40	0.011*
F	3.79 ± 0.89	3.38 ± 0.91	0.150
DI	6.14 ± 1.11	5.59 ± 1.31	0.137
DT	4.45 ± 0.57	3.79 ± 0.56	0.001*

*Statistically significant ($P < .05$)
(Courtesy of Kan JYK, Rungcharassaeng K, Umezu K, et al: Dimensions of peri-implant mucosa: An evaluation of maxillary anterior single implants in humans. *J Periodontol* 74:557-562, 2003.)

aspects of the implant restoration and the proximal aspects of the adjacent teeth on either side (MT, DT). In each case, the peri-implant biotype was classified as thin or thick.

Results.—The mean dimensions of the peri-implant mucosa were 4.20 mm at MT, 6.17 mm at MI, 3.63 mm at F, 5.93 mm at DI, and 4.20 mm at DT. The thick biotype was associated with significantly greater peri-implant mucosa dimensions at MT, MI, and DT (Table 1).

Conclusion.—The study provides new information on the dimensions of the peri-implant mucosa of maxillary anterior single implants after years of function. The facial dimension appears somewhat larger than the average dimension of the dentogingival complex. The interproximal papillary level is unaffected by the proximal bone level next to the implant but is affected by the level next to adjacent teeth. A thick peri-implant biotype is associated with greater peri-implant mucosal dimensions.

▶ This retrospective case series looking at 2-stage implants in function in the esthetic zone provides some very useful information on the dimensions of the peri-implant mucosa. Achieving an esthetic result is our goal, and knowing what parameters one can expect after healing is critical. While the differentiation of the thick versus thin gingival biotypes is very crude, it is nonetheless a particularly important observation. The implants were all of external hex design and primarily Branemark with some Sterioss fixtures. It will be interesting to see if future studies on single-stage implants of these and other manufacturers will show any difference in these dimensions.

A. Dentino, DDS, PhD

Periodontal Plastic Surgery for Treatment of Localized Gingival Recessions: A Systematic Review

Roccuzzo M, Bunino M, Needleman I, et al (Univ of Torino, Italy; Univ College of London; Univ Complutense of Madrid)
J Clin Periodontol 29(Suppl 3):178-194, 2002   4–5

Introduction.—Evidence concerning the efficacy of periodontal plastic surgery (PPS) for treatment of recession defects has yet to be systematically examined. The efficacy of PPS in achieving root coverage in the treatment of localized gingival recession was systematically reviewed.

Methods.—Randomized controlled trials, along with case series of at least 6 months' follow-up, were reviewed for guided tissue regeneration (GTR), free gingival grafts, connective tissue grafts (CTGs), and coronally advanced flaps (CAFs). The data sources included electronic databases and hand-searched journals. Screening, data abstraction, and quality assessment were performed independently and in duplicate.

Results.—A limited yet statistically significant greater benefit was seen for CTGs versus GTR (weighted mean difference, 0.43; 95% CI, 0.62-0.23). No differences were seen comparing either GTR with CAFs or resorbable versus nonresorbable GTR barriers. The gain in attachment was similar for each of the 3 comparisons. Analysis of single arms of trials and case series revealed that PPS can result in a substantial improvement in clinical variables. Heterogeneity was often high and only partially explained by the initial defect depth. The use of barrier membranes did not statistically significantly enhance root coverage as compared with the use of CAFs. Data were limited concerning free gingival grafts and laterally positioned flaps. Data do not support the use of root modification agents to enhance root coverage.

Conclusion.—Overall, PPS was effective in decreasing gingival recession and resulted in a concomitant improvement in attachment levels. Even though no single treatment may be considered superior, CTGs were statistically significantly more effective than GTR in recession reduction.

▶ This systematic review provides evidence that PPS procedures can be used to achieve root coverage and a gain in clinical attachment levels. The meta-analysis suggests that CTGs when compared with GTR to cover root surfaces were statistically significantly better due to less recession, and GTR membranes did not enhance root coverage compared with CAFs. This suggests that the additional cost of the membrane may be an unnecessary expense for our patients.

A. Dentino, DDS, PhD

A 3-Year Longitudinal Evaluation of Subpedicle Free Connective Tissue Graft for Gingival Recession Coverage

Lee Y-M, Kim JY, Seol Y-J, et al (Seoul Natl Univ, Korea; Univ of California, Los Angeles; Sungkyunkwan Univ, Seoul, Korea)
J Periodontol 73:1412-1418, 2002   4–6

Introduction.—Covering exposed root surfaces is an important component of surgical periodontal practice. A major concern regarding free gingival grafts is the color discrepancy between the graft and surrounding tissue that has been described as "keloid-like" in appearance. The decrease in gingival recession (GR) with the use of a subepithelial free connective tissue graft placed under a coronally advanced partial-thickness pedicle flap was examined during a 3-year longitudinal investigation.

Methods.—Twenty-one buccal recession defects (mean, 3.67 mm; range, 3-4.5 mm; Miller Class I, II, and III) from 15 patients were treated with the use of a subpedicle free connective tissue graft for GR coverage. The amount of GR, clinical attachment loss (CAL), and width of keratinized gingiva (WKG) were followed for 3 years postoperatively. Measurements were obtained before surgery and 1, 3, 6, 12, 18, 24, and 36 months postoperatively.

Results.—GR diminished from 3.67 mm at baseline to 0.33 mm at 36 months' follow-up, which represented a decrease of 3.33 mm; this corresponded to a 91.28% mean root coverage. The CAL was significantly reduced at 36 months from 5.26 mm to 2.14 mm. A mean of 3.12 mm of attachment gain was observed, and the WKG was increased significantly after 36 months. The GR, CAL, and WKG had the most positive outcomes at 12 months and were maintained at stable levels during the 36-month evaluation period.

Conclusion.—The connective tissue graft with a partial-thickness coronal advancement pedicle is a predictable approach for root coverage. In the presence of optimal maintenance care, the clinical outcomes gained by this approach can be well maintained.

▶ This article is one of the few that examine the long-term stability of subpedicle free connective tissue grafts. This procedure and its variants have become widely used for esthetic gingival augmentation. Moreover, with the recent controlled clinical trial by Goldstein and coworkers,[1] who demonstrated that successful gingival grafting for root coverage can predictably be carried out on areas previously affected by decay, the applicability of this therapy continues to expand. This case series provides some reassurance that the gains in root coverage can be long lasting when regular maintenance is provided.

A. Dentino, DDS, PhD

Reference

1. Goldstein M, Nasatzky E, Goultschin J, et al: Coverage of previously carious roots is as predictable a procedure as coverage of intact roots. *J Periodontol* 73:1419-1426, 2002.

Tissue Engineering

Gene Therapy of Bone Morphogenetic Protein for Periodontal Tissue Engineering

Jin Q-M, Anusaksathien O, Webb SA, et al (Univ of Michigan, Ann Arbor)
J Periodontol 74:202-213, 2003   4–7

Objective.—Bone morphogenetic proteins (BMPs) are multifunctional growth factors with potential value for periodontal regeneration. Problems with the concept of periodontal BMP therapy include the need to deliver high doses, their short-lived biological activity, and low bioavailability at the wound site. A gene transfer approach to BMP delivery to periodontal disease sites was investigated.

Methods and Results.—Ex vivo techniques were used to transduce syngeneic dermal fibroblasts with adenovirus-encoding green fluorescent protein, BMP-7, or the BMP antagonist noggin. After seeding on gelatin carriers, the adenovirus-transduced syngeneic dermal fibroblasts were transplanted into large alveolar defects created in the mandibles of Lewis rats. Osteogenesis was inhibited at sites treated with noggin-transduced adenovirus, compared with either BMP-7– or GFP-treated wounds. In contrast, sites receiving the BMP-7 gene showed fast chondrogenesis followed by osteogenesis, cementogenesis, and bridging of the bony defect. Bone bridging occurred by 5 weeks at most BMP-7–treated sites, compared with none of the GFP- or noggin-treated defects.

Conclusion.—Ex vivo BMP gene transfer offers a promising approach to periodontal tissue engineering. Fibroblasts transduced with BMP-7 stimulate formation of new bone, periodontal ligament, and cementum. With further development, BMP gene transfer could provide an effective new alternative for treatment of periodontal bone defects.

▶ This is a landmark article demonstrating that gene transfer of BMP is possible using a viral delivery system and fibroblasts in the rat mandibular bone defect model. These are the first successful steps in periodontal tissue engineering, and they have generated much excitement in the periodontal community.

A. Dentino, DDS, PhD

An Autologous Cell Hyaluronic Acid Graft Technique for Gingival Augmentation: A Case Series

Prato GPP, Rotundo R, Magnani C, et al (Univ of Florence, Italy; Florence, Italy; Fidia Advanced Biopolymers srl, Abano Terme (Padova), Italy)
J Periodontol 74:262-267, 2003   4–8

Introduction.—Tissue engineering is one of the most exciting advances in regenerative medicine. The ability to create new tissue and organs from a patient's own cells has enhanced treatments and prognoses for many patients.

An autologous cell hyaluronic acid (HA) graft was used for gingival augmentation in mucogingival surgery.

Methods.—Seven sites from 6 patients were used for an autologous cell HA graft for gingival augmentation. Five patients (5 sites) required gingival augmentation before prosthetic rehabilitation. One patient (2 sites) required augmentation because of pain during daily toothbrushing. The full-mouth plaque score, full-mouth bleeding score, probing depth, and clinical attachment level were documented for the sites at baseline and 3 months after surgery. The amount of keratinized tissue was determined in the mesial, middle, and distal sites of each involved tooth. A 2 × 1 × 1-mm section of gingiva (epithelium and connective tissue) was removed from every patient, placed in a nutritional medium, and transferred to the laboratory. The gingival tissue was processed by separating the keratinocytes and fibroblasts. Only the fibroblasts were cultivated. The fibroblasts were cultured on a scaffold of fully esterified benzyl ester HA. They were returned to the periodontal office under sterile conditions. During the gingival augmentation procedure, the periosteum of the affected teeth was exposed. The membrane containing cultivated fibroblasts was adapted to and positioned on the prepared site.

Results.—At 3 months after surgery, an increased amount of gingiva was observed. The histologic examination showed fully keratinized tissue on all treated sites.

Conclusion.—Tissue engineering technology and an autologous cell HA graft were used in gingival augmentation procedures. This approach provides an increase in gingiva in a very short time without any discomfort for the patient.

▶ This is another landmark article in tissue engineering and represents an interesting approach that takes advantage of advances in cell culture and polymer matrices to avoid the morbidity associated with a significant second surgical site.

A. Dentino, DDS, PhD

Guided Tissue Regeneration

Use of Barrier Membranes and Systemic Antibiotics in the Treatment of Intraosseous Defects

Loos BG, Louwerse PHG, van Winkelhoff AJ, et al (Univ of Amsterdam)
J Clin Periodontol 29:910-921, 2002   4–9

Introduction.—The current literature is not clear on the use of barrier membranes for regeneration of intraosseous defects. One reason for the ambivalent results may be associated with infection before, during, and after the surgical procedure. The use of both membranes (MEM) and antibiotics (AB) were assessed separately and in combination in a randomized controlled trial.

Methods.—Twenty-five patients with 2 intraosseous periodontal defects each were randomly assigned to receive either systemic antibiotics (AB+) or no antibiotics (AB–). After flaps were raised and after debridement, both defects in each patient were covered via a bioresorbable membrane (MEM+). Before the flaps were sutured in a coronal position, the membrane over 1 of the 2 defects was removed at random (MEM–). This protocol produced 4 groups of defects: MEM– AB–; MEM+ AB–; MEM– AB+; MEM+ AB+. Patients were followed up clinically. Microadjusted means for clinical variables were acquired from the final statistical model.

Results.—The decrease in probing pocket depth at 12 months postoperatively varied between 2.54 and 3.06 mm among the 4 treatment approaches; overall, no main effect of MEM or AB was detected. Gains in probing attachment level (PAL) at 12 months postoperatively varied from 0.56 to 1.96 mm for the 4 treatment methods. In the overall analysis for PAL, no main effect of MEM or AB was identified. Gains in probing bone level (PBL) 12 months postoperatively ranged from 1.39 to 2.09 mm. No main effects of MEM or AB were seen for PBL. Explorative statistical analyses revealed that smoking, but not MEM or AB, was a determining factor for a gain in PBL ($P = .0009$). Nonsmokers were estimated to have gained 2.04 mm PBL versus 0.52 mm for smokers. The prevalence of numerous periodontal pathogens on the day of surgery or postoperatively and specific defect characteristics were not determining factors for a gain in PAL or PBL.

Conclusion.—Neither the application of MEM nor the use of systemic AB demonstrated an additional effect over the control group on both soft and hard tissue measurements in the treatment of intraosseous defects. Smoking was a determining factor that severely restricted the gain in PBL in surgical procedures directed at regeneration of intraosseous defects.

▶ This elegantly designed randomized controlled trial set out to determine the efficacy of barrier membrane placement over intrabony defects with and without systemic AB coverage. Some of the features that make this study so good include the full treatment of each patient periodontally before the start of this study, with the exception of the sites entered into the protocol; the thorough preoperative and postoperative infection control; and the collection of microbiological data, as well as soft tissue and bone-sounding measurements. The data suggest that the results were unimpressive in this population when AB, or MEM, or both were used. The most significant factor affecting successful therapy was smoking. Nonsmokers saw an additional 1.5-mm gain of PBL over sites in patients who were still smoking at the 12-month evaluation. The slightly lower overall gains in attachment in these cases compared with previously published studies are likely explained by the treatment protocol, which ensured less inflammation in all treated sites at baseline.

A. Dentino, DDS, PhD

Efficacy of Controlled-Release Subgingival Chlorhexidine to Enhance Periodontal Regeneration

Reddy MS, Jeffcoat MK, Geurs NC, et al (Univ of Alabama, Birmingham; AstraZeneca Pharmaceuticals, LP, Wilmington, Del)

J Periodontol 74:411-419, 2003   4–10

Introduction.—The success of periodontal regeneration may be limited when bone grafts and membranes are placed in infected sites. The local application of controlled-release antimicrobials, such as chlorhexidine (CHX) gluconate, may potentially improve the clinical outcome after guided tissue regeneration (GTR) surgery. The ability of controlled-release subgingival CHX administration during initial periodontal therapy and just before regenerative surgical procedures to enhance periodontal regeneration was examined in a randomized, blind, 2-arm parallel design, controlled clinical trial.

Methods.—Forty-four patients with 1 or more sites with a probing depth and a clinical attachment loss of 5 mm or more after initial therapy and initial evidence of bone loss were randomly assigned to receive either CHX chip or sham chip placement 1 week before regenerative therapy that included graft placement and site coverage with guided tissue membranes. They also received CHX or sham chip placement, per their randomization, adjunctively to scaling and root planing or maintenance procedures. Periodontal examinations were performed at baseline (8 weeks before surgery), 1 week before surgery, and 3, 6, and 9 months after surgery. The primary outcomes were changes in bone height and bone mass, as determined from standardized radiographs used for quantitative digital subtraction radiography over the 11-month evaluation period.

Results.—Patients in the sham chip placement group gained a mean bone height of 1.49 mm compared with 3.54 mm for patients in the CHX chip placement group ($P < .001$). Patients who received CHX chips as an adjunct gained significantly more bone mass than did patients who received standard therapy (5.57 mg vs 2.59 mg; $P < .001$).

Conclusion.—Locally delivered controlled-release antimicrobial treatment may enhance the amount of bone gained during GTR procedures. It appears that infection control is important for successful regeneration.

▶ Predictable GTR is our goal as clinicians. Several articles have shown that bacterial colonization/infection of GTR-treated sites, either through membrane contamination or the incomplete disinfection during debridement, results in less attachment and bone gain. This randomized controlled clinical trial provides data supporting the presurgical use of PerioChip, a resorbable CHX-containing local antimicrobial, as a way to enhance the response to therapy, presumably by achieving a "cleaner" site just before surgery.

A. Dentino, DDS, PhD

Deproteinized Cancellous Bovine Bone (Bio-Oss) as Bone Substitute for Sinus Floor Elevation: A Retrospective, Histomorphometrical Study of Five Cases

Tadjoedin ES, de Lange GL, Bronckers ALJJ, et al (Academic Ctr for Dentistry Amsterdam)

J Clin Periodontol 30:261-270, 2003   4–11

Introduction.—Placement of dental implants in the distal edentulous maxillary area is often challenging because of the significant resorption in the posterior maxilla after tooth extraction. The histomorphometric performance of deproteinized cancellous bovine bone (DPBB, Bio-Osso) granules as a bone substitute was examined retrospectively in 5 patients undergoing reconstruction for severe atrophy in the maxilla.

Materials.—Several mixtures of DPBB containing between 20% and 100% DPB13 and autogenous bone particles were examined for their capacity to augment the sinus floor to such an extent that implant fixtures could be placed within a reasonable time of healing (about 6 months). Twenty vertical biopsy specimens were obtained at the time of the fixture installation and were used in histomorphometric analysis as undecalcified Goldner-stained sections.

Results.—In all 5 patients, the DPBB granules had been interconnected via bridges of vital newly formed bone. The volume of bone in the grafted area was inversely correlated with the concentration of DPBB grafted; it varied between 37% and 23%. The total volume of mineralized material (bone plus DPB13 granules) remained within the same range for all 5 participants (between 53% and 59%). The high values for osteoid and resorptive surface, along with the presence of tartrate-resistant acid phosphatase–positive multinucleated osteoclasts in resorption lacunae, suggested that bone remodeling was very active in all grafts. Osteoclasts were also seen in shallow resorption pits on DPBB surfaces. The percentage of DPBB surface in contact with the bone remained stable at about 35% and was not associated with the proportion of DPBB grafted.

Conclusion.—DPBB, preferably combined with autogenous bone particles, was a suitable material for sinus floor elevation in the 5 patients with severely atrophic human maxilla.

▶ This case series shows the efficacy of DPBB as a sinus augmentation material when used alone or, preferably, with some autogenous bone. After 5 to 8 months, all samples showed active resorption of the DPBB and increasing levels of osteoid in proportion to the percentage of autogenous bone mixed with DPBB. The total volume of mineralized material ranged from 53% to 59%, and the actual amount of bone ranged from 23% to 37% as autogenous bone increased in the original mixture from 0% to 80%. A case series is certainly not the highest level of scientific evidence, but this study does provide very useful human histologic data, and in all 20 samples from 5 patients, these data suggest that DPBB can be used as a safe, efficacious, and resorbable material to rehabilitate the atrophic maxilla with the use of sinus lifting and subsequent implant placement.

A. Dentino, DDS, PhD

Enamel Matrix Proteins in the Treatment of Periodontal Sites With Horizontal Type of Bone Loss

Yilmaz S, Kuru S, Altuna-Kiraç E (Marmara Univ, Istanbul, Turkey)
J Clin Periodontol 30:197-206, 2003   4–12

Background.—Conventional periodontal therapies are highly effective in eliminating periodontal infection, repairing defects related to the disease, and stopping the disease's progression, but they do not address the regeneration of tissues that were destroyed, which requires regenerative periodontal treatment. A new modality in regenerative periodontal treatment uses enamel matrix proteins (EMP), which are involved in forming acellular cementum during root and periodontal tissue development and may, therefore, be capable of inducing the regeneration of periodontal attachment structures. When horizontal bone loss occurs, regeneration is much less predictable and the use of EMP may not be as effective. A preliminary assessment of the clinical and radiographic results of the use of EMP in horizontal bone loss in adults with periodontitis was undertaken, involving periodontal surgery followed by the adjunctive use of EMP. A comparison was made with patients undergoing conventional flap debridement with the use of 2 types of incision.

Methods.—The study followed the principles of a controlled randomized trial with a split-mouth design. First, all patients had nonsurgical periodontal therapy; all exhibited radiographic horizontal bone loss and a probing depth (PD) of at least 4 mm at the maxillary incisor–canine segment. For each of the 20 patients (age range, 35-56 years), the maxillary anterior segment was randomly assigned as a test or control side. Test sides received EMP (Emdogain) as part of a crevicular flap, and control sides received a similar intracrevicular or a reverse bevel incision as part of a conventional flap debridement. Thus, 10 patients had Emdogain (T1) and flap debridement with an intracrevicular incision (C1), and 10 had Emdogain (T2) and flap debridement with a reverse bevel incision (C2). Outcomes were assessed statistically after 8 months.

Results.—Seven hundred twenty sites were treated in the 20 patients. The T1 and T2 sides showed no statistically significant difference in any of the variables before and after treatment. PD was significantly decreased after treatment in all groups, and the greatest progress was made in T1 and C2. A significant improvement in relative attachment level (RAL) over initial findings was noted in all groups except C1. Significant differences in deep pocket sites (4-6 mm) were noted between the T1 and C1 groups and between the T2 and C2 groups, and the RAL gain was greater with EMP application. Recession (REC) values were also significantly better when EMP was used. Conventional flap treatment in shallow sites (1-3 mm) tended to result in a loss of attachment, but use of EMP maintained the level of attachment. The degree of probing and radiographic bone levels were comparable between the 2 treatment approaches.

Conclusions.—The use of EMP as an adjunct to crevicular flap debridement produced better clinical results than using conventional procedures in terms of PD reduction, attachment gain, and REC. The results were especially improved in areas with deep pockets. Conventional treatment of shallow pockets tended to result in a loss of attachment, but the use of EMP adjunctively tended to maintain attachment levels in these shallow pocket areas. After 8 months, no significant differences were found between the 2 approaches with respect to the degree of probing and radiographic bone levels.

▶ This article represents the first randomized controlled trial assessing the use of Emdogain as an adjunct to surgical access flaps in areas with horizontal bone loss in the esthetic zone. Changes in probing measurements including RAL, REC, and radiographic assessments suggest that the use of Emdogain seems to enhance attachment gain, prevent postsurgical bone loss, and significantly reduce postsurgical REC. The finding regarding improvements in postsurgical REC is consistent with the previous findings of Sculean et al[1] and suggest that the use of Emdogain in the esthetic zone may have benefits, even when dealing with shallow pockets (4-6 mm) with no associated intrabony defects. More studies showing longer follow-up and human histologic findings would be helpful in this area.

A. Dentino, DDS, PhD

Reference

1. Sculean A, Donos N, Blaes A, et al: Comparison of enamel matrix proteins and bioabsorbable membranes in the treatment of intrabony periodontal defects. A split-mouth study. *J Periodontol* 70:255-262, 1999.

A Systematic Review of Guided Tissue Regeneration for Periodontal Furcation Defects: What Is the Effect of Guided Tissue Regeneration Compared With Surgical Debridement in the Treatment of Furcation Defects?
Jepsen S, Eberhard J, Herrera D, et al (Univ of Kiel, Germany; Univ Complutense of Madrid; Univ College of London)
J Clin Periodontol 29(Suppl 3):103-116, 2002   4–13

Introduction.—Furcation involvement poses challenging problems in periodontal treatment, with various regenerative techniques used to achieve furcation closure. Bone fill at reentry is the only indicator of periodontal regeneration that can be assessed clinically; other outcomes of interest include attachment levels, probing depths, and radiologic outcomes. Several recent trials have assessed the use of guided tissue regeneration (GTR) techniques. A meta-analysis of GTR for the periodontal furcation defects was reported.

Methods.—A literature review identified 14 randomized controlled trials of GTR for periodontal furcation defects. All studies compared GTR with open flap debridement and included at least 6 months of follow-up. The main outcome measure was reduction in horizontal furcation depth. Meta-analysis was performed on this and secondary outcome measures.

Results.—Reduction in horizontal furcation depth on reentry was significantly greater with GTR than with open debridement. Weighted mean differences were 1.51 mm (95% confidence interval, 0.39-2.26 mm) for mandibular Class II furcations and 0.87 mm for maxillary Class II furcations (95% confidence interval, −0.08 to 1.82) in trials combining the 2 types of furcations. Secondary outcomes also favored GTR, including gain in horizontal and vertical probing attachment and reduction of vertical probing depth. Because of a lack of data, meta-analysis of the furcation closure rate could not be performed.

Conclusion.—Randomized trial data support the effectiveness of GTR therapy for periodontal furcation defects, compared with open debridement. GTR is more effective in reducing open horizontal furcation depth and other outcomes than is open debridement, for both mandibular and maxillary Class II furcation defects. However, the advantage of GTR is variable and modest and is based on limited outcome data. More research is needed to assess the factors associated with consistent benefits of GTR over conventional open debridement.

▶ This systematic review is another confirmation that GTR is a more beneficial therapy than simple surgical access and debridement. However, it is critical for us to know when to apply this therapy since predictability is still an issue, and lack of complete furcation closure can limit the long-term success of this therapy. The Bowers case series[1] on combined grafting and GTR have helped to define conditions that will maximize predictability.

A. Dentino, DDS, PhD

Reference

1. Bowers GM, Schallhorn RG, McClain PK, et al: Factors influencing the outcome of regenerative therapy in mandibular Class II furcations. Part I. *J Periodontol* 74:1255-1268, 2003.

Prognosis and Maintenance

The Prognostic Value of Several Periodontal Factors Measured as Radiographic Bone Level Variation: A 10-Year Retrospective Multilevel Analysis of Treated and Maintained Periodontal Patients

Nieri M, Muzzi L, Cattabriga M, et al (Florence, Italy; Univ of Florence, Italy; Rome)
J Periodontol 73:1485-1493, 2002

4–14

Introduction.—Assigning a prognosis to a patient with periodontal disease is one of the greatest challenges in clinical practice. Many different factors can affect the outcome of periodontal disease. The prognostic values of some clinical, genetic, and radiographic variables in predicting bone level variation were examined in patients with periodontal disease, aged 40 to 60 years, who received treatment and maintenance for 10 years.

Methods.—Scaling and root planing was performed in 60 consecutive nonsmokers (mean age, 46.77 years) with moderate to severe chronic periodontitis, some of whom also underwent additional surgical treatments. All patients were followed up in the same private practice for 10 years. At baseline (T0) and at least 10 years later (T2), these clinical variables were assessed: probing depth (PD), tooth mobility (TM), presence of prosthetic restorations (PR), and molar teeth (MT). In addition, radiographic measurements were obtained of the mesial and distal distances from the cemento-enamel junction (CEJ) to the bottom of the defect (BD), to the bone crest (BC), and to the root apex (RA). All 60 patients underwent genetic testing to ascertain the interleukin (IL)-1 genotype and genetic susceptibility for severe periodontal disease at T2. Based on these findings, patients' genotypes were categorized as IL-1 positive or negative. The differences between the bone levels measured at T0 and T2, illustrating the bone level variation, acted as the outcome variable. Different predictor variables were examined with the use of a 3-level statistical model (multilevel statistical analysis; patient, tooth, and site level). At the patient level, the variables were age, sex, and the interaction between mean bone loss and the IL-1 genotype (mean $CEJ\text{-}BD_{T0} \times$ IL-1 genotype); for the tooth level, they were TM_{T0}, PR_{T0}, and MT_{T0}; and for the site level, they were the infrabony component of the defect ($CEJ\text{-}BD_{T0} - CEJ\text{-}BC_{T0}$), PD_{T0}, and the residual supporting bone ($BD\text{-}RA_{T0}$).

Results.—A significant correlation was observed between the outcome variable and the following: (1) mean $CEJ\text{-}BD_{T0} \times$ IL-1 genotype ($P = .0019$), (2) TM_{T0} ($P < .0000$), (3) $CEJ\text{-}BD_{T0}$ ($P < .0000$), (4) $CEJ\text{-}BD_{T0} - CEJ\text{-}BC_{T0}$ ($P < .0000$), (5) PD_{T0} ($P = .0010$). Deeper PDs at a site and TM_{T0} were linked with the worst prognosis. A greater $CEJ\text{-}BD_{T0}$ distance and the infrabony component at baseline were linked with a better prognosis. The interaction between the mean CEJ-BD measurement at baseline and the IL-1 genotype was significantly linked with both a good or a poor prognosis. The other assessed variables, that is, age, sex, MT, PR, and residual supporting bone, were not significantly correlated with bone level variation.

Conclusion.—Several traditional prognostic factors were ineffective in predicting future bone level variation and, thus, were of no prognostic value. A few specific factors emerged at every level as valuable prognostic factors. At the patient level, the prognostic factor was the initial mean bone level combined with a positive IL-1 genotype; at the tooth level, it was TM; and at the site level, they were the initial bone level at a site, the infrabony component of a defect, and initial PD at a site. These factors may be useful to clinicians as predictors of bone level variation when determining a prognosis for a patient, a tooth, or a site.

▶ Establishing an accurate prognosis is one of the more difficult aspects of our jobs as clinicians. In recent years, studies by McGuire and coworkers[1-3] have begun to provide some insight on the most relevant variables to consider in making a prognosis. This is another retrospective private practice study that provides additional data on the usefulness of specific factors at the patient, the tooth, and the site levels. Although it uses surrogate variables rather than tooth loss as the measure of successful prediction of prognosis, the study has value in that it covers a 10-year follow-up period in real patients in a clinical practice.

A. Dentino, DDS, PhD

References

1. McGuire MK: Prognosis versus actual outcome: A long-term survey of 100 treated periodontal patients under maintenance care. *J Periodontol* 62:51-58, 1991.
2. McGuire MK, Nunn ME: Prognosis versus actual outcome: II. The effectiveness of clinical parameters in developing an accurate prognosis. *J Periodontol* 67:658-665, 1996.
3. McGuire MK, Nunn ME: Prognosis versus actual outcome: IV. The effectiveness of clinical parameters and IL-1 genotype in accurately predicting prognoses and tooth survival. *J Periodontol* 70:49-56, 1999.

The Effect of Triclosan-Containing Dentifrice on the Progression of Periodontal Disease in an Adult Population
Cullinan MP, Westerman B, Hamlet SM, et al (Univ of Queensland, Brisbane, Australia; Univ of Birmingham, England)
J Clin Periodontol 30:414-419, 2003   4–15

Background.—Except for chlorhexidine, antibacterial additives to toothpastes and mouthwashes have had little success in reducing the progression of periodontal disease. Dentifrices containing triclosan and other agents have been shown effective in reducing plaque and gingivitis. The effects of a triclosan/copolymer–containing toothpaste on periodontal disease progression among patients performing unsupervised plaque removal were evaluated.

Methods.—The controlled trial included 504 adult subjects with periodontal disease. Probing depths and attachment levels were assessed, then the subjects were assigned to use a 0.3% triclosan/2% copolymer toothpaste (Colgate Total) or a placebo toothpaste. The 2 groups were matched for disease status, plaque index, age, and sex. Follow-up examinations were performed at intervals of from 6 to 60 months, including bacteriologic assays of subgingival plaque samples.

Results.—For patients with initial probing depths of 3.5 mm or greater, the number of such sites at subsequent examinations was significantly lower with the triclosan/copolymer–containing dentifrice than with the control toothpaste. The larger the number of sites affected, the greater this protective effect. However, for patients with no sites with probing depths of 3.5 mm or greater, the active dentifrice had no significant effect. Probing depths were affected by various other factors including older age, smoking, and the presence of *Porphyromonas gingivalis* in the subgingival plaque. Patients with initial probing depths of 3.5 mm or greater were at increased risk of attachment loss at 2 years' follow-up.

Conclusion.—When used for unsupervised plaque removal, a triclosan/copolymer–containing toothpaste can slow the progression of adult periodontitis. The effect is more marked for patients with initial probing depths of 3.5 mm and for those with many involved sites. With long-term use, this type of dentifrice could have an important impact on periodontal disease outcomes.

▶ This long-term intervention study demonstrates that triclosan copolymer slows attachment loss in a compliant periodontal maintenance population. The effect was small but consistent over a 5-year observation period. This finding adds to the already impressive body of literature supporting the safety and efficacy of this antiseptic-containing dentifrice.

A. Dentino, DDS, PhD

A Systematic Review of Powered vs Manual Toothbrushes in Periodontal Cause-Related Therapy
Sicilia A, Arregui I, Gallego M, et al (Univ of Oviedo, Spain)
J Clin Periodontol 29(Suppl 3):39-54, 2002   4–16

Introduction.—It is not clear how the efficacy of power-driven toothbrushes (PDTs) compares with the efficacy of manual toothbrushes (MTs) in cause-related periodontal therapy. The effectiveness of PDTs versus MTs was compared by measures of gingival bleeding or inflammation resolution in a systematic review.

Methods.—Both electronic (MEDLINE and Cochrane Oral Health Group Specialized Trials Register) and manual searches were performed to identify trials that allowed the assessment of the efficacy of PDTs in decreasing gingival bleeding or inflammation and its effect on other secondary variables. The only trials that were included were randomized trials in adults that were published in English up to June 2001, that compared PDTs with MTs, and that assessed the evolution of gingival bleeding or inflammation. Selection of articles, extraction of data, and evaluation of validity were made independently by several reviewers.

Results.—Twenty-one trials were included. The heterogeneity of data hindered quantitative analyses. A higher efficacy in the reduction of gingival bleeding or inflammation in the research subjects using PDTs was identified in 10 trials. This effect seems to be associated with the capacity to diminish plaque and is more evident in counter-rotational and oscillating–rotating brushes. No definitive evidence exists for a higher efficacy of sonic brushes. In short-term trials with prophylaxis after the initial assessment, independently of the type of PDT used, no significant differences were seen.

Conclusion.—The use of PDTs, particularly counter-rotational and oscillating–rotating brushes, can be useful in decreasing the levels of gingival bleeding or inflammation.

▶ This systematic review is in partial agreement with the most recent Cochrane Collaboration Review on powered toothbrushing. Both independent analyses of the literature show that the oscillating–rotating PDT gave consistently better clinical outcomes regarding plaque and gingivitis than did the MT. Several other good PDTs are on the market, but their performance has not been as well documented as the oscillating–rotating toothbrush, based on independent systematic reviews of the available literature. One caveat for those who recommend PDTs is that the patient must be using the brush properly to get the maximum benefit, so it is incumbent on us to teach the proper use of any oral hygiene devices that we recommend.

A. Dentino, DDS, PhD

5 Endodontics

Introduction

For the 2004 edition, I have selected a variety of articles addressing primarily clinical topics that are likely to be frequently encountered in clinical practice. For example, the first 9 articles address root canal preparation and obturation. These procedures are done by everyone who does endodontic therapy in their practice. Most dentists would acknowledge that there is not one "right" technique for most of the things we do in dentistry. Endodontics is no exception. Each practitioner must try various accepted techniques for both the preparation and obturation of root canals and find what works best in their hands. The articles I have selected address a variety of techniques that will help practitioners find what works best for them.

After the above articles are several articles addressing root canal posts and cores, and postendodontic restorations. This particular area is constantly in a state of flux because new techniques and materials are continuously being developed. Ideally, posts, cores, and other types of restoration will provide maximum retention and strength without weakening the tooth structure itself.

We then move on to microbiological considerations, always a major consideration in the etiology, nature of the pathology, and outcomes of root canal and periapical involvement. As we also observe with periodontal disease, we are increasingly seeing more effective local agents for controlling microbes. We then move on to 2 articles on pain, a frequent sequella of endodontic involvement, but also a clinical symptom that can easily be ascribed to pulpal involvement when it in fact does not exist.

And finally, we complete the chapter with articles on the effect of radicular lesions adjacent to dental implants, diabetes and the dental pulp, and an article that looks at the validity of dye penetration studies in comparing the effectiveness of different canal obturating techniques.

Kenneth L. Zakariasen, DDS, MS, MS(ODA), PhD

Root Canal: Preparation and Obturation

Comparison of Apical Transportation in Four Ni-Ti Rotary Instrumentation Techniques

Iqbal MK, Maggiore F, Suh B, et al (Univ of Pennsylvania, Philadelphia)
J Endodont 29:587-591, 2003   5–1

Introduction.—The advent of Ni-Ti rotary instrumentation has revolutionized root canal treatment by decreasing operator fatigue, time needed to finish the preparation, and procedural errors. Described was a new radiographic technique used to compare apical transportation in 4 Ni-Ti rotary instrumentation sequences.

Methods.—Mesiobuccal canals of 60 extracted mandibular molars were randomly assigned to 1 of 4 groups. Groups 1 and 3 were instrumented by crown-down. Groups 2 and 4 were instrumented by step-back technique using 0.06 ProFiles series 29 to size 6. For groups 3 and 4, Greater Taper files were initially used in a crown-down fashion. The central axes of initial and final instruments were radiographically superimposed to ascertain loss of working length (WL) and transportation at 0, 0.5, 1, 3, and 5 mm from WL.

Results.—Three teeth in group 1 and 2 teeth in group 2 were lost due to separated instruments. The analysis of variance test revealed that there were no significant differences among groups concerning the extent of transportation or loss of WL. Transportation was negatively associated with the radius of curvature at 0.5 and 5 mm from WL.

Conclusion.—The operational sequence of ProFiles or preinstrumentation with Greater Taper files had no impact on the extent of transportation or loss of WL. The technique used for assessing instrumentation or root canals may be a valid tool for comparing instruments or instrumentation methods.

▶ For many decades, stainless steel endodontic hand-manipulated files were the primary instruments used in root canals. Those dentists who frequently performed endodontic therapy quickly found that the use of such instruments was very technique sensitive, particularly in small, significantly curved root canals. For example, forcing instruments rather than using them with finesse, or moving quickly to larger and larger sizes, would very frequently result in ledges being formed or in canals being blocked with debris. In response to this technique sensitivity, step-back and crown-down instrumentation techniques were developed to make consistent efficient and effective instrumentation possible while avoiding procedural errors.

The advent of Ni-Ti engine-driven files has not only made root canal instrumentation easier, and in most instances quicker, but appears to—as supported by the results of this study—have made root canal instrumentation less susceptible to many of the old procedural errors that necessitated step-back or crown-down instrumentation. However, practitioners must be cognizant of the fact that abuse of any instrumentation technique can lead to procedural errors. In the case of engine-driven rotary instrumentation with

Ni-Ti files, over-aggressive use of instruments in a manner not intended by the manufacturers can lead to instrument breakage, and this is an occurrence that can often be hard to recover from. A good principle during endodontic instrumentation is to favor the use of finesse rather than force. With any technique-sensitive procedure, training and experience are invaluable in learning how to use the instruments and techniques in ways that will avoid abuse. Likewise, learning the concept of finesse instead of force comes with practice, ie, much experience.

K. L. Zakariasen, DDS, MS, MS(ODA), PhD

Influence of Torque Control Motors and the Operator's Profiency on ProTaper Failures

Yared G, Dagher FB, Kulkarni K (Univ of Toronto; Lebanese Univ, Beirut)
Oral Surg Oral Med Oral Pathol Oral Radiol Endod 96:229-233, 2003   5–2

Introduction.—Instrument separation and deformation during root canal treatment are important concerns. Proper education and experience are necessary to minimize the incidence of instrument failure. The influence of 2 electric torque control motors and operator experience with a specific nickel-titanium rotary instrumentation method on the incidence of deformation and separation of instruments was examined.

Methods.—ProTaper (PT) nickel-titanium rotary instruments, which are manufactured in different sizes and variable tapers, were used at 300 rpm. In part of this 2-part trial, electric high torque control (group 1) and low torque control (group 2) motors were compared. In part 2, 3 operators with varying experience (groups 3, 4, and 5) were also compared. All sets of PT instruments were used in up to 5 canals and were sterilized between cases. During shaping, 2.5% NaOCl was used for irrigation. The number of deformed and separated instruments among the groups (within each part of the trial) was statistically examined for significance.

Results.—In part 1, instrument deformation and separation were not observed in groups 1 and 2. In part 2, 25 instruments were deformed and 12 were separated by the least experienced operator. The most experienced operator did not experience instrument deformation or separation. There was a significant difference between groups 3 and 4 concerning instrument deformation ($P = .0296$). The rate of instrument deformation was significantly different between groups 3 and 5 ($P < .0001$) and groups 4 and 5 ($P = .0018$). The rate of instrument separation was significantly higher in group 5, compared with groups 3 and 4 ($P = .0010$).

Conclusion.—Preclinical education and experience in the use of PT technique at 300 rpm is critical for preventing instrument separation and for decreasing the rate of instrument deformation. Use of an electric high torque control motor is safe in the hands of an experienced operator.

▶ This article demonstrates that both low- and high-torque electric motors used for rotary instrumentation in endodontics can be utilized safely by experienced operators. However, the most important point made by this article is the importance of operator proficiency in safely utilizing rotary instrumentation techniques. Instrument breakage, as discussed regarding the previous article (Abstract 5–1), can have very serious consequences for obtaining satisfactory results during endodontic therapy.

In this study, the experienced operator had no instrument deformation or instrument breakage. The inexperienced operator had significant numbers of instruments break and many instruments deform. If this operator had continued to utilize the deformed instruments—as is entirely possible if the deformation goes unnoticed—more instrument breakage would have occurred. It is the inexperienced operator who is more likely to not notice that deformations are occurring.

K. L. Zakariasen, DDS, MS, MS(ODA), PhD

Crown-Down Tip Design and Shaping
Ponce de Leon Del Bello T, Wang N, Roane JB (Oklahoma Univ, Oklahoma City)
J Endodont 29:513-518, 2003   5–3

Introduction.—There are currently 3 different file tip designs for endodontic files: (1) pyramidal with sharp transition angles and a forward-cutting ridge on the face (Fig 1); (2) conical with sharp transition angles and a smooth face (Fig 2); and (3) biconical with decreased transition angles and

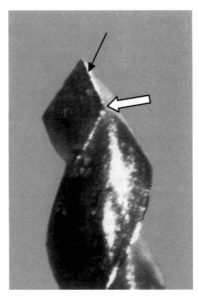

FIGURE 1.—A pyramidal design tip has ridges on the face, which enable it to cut in a forward direction (*small arrow*). These ridges intersect with the cutting edges to form shape points at the transition angles (*large arrow*). These points cut away the canal structure when a curvature is present and enable the file to follow a straightened path. (Courtesy of Ponce de Leon Del Bello T, Wang N, Roane JB: Crown-down tip design and shaping. *J Endodont* 29[8]:513-518, 2003.)

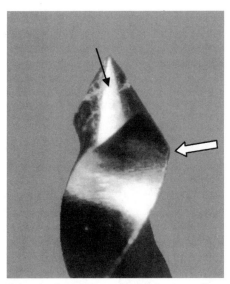

FIGURE 2.—A conical-shaped tip has no ridges on the face of its tip (*small arrow*); however, the intersection of the face and the cutting edges form sharp points at the transition angles (*large arrow*). These points cut away the canal wall when a curvature is present and allow the instrument to follow a straightened path. (Courtesy of Ponce de Leon Del Bello T, Wang N, Roane JB: Crown-down tip design and shaping. *J Endodont* 29[8]:513-518, 2003.)

dual-guiding faces (Fig 3). Tip shape may be important during crown-down shaping. The effect of file tip design on the prevalence of instrument damage, breakage, extent of transportation, and ledge formation during canal shaping was examined during canal shaping using the crown-down technique.

Methods.—Ninety curved canals were sorted by degree of curvature into 3 equal groups of 30. Canals in each group were shaped via a crown-down technique with the use of 1 of the 3 different tip shapes: biconical tip (Flex-R, Union Broach, York, Pa), conical tip (Mor-Flex, Union Broach), and pyramidal tip (Flex-O, Dentsply Maillefer, Ballaigues, Switzerland). There were 2 operators. The canals were photographed at baseline and after shaping. The finished shape was analyzed. The rates of transportation, ledging, and instrumentation damage were documented during instrumentation. National Institutes of Health image software was used to determine the longitudinal cross-sectional areas and cross-sectional diameters at specified canal depths.

Results.—Preparations varied significantly by which of the 3 tip shapes was used during the crown-down technique. The biconical tip files (Flex-R) caused the least transportation and no ledges. The pyramidal tip files (Flex-O) caused the most transportation, ledges, and damaged files. Only the pyramidal tip files developed ledges and encountered separation. Both operators reported less difficulty in shaping with a biconical-tipped file and the greatest technical difficulty using a pyramidal-shaped tip.

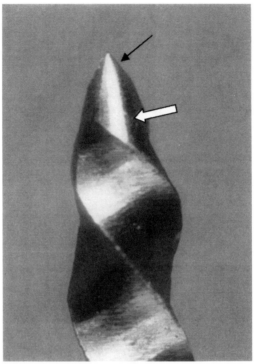

FIGURE 3.—A biconical tip has a smooth surface on the primary (*small arrow*) and secondary cones (*large arrow*). The secondary cone removes the points at the transition angles and provides a smooth surface that guides the tip through a curve. (Courtesy of Ponce de Leon Del Bello T, Wang N, Roane JB: Crown-down tip design and shaping. *J Endodont* 29[8]:513-518, 2003.)

Conclusion.—During crown-down rotational instrumentation, biconical file tips maintain the original canal curvature better and more frequently, compared with conical and pyramidal file tips.

▶ While the previous 2 articles (Abstracts 5–1 and 5–2) discussed the use of engine-driven Ni-Ti instrumentation systems, which indeed are becoming very popular, it should be recognized that many practitioners still utilize and feel comfortable with hand instrumentation with stainless steel files. We know that many procedural errors—eg, instrument breakage, instrument deformation, and canal ledging—can occur. Through experience and good technique, such procedural errors can be minimized. However, as this article demonstrates, instrument design, such as in the shape of the instrument tip, can also make a significant difference in the avoidance of procedural errors. If you examine the photographs of the 3 tip designs, it is quite evident why the biconical tip design produces superior results, ie, fewer procedural errors. Something to think about as you select your hand files.

K. L. Zakariasen, DDS, MS, MS(ODA), PhD

An In Vivo Comparison of Two Frequency-Based Electronic Apex Locators

Welk AR, Baumgartner JC, Marshall JG (Oregon Health & Sciences Univ, Portland)
J Endodont 29:497-500, 2003

5–4

Introduction.—Establishing the length of the root canal system at the apical constriction is regarded as the ideal working length for endodontic treatment. A working length established beyond the minor diameter may produce apical perforation and overfilling of the root canal system. One that is established short of the minor diameter may lead to insufficient debridement and underfilling of the canal. The accuracies of a 2-frequency (Root ZX, J Morita Co, Tustin, Calif) and a 5-frequency (Endo Analyzer Model 8005, Analytic, Sybron Dental, Orange, Calif) electronic apex locator were examined.

Methods.—Thirty-two teeth planned for extraction were used from 7 healthy adult patients having teeth extracted for prosthodontic reasons (age range, 37-82 years; mean age, 53 years). The coronal portion of each canal was flared utilizing Gates Glidden drills and Orifice Shapers. Canals were irrigated with 2.6% sodium hypochlorite. A K-type file was used to ascertain a separate working length in every canal using the electronic apex locators.

The teeth were extracted. The apical 4 mm of each root canal was exposed along the long axis of the tooth. Photographic slides of each canal were projected. The file position in relation to the minor diameter was ascertained by 2 observers.

Results.—The mean distances between the electronic apex locator working length and the minor diameter were 1.03 mm and 0.19 mm for the Endo Analyzer and the Root ZX, respectively (Table 2). The Endo Analyzer had significantly longer readings beyond the minor diameter, compared with the Root ZX ($P < .0001$). The ability to locate the minor diameter was 90.7% and 34.4% for the Root ZX and the Endo Analyzer Model 8005, respectively.

Conclusion.—The Root ZX was able to predictably locate the minor diameter more often than the Endo Analyzer Model 8005 (90.7% vs 34.4% accuracy).

▶ In today's world of emphasis on evidence-based dentistry, this study represents the type of research we need in much greater frequency: a well-con-

TABLE 2.—Distance From the Tip of the File Relative to the Minor Diameter

	Mean	SD	Minimum	Maximum	Range
Endo Analyzer Model 8005 ($n = 32$)	1.026*	0.945	0.095	4.577	4.482
Root ZX ($n = 32$)	0.189	0.398	−0.525	1.730	2.255

Note: Distances are in millimeters.
*Paired samples *t* test: statistically significantly longer readings beyond the minor diameter ($P < .0001$).
(Courtesy of Welk AR, Baumgartner JC, Marshall JG: An in vivo comparison of two frequency-based electronic apex locators. *J Endodont* 29[8]:497-500, 2003.)

trolled clinical trial whose results can be applied directly to clinical practice with meaningful positive outcomes. While the goals of these 2 electronic apex locators are the same—ie, accurate location of the root canal minor diameter—the results are distinctly different. This points out the significant need for practitioners to request credible research results to support a specific device or material they are considering using in their practices. When the success or failure of our treatment can be significantly influenced by the accuracy of a diagnostic device, we owe it to our patients to use those devices that are proven to consistently be accurate.

K. L. Zakariasen, DDS, MS, MS(ODA), PhD

Efficacy of Various Concentrations of Citric Acid at Different pH Values for Smear Layer Removal
Haznedaroğlu F (Istanbul Univ, Turkey)
Oral Surg Oral Med Oral Pathol Oral Radiol Endod 96:340-344, 2003   5–5

Introduction.—Several investigators who have examined the effects of various irrigants on smear layer have concluded that its elimination necessitates both organic (eg, sodium hypochlorite) and inorganic (eg, EDTA, citric acid) solvents. Scanning electron microscopy was used to ascertain the efficacy of various concentrations of citric acid at various pH values for removal of the superficial smear layer from dentinal surfaces.

Methods.—Fifty freshly extracted human maxillary canine teeth with fully developed apices were irrigated with sodium hypochlorite. Citric acid solutions at 50%, 25%, 10%, and 5% (weight/volume) concentrations were formulated. Additionally, similar solutions were buffered at pH 6. Citric acid solutions with original and buffered pH values were employed for final rinses.

Results.—Lower concentrations with lower pH values removed smear layer more efficiently, compared with those with higher pH values ($P < .05$)

TABLE 2.—Scores Allocated to the Specimens in Each Group

Group	Scores 0	1	2
Control 1 (2.5% NaOCl)	—	—	10
Control 2 (bidistilled water)	—	—	10
1 (5% citric acid, pH = 1.9)	7	3	—
2 (5% citric acid, pH = 6.0)	—	6	4
3 (10% citric acid, pH = 1.8)	9	1	—
4 (10% citric acid, pH = 6.0)	2	5	3
5 (25% citric acid, pH = 1.5)	9	1	—
6 (25% citric acid, pH = 6.0)	4	4	2
7 (50% citric acid, pH = 1.1)	10	—	—
8 (50% citric acid, pH = 6.0)	6	4	—

Note: 0, No smear layer, clean, with open tubule; 1, partial smear layer, scattered debris, some tubules partially occluded; 2, total smear layer, debris present, very few or no open tubules.

(Reprinted by permission of the publisher from Haznedaroğlu F: Efficacy of various concentrations of citric acid at different pH values for smear layer removal. *Oral Surg Oral Med Oral Pathol Oral Radiol Endod* 96:340-344, 2003. Copyright 2003 by Elsevier.)

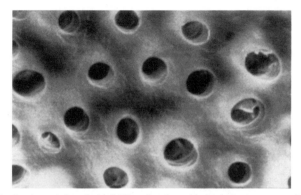

FIGURE 1.—Specimens irrigated with 2.5% sodium hypochlorite during instrumentation followed by 5% citric acid with a pH of 1.9 as final rinse. At high magnification, the smear layer is totally removed. Dentin tubular orifices are clearly visible; original magnification, × 5000. (Reprinted by permission of the publisher from Haznedaroğlu F: Efficacy of various concentrations of citric acid at different pH values for smear layer removal. *Oral Surg Oral Med Oral Pathol Oral Radiol Endod* 96:340-344, 2003. Copyright 2003 by Elsevier.)

(Table 2 and Fig 1). No significant differences for higher concentrations were identified between low and high pH values. More destruction of peritubular dentin was seen at higher concentrations with lower pH values.

Conclusion.—Lower concentrations of citric acid with its original pH were as effective as higher concentrations in the removal of the superficial smear layer.

▶ This article demonstrates, as have previous articles, that citric acid can be utilized to remove the smeared layer from prepared root canals. It is interesting to note that relatively low concentrations of the citric acid, at their natural pH, appear to be as effective as much higher concentrations, thus making the higher concentrations unnecessary. However, it should also be noted that the sample sizes in this study are relatively small and may not be picking up real differences between higher and lower concentration groups if they do in fact exist. That being said, even if the differences exist, the clinical significance of such differences may be negligible. As in a subsequent article (Abstract 5–9), we must ask whether removing the smeared layer will enhance the obturation effectiveness. Another question one could ask is whether the smeared layer includes components that are pulpal tissue and/or bacterial in nature that could help support bacterial growth. If so, we should indeed be attempting to remove the smeared layer.

K. L. Zakariasen, DDS, MS, MS(ODA), PhD

The Effect of Insertion Rates on Fill Length and Adaptation of a Thermoplasticized Gutta-Percha Technique

Levitan ME, Himel VT, Luckey JB (Univ of Tennessee, Memphis)
J Endodont 29:505-508, 2003   5–6

Background.—Ideally, obturation material must be easily manipulated, insoluble in tissue fluids, nonirritable, nontoxic, nonstaining, bactericidal, radiopaque, and able to adapt to root canal walls, with dental gutta-percha remaining the material of choice. However, use with thermoplasticized techniques may increase the tendency for sealer and gutta-percha extrusion from the apex. Whether insertion rate has an effect on the quality of the root canal obturation was explored.

Methods.—A single model root canal system replicating a maxillary central incisor was constructed so that it could be obturated repeatedly. Three groups were formed, one with an insertion rate of 18 mm/s, one at 6 mm/s, and one at 3 mm/s. The obturation's quality was evaluated by measuring the length of fill and the replication of induced canal irregularities (dimples and grooves).

Results.—The length of fill declined with decreasing insertion rate, with a statistically significant difference between the groups with the fastest insertion rate and the slowest rate. There was a mean overextension of +0.88 mm with the fastest rate and a mean underfill of −0.13 mm with the slowest rate (Table 1). Fifteen of the insertions at the rate of 18 mm/s had overextensions, whereas only 9 of those at the rate of 6 mm/s and 4 of those at the rate of 3 mm/s did. The slowest rate proved to be most likely to have a result short of the desired length. As the rate of insertion decreased, the replication of induced irregularities also declined.

Discussion.—Rate of insertion affected the length of the fill, most likely as the result of the cooling that occurs with the slower rate of insertion. The lower viscosity of the gutta-percha at the faster rate was associated with a greater potential for overextension. In addition, the use of gutta-percha at the fastest rate was best able to replicate the grooves and dimples of the model. However, this greater degree of replication was accompanied by a

TABLE 1.—Quality of Obturation With Data for Length of Fill and Replication of Surface Irregularities

Group	Duration of Insertion	Length of Fill from WL (mm)	Mean Replication of No. of Irregularities	
			Dimples ($n = 4$)	Grooves ($n = 3$)
A	1s (0.51-1.09)	+0.88[a]	3.95 (99%)[a]	3.0 (100%)[a]
B	3s (2.02-4.14)	+0.5[a,b]	3.85 (96%)[a,b]	2.65 (88%)[b]
C	6s (6.05-6.92)	−0.13[b]	3.60 (90%)[a]	2.76 (97%)[a,b]

Note: Different superscript letters are statistically significant at *P* < .05.
Abbreviations: WL, Working length; +, overextension; −, underfill.
(Courtesy of Levitan ME, Himel VT, Luckey JB: The effect of insertion rates on fill length and adaptation of a thermoplasticized gutta-percha technique. *J Endodont* 29[8]:505-508, 2003.)

loss of control over the length of fill, which produced a tendency toward overextension.

▶ The results of this study, as supported by the data presented, also intuitively make sense. As gutta-percha cools, it becomes thicker and flows with more difficulty. However, the authors clearly identify that there are limitations to this study. For example, the insertion forces at the various rates of insertion were not measured, and would most certainly increase as the gutta-percha cooled. At what point do the insertion forces required approach the root fracture threshold? If, in using this system, root fracture forces are not approached, one could speculate that using more insertion force when approaching working length with the slowest insertion speed may improve replication rates and still limit overfills. One potential advantage of the slowest insertion rate is that the temperature differential between the temperature of the gutta-percha at the completion of full insertion and its temperature when it has cooled to body temperature would be minimized, theoretically allowing less contraction on cooling. However, since this has not been measured it is only conjecture, and even if true, may not be of clinical significance. Then again, we have no idea whether the results reported in this study have any clinical significance. Perhaps when canal sealability is measured, all 3 insertion speeds result in similar sealability. . . and even if the sealabilities are somewhat different, would that make a difference in clinical success rates?

An important point from this discussion is that many of the results of our in vitro research are simply used to infer that better clinical results will be obtained. From an analytic point of view, such inferences are on very shaky ground. However, as a clinician, my intuitive sense is that I should attempt to obtain the best canal replications possible, as well as root canal obturations as close to working length as possible, because these could make a difference in clinical success. Wouldn't it be nice to have all the answers? The reality is that we don't have all the answers, and, as professionals, we are expected to weigh all the best evidence we do have, synthesize it, and deliver what we believe is the most effective care possible.

K. L. Zakariasen, DDS, MS, MS(ODA), PhD

Analysis of Continuous-Wave Obturation Using a Single-Cone and Hybrid Technique

Guess GM, Edwards KR, Yang M-L, et al (Univ of Pennsylvania, Philadelphia)
J Endodont 29:509-512, 2003   5–7

Introduction.—Obturation of the cleaned and shaped root canal system has been performed by various approaches, most of which have been successful. Most of the new techniques are compared against the standard obturation approach: lateral condensation, which has the advantage of producing a tight apical seal through compaction of many gutta-percha points via a spreader in the apical area.

A hybrid technique of root canal obturation that uses an initial lateral condensation of cones followed by a continuous-wave down-pack with a System-B plugger was compared with the single-cone continuous-wave obturation technique by examining the ability of both approaches to adapt gutta-percha to the prepared root canal walls in the apical 1 mm and 3 mm of the root. Additionally, the effect of various System-B heated plugger depths on the adaptation of the gutta-percha to the root canal walls during continuous-wave obturation was evaluated both hybrid and single-cone techniques.

Methods.—Profile NiTi rotary instruments were used to instrument 56 extracted human mandibular molars. Teeth were stratified based on curvature, then randomly assigned to 1 of 2 groups. Group 1 teeth were obturated by means of the single-cone continuous wave technique and group 2 was obturated by means of a hybrid technique (lateral condensation followed by a continuous-wave down-pack). Based on System-B plugger penetration, teeth were placed in 1 of 3 subgroups: less than 3.5 mm, 3.5 to 4.5 mm, and over 4.5 mm. The roots were horizontally sectioned at 1 mm and 3 mm coronal to the apical foramen, then stained and photographed. The adaptation of gutta-percha to the prepared canal walls was assessed by 4 evaluators.

Results.—There was no statistically significant difference between the 2 obturation methods at 1 mm (x = 1.80) or 3 mm (x = 1.804) sections. Optimal results were obtained with a plugger depth 3.5 to 4.5 mm from the working length.

Conclusion.—It appears that having a single cone with sealer in the apical region is as effective as several smaller cones laterally compacted together in filling the root canal space. This is in agreement with earlier findings.

▶ Here is another example of a study comparing root canal obturation techniques by visually comparing cross sections of canals obturated by different techniques, in this case with no difference between the techniques being observed. However, as in the previous study (Abstract 5–6), there are serious limitations as to what these results mean. If you were to compare these 2 techniques in fluid leakage studies, or put another way, comparing the sealing effectiveness of each technique, would there be statistically and clinically significant differences in the leakage? This would be far more relevant information to the clinical situation than the cross-sectional gutta-percha adaptation results.

However, statistically significant differences in leakage do not translate directly into being clinically significant. Only well-designed, long-term clinical trials could provide the hard evidence regarding clinical significance. It is my opinion that, given the emphasis today on evidence-based dentistry, we will see increasing numbers of such clinical trials.

K. L. Zakariasen, DDS, MS, MS(ODA), PhD

The Effect of Using an Inverted Master Cone in a Lateral Compaction Technique on the Density of the Gutta-Percha Fill

Wu M-K, de Groot SD, van der Sluis LWM, et al (Academic Ctr for Dentistry, Amsterdam)
Oral Surg Oral Med Oral Pathol Oral Radiol Endod 96:345-350, 2003   5–8

Introduction.—A good adaptation of gutta-percha (GP) to the canal wall enhances the complete obturation of the root canal space. There are advantages to using warm GP, but it may elevate the temperature of the external surface of the root to the extent of adversely affecting periodontal tissues. Cold lateral compaction root fillings in the apical root canal contain significantly less GP and more sealer, compared with the warm vertical compaction root fillings. It is assumed that if an inverted master GP cone is placed to the working length (Fig 1), the space available in the coronal root canal to accommodate accessory GP cones will be considerably larger.

This may facilitate the apical placement of more accessory cones and result in an apical root filling that contains more GP and less sealer. The per-

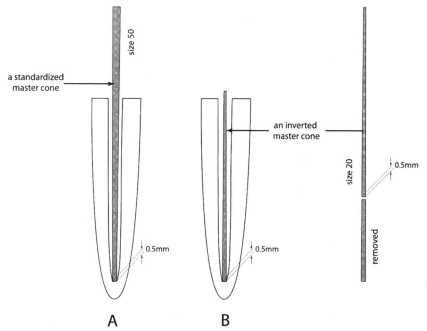

FIGURE 1.—Schematic representation of 2 types of master cones. A, A standardized size 50 gutta-percha master cone in the canal with its narrow end in an apical position. B, An inverted master cone in the canal with its large end in an apical position. The wide part of a standardized size 20 cone was removed, the remaining portion (large end, 0.5 mm in diameter) used as an inverted master cone. The standardized and inverted master cones had the same apical diameter and fit in the apical canal. (Reprinted by permission of the publisher from Wu M-K, de Groot SD, van der Sluis LWM, et al: The effect of using an inverted master cone in a lateral compaction technique on the density of gutta-percha fill. *Oral Surg Oral Med Oral Pathol Oral Radiol Endod* 96:345-350, 2003. Copyright 2003 by Elsevier.)

TABLE.—Mean and Standard Deviation of the Percentage of Gutta-Percha–Filled Areas in the Root Canals of Mandibular Premolars

| | 3 mm From the Apex | | 5 mm From the Apex | |
Master Cone	Area of Canal (mm²)	% of GP-Filled Area	Area of Canal (mm²)	% of GP-Filled Area
Standardized (n = 34)	0.42 ± 0.07	86.3 ± 10.4	0.50 ± 0.08	91.5 ± 9.0
Inverted (n = 35)	0.43 ± 0.09	91.1 ± 6.6	0.52 ± 0.13	94.6 ± 6.2

(Reprinted by permission of the publisher from Wu M-K, de Groot SD, van der Sluis LWM, et al: The effect of using an inverted master cone in a lateral compaction technique on the density of gutta-percha fill. *Oral Surg Oral Med Oral Pathol Oral Radiol Endod* 96:345-350, 2003. Copyright 2003 by Elsevier.)

centage of GP-filled area in the apical root canal after the use of a standardized or inverted master cone in cold lateral compaction was calculated.

Methods.—Two groups of extracted mandibular premolars with a single canal were instrumented with instruments of the same size and were obturated using laterally compacted GP cones with AH26 as a sealer. In the first group, a standardized master cone was utilized with its wide end in an apical position. The 2 master cones had corresponding apical diameters and fit in the apical canal. After lateral compaction, horizontal sections were cut at a level 3 mm and 5 mm from the apex of every filled tooth. Photographs of the sections were obtained via a microscope equipped with a digital camera. The photographs were scanned as tagged-image file format images. The cross-sectional area of the canal and the GP were ascertained with the use of an image-analysis program, The percentage of GP-filled area was determined.

Results.—At both the 3 mm and 5 mm levels, the inverted master cone generated a statistically significantly higher percentage of GP-filled area than did the standardized master cone ($P = .001$ at 3 mm; $P = .012$ at 5 mm) (Table).

Conclusion.—The use of an inverted master cone in cold lateral compaction may enhance the apical placement of accessory cones, significantly increasing the volume of GP while diminishing the volume of sealer in the apical root canal.

▶ The concept of using an inverted master cone to create a more favorable space for effective lateral condensation is a very clever one. Apparently, the inverted master cone allows very effective spreader penetration and facilitates effective apical placement of accessory cones. This seems to permit more complete and consistent lateral condensation of the root canal space. One concern I would have with this technique is that I believe it would be more technique sensitive regarding the fitting of the master cone. If the apical foramen is naturally relatively large or has been inadvertently enlarged greater than its normal size, an inverted master cone could be more easily overextended than a noninverted master cone during condensation.

One way to ensure that this does not happen is to custom fit the inverted master cone to be a snug fit slightly short—eg, approximately 1/2 mm—of full working length. Alternatively, a mild solvent for GP, such as eucalyptol, could be utilized to custom fit a slightly short-of-full-working-length, tight-fitting inverted master cone to full working length. The technique described in this article—perhaps with some interesting modifications as discussed here—may have some potential for improving the lateral condensation technique.

K. L. Zakariasen, DDS, MS, MS(ODA), PhD

Adhesion of Endodontic Sealers: Scanning Electron Microscopy and Energy Dispersive Spectroscopy
Saleh IM, Ruyter IE, Haapasalo MP, et al (NIOM-Scandinavian Inst of Dental Materials, Haslum, Norway; Univ of Oslo, Norway)
J Endodont 29:595-601, 2003   5–9

Introduction.—The role of the smear layer in endodontics has been the focus of considerable debate. Documenting the mode of failure of sealers to different dentin surfaces and gutta-percha (GP) may improve understanding of the significance of the smear layer. The microscopic details of the debonded interfaces between endodontic sealers and dentin or GP were examined.

Methods.—Dentin from human single-rooted teeth was conditioned with either 37% H_3PO_4 for 30 seconds, 25% citric acid for 30 seconds, 17% EDTA for 5 minutes, or a rinse with 10 mL of distilled H_2O (control). The GP surfaces were coated with freshly mixed sealer as follows: Grossman's sealer (GS), Apexit, Ketac-Endo, AH Plus, RoekoSeal Automix, or RoekoSeal Automix with an experimental primer. The surfaces were pressed together and the sealers were given time to set. After tensile bond strength testing, the morphological aspects of the fractured surfaces were examined by scanning electron microscopy and energy dispersive spectroscopy.

Results.—Energy dispersive spectroscopy successfully traced sealer components to the debonded surfaces. Some of the sealers infiltrated the dentinal tubules when the dentin surface had been pretreated with acids. These sealer tags continued to occlude the tubules after bond failure in some instances with GS, RoekoSeal Automix with an experimental primer, AH Plus/EDTA). Penetration of the endodontic sealers into the dentinal tubules when the smear layer was removed was not linked with higher bonding strength. Pretreatment of dentin with phosphoric acid yielded the highest bond strength for GS.

Conclusion.—The highest bond strengths for all sealers, excluding GS, were observed when the smear later was not removed.

▶ There has been discussion for years regarding the effects of the smeared layer found on the root canal wall following instrumentation. Some investigators have noted that when the smeared layer is removed with acids, eg, citric acid, sealer cements can enter the dentinal tubules and potentially enhance the obturation of the root canal system. This study examined removal and nonremoval of the smeared layer, penetration of sealers into the tubules, and the resulting strength of sealer adhesion. The authors found that penetration of the sealer into the tubules did not improve bond strengths. The authors acknowledge that micromechanical retention by sealer tags in the tubules may not be an important factor in sealer adhesion. My question would be: Why measure the bond strengths at all regarding endodontic sealers? The real question is whether the sealers can create a barrier to leakage. If not, when leakage occurs, a potential route for infection is created. Thus, we would want to ask the question: Are there conditions under which the radicular seal is enhanced when sealers can flow into dental tubules? If so, this may enhance the barrier for the exchange of bacteria between the root canal system and the periapical tissues.

K. L. Zakariasen, DDS, MS, MS(ODA), PhD

Root Canal: Posts and Cores and Restorations

Comparison of Two Methods for the Removal of Root Canal Posts
Chandler NP, Qualtrough AJE, Purton DG (Univ of Otago, Dunedin, New Zealand; Univ Dental Hosp of Manchester, England)
Quintessence Int 34:534-536, 2003   5–10

Introduction.—The failure rate of post-and-core-retained restorations is high and clinicians are faced with the need to atraumatically remove posts. Popular techniques for removing posts include the use of a trephining bur to cut a channel around the coronal aspect of the post and US vibration applied to the post to disrupt the luting agent. Trephination and US were compared in the removal of parallel-sided root canal posts.

Methods.—Thirty recently extracted, single-rooted human canine teeth were decoronated and prepared to receive preformed titanium posts, which were cemented with Panavia F resin cement (Kuraray). Ten teeth were used as controls, 10 had a 4-mm-deep gutter cut around the post using a Masserann trephining bur, and 10 underwent 10 minutes of US. The forces needed to dislodge the posts were ascertained with a universal testing machine.

TABLE 1.—Forces Required to Dislodge Posts (in Newtons)

Post	Control	Trephination	Ultrasound
1	127.5	16.7	36.8
2	188.8	47.6	401.7
3	134.9	94.2	202.6
4	69.65	97.6	107.4
5	89.7	21.6	234.0
6	175.1	68.7	150.6
7	38.75	124.1	67.7
8	159.9	73.6	66.2
9	113.8	212.4	200.1
10	160.1	46.1	334.5
Mean	125.8	80.3	180.2
SD	48	57	120

Abbreviation: SD, Standard deviation.
(Courtesy of Chandler NP, Qualtrough AJE, Purton DG: Comparisons of two methods for the removal of root canal posts. *Quintessence Int* 34:534-536, 2003.)

Results.—The only significant difference was between the trephined and US-energized post groups ($P = .032$), with the US-treated posts needing higher forces for dislodgement (Table 1).

Conclusion.—Resin composite cement could be removed from around the posts with the trephine bur with considerable difficulty. Neither cement removal from 40% of the post length or 10-minute exposure to US significantly diminished the force needed to remove posts.

▶ This study investigated the effectiveness of 2 popular techniques for removing posts from prepared root canals, an engine-driven trephine bur and US energy. While many practitioners have used these techniques with considerable success in the past (probably most effectively when used together), the use of resin composite cements rather than the more traditional zinc phosphate cement adds a complicating factor that seems to make both techniques largely ineffective. However, it would have been interesting to have a third experimental group, one in which the trephine bur was utilized first, as in the first experimental group, followed by the application of US energy, as in the second experiment group.

While the authors of this article discussed this combination, they unfortunately did not include it in this study. While the authors' discussion would lead us to believe that such a combination of the 2 techniques would probably be ineffective, it would have required only 1 more experimental group to actually test it. With so many unexplained factors potentially at work here, the results of having this third experimental group included may have helped to answer some important questions.

K. L. Zakariasen, DDS, MS, MS(ODA), PhD

Depth of Light-Initiated Polymerization of Glass Fiber–Reinforced Composite in a Simulated Root Canal

Le Bell A-M, Tanner J, Lassila LVJ, et al (Univ of Turku, Finland)

Int J Prosthodont 16:403-408, 2003   5–11

Background.—Fiber-reinforced composite (FRC) root canal posts were introduced in the 1990s and consist of continuous unidirectional reinforcing fibers embedded in a polymer matrix. Made of carbon/graphite, glass, or silica, their elastic modulus resembles that of dentin. The use of in situ–polymerized FRC posts requires an adequate degree of conversion of polymer matrix in the root canal. The depth of light-initiated conversion achieved in a simulated in situ–polymerized FRC post was assessed, along with the time needed to achieve adequate conversion.

Methods.—Polymer-preimpregnated E-glass fiber reinforcement was used and underwent further impregnating with light-polymerizable dimethacrylate monomer resin. A control sample of the resin without fiber reinforcement was used for comparison. Light-protected cylinders filled with the test materials were light polymerized from one end; these cylinders measured 4 to 24 mm in length. Fourier transform infrared spectrometry was used to determine the degree of monomer conversion that occurred, with infrared spectra measured at 6 time points from the beginning of polymerization. Test material microhardness was also documented along the length of each cylinder.

Results.—With increasing time, the mean degree of conversion after polymerization increased regardless of cylinder length. The degree of conversion for the FRC groups was 70% in the 4-mm cylinder and 33% in the 24-mm cylinder at 15 minutes. For the plain resin groups, the degree of conversion was 72% and 15%, respectively. With longer cylinders, conversion declined. A slightly higher degree of conversion was present in the longest cylinders made of FRC than those of the plain resin. The degree of conversion was significantly related to cylinder length and material. The Vickers hardness number (VHN) decreased with increased distance from the light-exposure surface, indicating less hardness. The resin group had a higher VHN than the FRC group. A statistically significant, although slight, increase in VHN values was documented measuring from the 0-mm to the 4-mm point.

Discussion.—The glass FRC and monomer resin without fibers had nearly equal degrees of conversion after light curing. FRC showed a slightly higher degree of conversion for the longest cylinders than was noted with the resin without fibers, which may be attributable to the fibers' light-conducting ability.

▶ The intent and recommendations for root canal posts have changed dramatically over the years. The long rigid posts that were recommended for so many years were very good at retaining crowns, but had a propensity to fracture roots if significantly traumatized. The glass fiber–reinforced composite post, with an elastic modulus similar to dentin, was introduced to obviate this problem while still providing good retention. This article begins the needed comparisons between prefabricated FRC posts and those individually formed in the tooth being treated. The initial data indicate that sufficient polymerization can occur in the root canal space, and that the fibers may actually help conduct light to greater depths than composite cylinders without fibers. This research is promising and indicates that, with more positive research findings to support it, individually formed FRC posts (ie, customized) may be a better direction to take than preformed FRC posts.

K. L. Zakariasen, DDS, MS, MS(ODA), PhD

It Is Unclear Whether Endodontically Treated, Single-Rooted Teeth Need Cast or Direct Posts and Cores
Caplan D (Univ of North Carolina, Chapel Hill)
J Evid Base Dent Pract 1:13-14, 2003   5–12

Introduction.—Cast post-and-core restorations have long been considered to provide the best long-term restorative therapy for severely broken down endodontically treated anterior teeth. Improvements in restorative materials and the desire of both patients and dentists to avoid a 2-visit procedure have prompted this systematic comparison between cast and direct post-and-core restorations.

Methods.—A systematic review was performed of the success rates of reports that evaluated endodontically treated, single-rooted teeth restored with cast versus direct post-and-core in humans, both in vitro and in vivo. Six trials qualified for inclusion. None were randomized controlled trials. Five trials did not compare the 2 techniques at all; 3 were case series descriptions of restorations and 2 were case series descriptions of direct restorations. Only 1 trial reported on the success of both restoration types and described a 90% success rate in both groups over a 3-year period.

Results.—Success rates in the 6 reports ranged from 87% to 93% for cast restorations and from 68% to 93% for direct restorations. Follow-up ranged from 3 to 8 years. Definitions of failure varied among reports.

Conclusion.—There was no conclusive evidence that favored cast over direct post-and-core restorations or vice versa. Randomized controlled trials now are needed for this comparison.

▶ This is a very interesting article in that it analyzes and evaluates an extensive systematic review of cast post-and-cores versus direct post-and-cores. This review found 1773 publications on this topic, only 6 of which were relevant for inclusion in the systematic review. Of these 6, none were randomized controlled trials. The author concluded that "No conclusive evidence favors cast over direct post-and-core restorations. . ." This is really amazing given the amount of research that has been done on this topic but is certainly not uncommon when one looks for definitive clinical evidence—particularly in the form of randomized controlled trials—in most areas of clinical dentistry.

While much in vitro research is available in many areas of dentistry to indicate possible effectiveness differences between various techniques and materials, we are woefully short of real clinical research that verifies whether such in vitro differences have any clinical significance. There may be very real differences of clinical significance between cast and direct post-and-cores, but, as shown by this review and analysis, we can't really tell from the evidence available.

K. L. Zakariasen, DDS, MS, MS(ODA), PhD

Assessment of the Resistance to Fracture of Endodontically Treated Molars Restored With Amalgam
Assif D, Nissan J, Gafni Y, et al (Tel Aviv Univ, Israel)
J Prosthet Dent 89:462-465, 2003   5–13

Introduction.—Restoration of endodontically treated molars is challenging. There is controversy concerning the optimal restoration of these teeth and their resistance to fracture under occlusal load. The resistance to fracture of endodontically treated molars with various degrees of tooth structure loss restored with amalgam under simulated occlusal load was examined.

Methods.—Ninety noncarious, nonrestored molars stored in physiologic saline solution were endodontically treated and randomly divided into 9 experimental groups of 10 specimens each with varying degrees of tooth loss. Tooth loss ranged from a conservative orthodontic access to removal of all cusps (Fig 1). All molars were restored to their original contour with amalgam by a standardized technique. Every specimen was mounted on a specialized jig for loading at the central fossa at a 30° angle to the long tooth axis. The resistance to fracture was applied by means of a universal testing machine and was documented. Continuous compressive force at a cross-head speed of 2 mm/min was used.

Results.—The group with a conservative endodontic access (1137.6 newtons) and the group in which all cusps were removed (1261.4 newtons) had significantly higher resistance to fracture, compared with the other groups ($P < .05$). No significant differences in resistance to fracture under the simu-

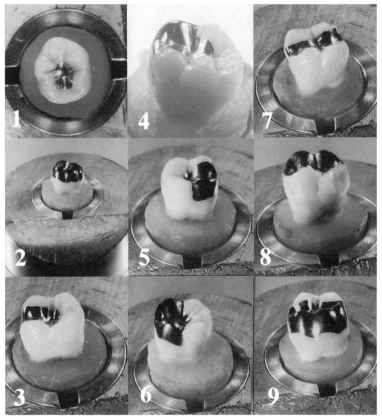

FIGURE 1.—Tested teeth with various degrees of tooth structure loss restored with amalgam. (Reprinted from Assif D, Nissan J, Gafni Y, et al: Assessment of the resistance to fracture of endodontically treated molars restored with amalgam. *J Prosthet Dent* 89:462-465, 2003. Copyright 2003, with permission from The Editorial Council of The Journal of Prosthetic Dentistry.)

TABLE 1.—Mean and Standard Deviation of Resistance to
Failure Force for All Groups

Group	Mean	SD
1	1137.6*	311.6
2	1261.4*	195.1
3	823.4	184.2
4	768.8	279.5
5	906.3	168.1
6	730.2	304.2
7	655.8	229.4
8	799.7	247.2
9	825.6	163.2

Note: Figures are in newtons.
*$P < .05$.
(Reprinted from Assif D, Nissan J, Gafni Y, et al: Assessment of the resistance to fracture of endodontically treated molars restored with amalgam. *J Prosthet Dent* 89:462-465, 2003. Copyright 2003, with permission from The Editorial Council of The Journal of Prosthetic Dentistry.)

lated load was observed among the other 7 groups (range, 655.8 N to 906.3 N) ($P < .05$) (Table 1).

Conclusion.—The endodontically treated molars with a conservative endodontic access and those in which all cusps were removed, then restored to their original contour with amalgam, had the highest resistance to fracture under a simulated occlusal load.

▶ As we can see from this and other articles from the literature, the discussions about the most appropriate techniques and materials for restoring endodontically treated teeth are far from over. If we look at making clinical decisions based on scientific evidence, we are still short of the evidence we require, both in vitro and especially in vivo research. This article is most interesting in that the most conservative and most extensive restorations gave the greatest resistance to fracture. While the most conservative restoration—basically the restoration of the endodontic access opening—makes sense to most of us, when something more extensive is needed because of destruction by caries, our logic and training usually tell us to use the most conservative restoration possible. This research would indicate that this may be faulty thinking. However, the authors are very cognizant of the limitations of this study and the fact that further research is needed to confirm and expand on these findings. Still, here is another example of "hard data" challenging what has in the past been "conventional wisdom."

K. L. Zakariasen, DDS, MS, MS(ODA), PhD

Microbiologic Considerations

Bacteriological Study of Root Canals Associated With Periapical Abscesses

de Sousa ELR, Ferraz CCR, de Almeida Gomes BPF, et al (Univ of Campinas, Piracicaba, Brazil)

Oral Surg Oral Med Oral Pathol Oral Radiol Endod 96:332-339, 2003   5–14

Background.—Antibiotic therapy to complement dental treatments can be overused and result in allergic reactions, the development of superinfection promoted by resistant bacterial species, and the unneeded exposure to the toxicity and side effects of these medications. Periapical abscesses in root canals do not usually require antibiotic therapy or bacteriologic investigation, and when antibiotics are required, empirical treatment not predicated on the results of culture and susceptibility tests is usually sufficient. In general, multiple bacteria are present in periapical abscesses. The microorganisms found in root canals with periapical abscesses were identified, and their susceptibility to specific antibiotics was assessed.

Methods.—Sterile paper points were used to sample 30 root canals, and the samples were then subjected to microbiologic identification methods. With the use of the E test system, a plastic strip with a continuous gradient of antibiotic with 15 minimum inhibitory concentration (MIC) dilution, the susceptibility of *Peptostreptococcus prevotii* and *Fusobacterium necrophorum* to the following antibiotics was assessed: benzylpenicillin (the parenteral antibiotic of choice when rapid effect or high serum concentration is needed); amoxicillin (often recommended as a first-choice antibiotic because of its broader spectrum, longer action, and ability to compete with food for absorption, although drawbacks include gastrointestinal side effects, hypersensitivity, and the development of resistant strains, plus its inactivation by β-lactamase); amoxicillin and clavulanate potassium; metronidazole; clindamycin (which exerts a bacteriostatic effect except at high doses, when it becomes bactericidal); erythromycin (used when patients are allergic to penicillin but is not effective against *Fusobacterium* and does not achieve high concentrations in blood, nor is it as effective against important anaerobes); and azithromycin.

Results.—A mean incidence of 3.9 bacteria per root canal was found, with 117 cultivable isolates retrieved from the 30 root canals. Seventy-five isolates were strict anaerobes; 42, facultative anaerobes; 29, gram-negative species; and 88 gram-positive species. *P prevotii* was the predominant strict anaerobic bacteria found, followed by *Peptostreptococcus micros, F necrophorum, Streptococcus constellatus,* and *Prevotella intermedia/Prevotella nigrescens.* The *P prevotii* and *F necrophorum* strains were susceptible to benzylpenicillin, amoxicillin, amoxicillin plus clavulanic acid, metronidazole, and clindamycin. Eighty percent of the *F necrophorum* strains were not susceptible to erythromycin, and 60% of them were not susceptible to azithromycin; both of these antibiotics exhibited activity against 80% of the *P prevotii* species found. The MICs of the antibiotics to *P*

TABLE 3.—MIC of the Antibiotics to *P prevotii*

Peptostreptococcus Prevotii (*n* = 5)

Antimicrobial Agents	MIC (µg/mL)* 50%	90%	Range of MIC	Susceptibility Rate %
Benzylpenicillin	0.016	0.38	<0.016-0.38	100%
Amoxicillin	0.19	0.25	0.032-0.25	100%
Amoxicillin + clavulanic acid	0.125	0.19	0.064-0.19	100%
Metronidazole	0.016	0.38	<0.016-0.38	100%
Clindamycin	0.38	0.125	<0.016-0.125	100%
Erythromycin	1.0	1.0	0.016-1.0	80%
Azythromycin	1.5	8.0	0.016-8.0	80%

*Fifty percent and 90%, at which 50% and 90% of the isolates are inhibited, respectively.
Abbreviation: MIC, Minimum inhibitory concentration.
(Reprinted by permission of the publisher from De Sousa ELR, Ferraz CCR, de Almeida Gomes BPF, et al: Bacteriological study of root canals associated with periapical abscesses. *Oral Surg Oral Med Oral Pathol Oral Radiol Endod* 96:332-339, 2003. Copyright 2003 by Elsevier.)

prevotii and those of the antibiotics to *F necrophorum* were determined (Table 3).

Discussion.—Periapical abscesses are infected with several bacteria, with the most predominant being anaerobic gram-positive cocci, which were found in 80% of the samples. The microorganisms tested were highly susceptible to benzylpenicillin and particularly susceptible to amoxicillin. All the species tested were susceptible to the penicillins. Erythromycin had poor antimicrobial activity against *F necrophorum* but may be effective against mild or moderate infections in persons with penicillin allergy. Clindamycin was effective against the strict anaerobes tested; its use has been limited because it tends to cause antibiotic-associated colitis. Penicillin would appear to be the drug of choice in treating oral infections, with clindamycin given to patients allergic to penicillin.

▶ This article reinforces the seriousness of periapical infections, the polymicrobial nature of such infections, and the need for early recognition of the etiology of such infections as essential in arriving at appropriate therapy. The article reviewed many types of organisms found, and their susceptibility to the various antibiotics, most of which are very familiar to practicing dentists. Fortunately, most of the bacteria with which we deal are susceptible to one or more of these antibiotics. However, it must be recognized that the indiscriminate use of antibiotics where they are not really required will continue to lead to more and more resistant organisms, certainly something that will complicate the future treatment of patients.

K. L. Zakariasen, DDS, MS, MS(ODA), PhD

Antibacterial Efficacy of a New Chlorhexidine Slow Release Device to Disinfect Dentinal Tubules

Lin S, Zuckerman O, Weiss EI, et al (Tel-Aviv Univ, Israel; Hebrew Univ, Jerusalem)
J Endodont 29:416-418, 2003   5–15

Introduction.—Since mechanical preparation cannot effectively eradicate bacteria from dentinal tubules and other irregularities in the root canal, remnant microorganisms can multiply between patient visits and can reach the same level as at the beginning of the previous appointment. An effective intracanal medication could help sterilize the root canal system. The antibacterial effect of chlorhexidine (CHX) was evaluated as an intracanal medication and as an irrigation solution. An in vitro model for dentinal tubule infection of root canals was used.

Methods.—Dentinal tubules of 27 cylindrical bovine root incisors were infected with *Enterococcus faecalis*. In 9 specimens each, 5% CHX in a slow-release device (Activ Point, Roeko, Langenau, Germany), 10 mL of 0.2% CHX (Tarodent, Taro, Haifa, Israel), or no medication (positive control) were incubated for 7 days at 37°C under humid conditions. Triplicate samples of 0.01 mL were incubated for 48 hours at 37°C. Growing colonies were counted and documented.

Results.—Heavy bacterial infection was seen at the layer close to the lumen in the control specimens, diminishing rapidly by layer to the deepest layer tested (400-500 μm), which contained several hundred colony forming units (Table 1). Viable bacteria in each layer of dentin were significantly decreased with CHX irrigation solution ($P < .01$) and were completely eradicated with the CHX slow-release device ($P < .01$).

Conclusion.—The Activ Point CHX slow release device appears to be an effective intracanal medication with high penetration abilities and strong antibacterial properties.

TABLE 1.—Logarithmic Transformation of the Number of Colony-Forming Units (CFU + 1) at Different Dentine Layer Depths

Dentin Depth (μm)	Activ-Point®	CHX-Irrigation	Control	Significance*
0-100	0	8.4 ± 1.7	12.2 ± 1.4	p < 0.001
100-200	0	7.8 ± 1.6	10.2 ± 0.77	p < 0.001
200-300	0	8.2 ± 0.8 ------------ 9.6 ± 0.8		p < 0.001
300-400	0	7.9 ± 0.4 ------------ 8.9 ± 0.9		p < 0.001
400-500	0	5.9 ± 0.3 ------------ 7.0 ± 0.8		p < 0.001

*One-way analysis of variance was performed on log transformation of colony-forming units for each layer. *Horizontal lines* connect data that do not show significant differences (Tukey's method).

(Courtesy of Lin S, Zuckerman O, Weiss EI, et al: Antibacterial efficacy of a new chlorhexidine slow release device to disinfect dentinal tubules. *J Endodont* 29(6):416-418, 2003.)

Efficacy of Calcium Hydroxide: Chlorhexidine Paste as an Intracanal Medication in Bovine Dentin

Evans MD, Baumgartner JC, Khemaleelakul S-u, et al (Oregon Health & Science Univ, Portland)

J Endocrinol 29:338-339, 2003   5–16

Introduction.—Several reports have documented the antimicrobial efficacy of chlorhexidine (CHX) gel and sustained release vinyl ribbons containing CHX as intracanal medications. The antibacterial efficacy of an intracanal paste composed of calcium hydroxide mixed with 2% CHX was evaluated.

Methods.—Twenty-four extracted bovine incisors were made into standardized cylindrical segments of dentin and infected with *Enterococcus faecalis*. The incisors were treated with an intracanal paste of calcium hydroxide and sterile water (group A) or calcium hydroxide and 2% CHX (group B) for 1 week. Dental shavings were obtained, suspended in solution, and spread on brain-heart infusion agar. The number of colony-forming units (CFUs) was counted and the amount of bacteria per milligram of dentin was determined after incubation.

Results.—The total number of colony-forming units of *E faecalis* per milligram of dentin shavings was higher in group A than in group B (1040 CFU/mg vs 23 CFU/mg; $P < .001$). The paste used for group B was more effective in killing *E faecalis* in the dentinal tubules than the paste used for group A.

Conclusion.—Calcium hydroxide paste with 2% CHX was significantly more effective in killing *E faecalis* in the dentinal tubules, compared to calcium hydroxide with water.

▶ Success in endodontic therapy depends on many factors. Given that we know that root canal failures most often occur because of bacterial involvement, we stress strongly the debridement and enlargement of the root canal system to eliminate bacteria and the substrates that support bacterial growth, and to facilitate effective obturation of the root canal system so that bacteria can neither escape nor re-enter the canal space. In addition, we have used a variety of intracanal medications to help eliminate microorganisms from the root canal system (CMCP, sodium hypochlorite, antibiotics, calcium hydroxide, etc). Ideally, such medications will effectively kill microorganisms, while at the same time not be damaging to host tissues.

While calcium hydroxide has found much favor as an intracanal medication and is currently used extensively, the extent of its bactericidal properties and its ability to penetrate dentinal tubules can certainly be questioned. We also know that chlorhexidine is an effective antibacterial agent that is effectively used directly in contact with tissues, eg, in periodontal pockets.

The research reported in these 2 articles (Abstracts 5–15 and 5–16) clearly points out the potential antibacterial efficacy of CHX in endodontic applications and, in the second article (Abstract 5–16), contrasts this efficacy with calcium hydroxide used alone. These research articles point to increased endodontic therapy effectiveness through a strengthening of the antibacterial capabilities of our treatment regimen. However, it is also clear from these articles that antibacterial efficacy can be significantly affected by the manner in which the antibacterial agent is applied. Undoubtedly, more research in this important area will be forthcoming.

K. L. Zakariasen, DDS, MS, MS(ODA), PhD

Pain

Toothache of Nonodontogenic Origin: A Case Report

Mascia P, Brown BR, Friedman S (State Univ of New York, Stony Brook)
J Endodont 29:608-610, 2003   5–17

Background.—Tracking down the origin of a patient's oral pain may require evaluation of the patient's medical history, dental history, and psychological state, as well as radiographs, thermal testing, percussion, palpation, occlusal sensitivity, and electric pulp testing. With diffuse pain or pain radiating to other areas, nonodontogenic causes should be strongly considered. In addition, more than one source may be at play, requiring careful assessment of each possible cause.

Trigger Points and Referred Pain.—A regional, dull, aching muscle pain plus localized tender sites or trigger points characterize myofascial pain. Trigger points involve a taut band within muscle that produces a regional referred pain, autonomic symptoms, or both when palpated. Trigger points can be active, causing reproducible pain over an extensive area when palpated, or latent, present but not causing symptoms. Active trigger points may not produce pain in the muscle where they are located. Trigger points can occur with overstretching or overcontracting a muscle. Referred pain is believed to result from a misinterpretation of nociceptive afferent input. Both the cervical region and areas supplied by the trigeminal nerve send afferent input to the CNS, with secondary neurons carrying peripheral input to higher CNS centers. These secondary neurons lie close to one another, which can permit neurotransmitters from one pathway to stimulate a closely related pathway, leading to misinterpretation in the cortex. Trigger points at the zygomatic origin can refer pain to the maxillary posterior teeth, causing a maxillary "toothache"; those in the mandibular angle can refer pain to the mandibular posterior teeth. Pain referral patterns of the medial pterygoid can create similar findings, plus a "sore throat." Anterior temporalis referred pain can affect the maxillary anterior teeth and cause headache. Trapezius muscle referred pain can be experienced in the mandibular angle and ear area.

Case Report.—Woman, 25, complained of spontaneous pain on the left side of the face that radiated to the ear and temporal region and began several hours previously. A 650-mg dose of acetaminophen produced no relief. Caries and periodontal sources were ruled out; radiographs found no pathologic conditions. Pericementitis of tooth #18 was eliminated by selective anesthesia, but the diffuse pain was not relieved. On myofascial pain assessment, the left masseter muscle was tender to palpation at the mandibular angle, and a trigger point was found in the muscle belly. When stimulated, the trigger point produced pain referred to the oral cavity that corresponded to the patient's chief complaint. In addition, tenderness was found in the left medial pterygoid muscle and the anterior segment of the left temporalis muscle, with moderate pain in the left temporal tendon. Myofascial pain with a trigger point in the masseter muscle referring pain into the dentition was diagnosed; injection of 3% carbocaine into the area relieved the pain.

Discussion.—Oral pain may be produced by nonodontogènic sources in a significant number of cases. Myofascial examination is in order when a patient complains of diffuse pain, but no etiology can be identified on standard testing or radiographs.

▶ The etiology of pain of the head and neck region can be very difficult to diagnose. Given the frequency with which referred pain can occur, the dentist must be very good at differential diagnosis. Unfortunately, it is very easy to assume an odontogenic etiology when patients complain of oral pain. This can easily lead to inappropriate and unneeded therapy, such as root canal therapy. After such treatment, the patient will still be left with their pain problem. The case described in this article is one that could easily be misdiagnosed. . . a case with dental symptoms, no clear dental etiology, but with a pain trigger point in the masseter muscle. Fortunately, the authors recognized the possibility of referred pain with a nonodontogenic origin, did not administer any dental therapy, and found the masseter trigger point. I have seen similar cases in my own endodontic practice, cases in which the patients were so sure that a tooth was responsible for their pain that they demanded root canal therapy. Not finding a dental origin, I refused to render endodontic therapy and eventually found the nondental origin for the referred pain. Such patients go from being initially mad at the caregiver for not rendering dental treatment to delighted with having their pain alleviated properly and not receiving treatment they didn't need. I've often thought that in dental school we have stressed excellence in technical procedures, as we should, but have underemphasized the need to become excellent diagnosticians. Cases as described in this article emphasize the need for superb differential diagnostic skills.

K. L. Zakariasen, DDS, MS, MS(ODA), PhD

Comparison of Preoperative Pain and Medication Use in Emergency Patients Presenting With Irreversible Pulpitis or Teeth With Necrotic Pulps
Nusstein JM, Beck M (Ohio State Univ, Columbus)
Oral Surg Oral Med Oral Pathol Oral Radiol Endod 96:207-214, 2003   5–18

Background.—Pain has been reported as the primary cause for persons to seek endodontic treatment. One study reported that 66% of patients who sought care at an emergency dental clinic were in pain and that 89% of these patients had been in pain for more than 1 week. The symptoms of teeth with irreversible pulpitis and necrotic pulps with periapical pathosis have been well described. However, the histopathologic status of the pulp in vital teeth cannot be determined by consideration only of a patient's pain symptoms. The main diagnostic regimen comprises subjective questioning of the patient regarding symptoms, a clinical examination, and pulp testing.

The preoperative factors involved in pain and the use of medications to relieve preoperative pain have been described in previous studies. However, further study is warranted. The purpose of this retrospective study was to compare differences in preoperative pain and medication use in patients with moderate to severe pain who sought emergency endodontic treatment for teeth with irreversible pulpitis and for symptomatic teeth with necrotic pulps.

Methods.—The study group included 323 patients who sought emergency endodontic treatment and completed questionnaires regarding biographic information, pain, pain history, and medications. Their teeth were tested for vitality, mobility, percussion, and pain on palpation. Lymphadenopathy was also evaluated.

Results.—Patients with irreversible pulpitis waited significantly longer to seek emergency care than did patients with symptomatic teeth with necrotic pulps (9 days vs 4 days). There were no differences between the 2 groups in terms of analgesic or antibiotic use and pain relief from preoperative narcotic medications. Nonnarcotic analgesics were reported to provide significant pain relief more often in patients with symptomatic teeth with necrotic pulps. More women than men used analgesic medications, and in the group with symptomatic teeth with necrotic pulps, more men than women reported relief of pain from their analgesic medications.

Conclusion.—Patients with irreversible pulpitis wait longer before seeking emergency treatment, and most emergency patients (81% to 83%) with moderate to severe pain will take some type of medication for pain relief. More women than men with irreversible pulpitis will take an analgesic. This group of patients will obtain relief in 62% to 65% of cases by taking preoperative medications, and more men than women with symptomatic teeth with necrotic pulps will obtain relief of pain.

▶ Pain is both a very difficult phenomenon to study for researchers and a difficult sensation to live with for patients. This is evidenced by the difficulty the authors experienced in attempting to compare endodontic pain studies and by the fact that over 80% of patients with moderate to severe pain utilized some analgesic in an attempt to relieve the pain.

However, in dealing with endodontic-origin pain problems, once the pain has begun, it usually gets progressively worse whether the pain is of irreversible pulpitis origin or of periapical origin. It is better to get the patient in for treatment as soon as possible before the condition has a chance to progress further—eg, worsening infection—and before the patient has lived with significant pain for an extended period. If this can be done, the patients are usually easier to treat and make comfortable, and the patient lives with pain for a shorter overall period of time.

K. L. Zakariasen, DDS, MS, MS(ODA), PhD

Other Topics

Effect of Teeth With Periradicular Lesions on Adjacent Dental Implants
Shabahang S, Bohsali K, Boyne PJ, et al (Loma Linda Univ, Calif; Nice, France)
Oral Surg Oral Med Oral Pathol Oral Radiol Endod 96:321-326, 2003   5–19

Background.—Advances in dental implant technology have made possible new treatment options for edentulous areas. Dental implants offer a viable alternative to fixed partial dentures in partially edentulous patients, and fully edentulous patients now have an opportunity to obtain more stable and functional prostheses. However, a variety of complications have been reported in association with implant placement. One of these complications is the presence of inflammation near the root-form implant. It is generally accepted that dental implants should not be placed in areas of infection. However, the effects of periradicular infections of natural teeth on adjacent osseointegrated implants is less understood. The effects of periradicular lesions on osseointegration of existing implants were more clearly elucidated.

Methods.—In this canine model, a total of 40 titanium solid root-form implants were placed close to premolars. After healing, the adjacent premolars were treated in 1 of 4 ways as follows: Group A received no treatment of the adjacent premolar; group B underwent induction of a periradicular lesion followed by nonsurgical root canal therapy of the premolar; group C underwent induction of a periradicular lesion followed by nonsurgical root canal therapy of the premolar and surgical detoxification of the implant surface; and group D underwent induction of a periradicular lesion and no treatment

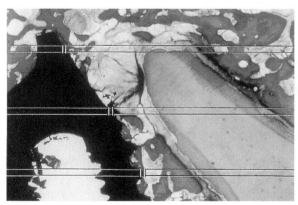

FIGURE 3.—Photomicrograph demonstrating the histologic appearance of an implant in direct contact with the periapical lesion of an adjacent tooth. Histomorphometric analysis of bone apposition around the implant was performed at the apical 2 mm of the implant-tooth interface by using computer-assisted lineal analysis, as denoted with the *white lines*. (Reprinted by permission of the publisher from Shabahang S, Bohsali K, Boyne PJ, et al: Effect of teeth with periradicular lesions on adjacent dental implants. *Oral Surg Oral Med Oral Pathol Oral Radiol Endod* 96:321-326, 2003. Copyright 2003 by Elsevier.)

of the tooth. Block sections were prepared after 7.5 months, and the percentage of osseointegration was assessed.

Results.—The average integration was 54% for group A, 74% for group B, 56% for group C, and 68% for group D (Fig 3). One-way analysis of variance showed no differences among the 4 groups.

Conclusion.—Teeth with periradicular lesions have no adverse effect on adjacent titanium solid root-form implants.

▶ It appears in reading this article that there is considerable disagreement regarding the effect and treatment of periradicular lesions adjacent to dental implants. However, it would seem logical that in a closed system—ie, no oral connection to the periradicular lesion—the lesion would heal following treatment without any lasting detrimental effect on the implant.

A puzzling situation here is that even group D, the group where lesions were induced but not treated, did not show detrimental effects on osseointegration. However, if the study had been run sufficiently long that the periapical lesion continued to remain active and to expand, the outcome may have been different. Clearly, this study is a good start but is not definitive in itself, as the authors acknowledge. But the results are encouraging, and certainly merit further study. Given the popularity of dental implants today, the topic addressed by these authors is an important one.

K. L. Zakariasen, DDS, MS, MS(ODA), PhD

Diabetes Mellitus and the Dental Pulp
Bender IB, Bender AB (Dr I B Bender Academy House, Philadelphia)
J Endodont 29:383-389, 2003   5–20

Background.—In diabetes mellitus (DM), impaired secretion or function of insulin causes glycemic levels to rise and creates a generalized circulatory disorder so that the blood supply may be inadequate. This effect plus the increased level of blood glucose at an injury site puts the diabetic patient at risk for more serious infections, including those of the oral cavity. In type 1 DM, insulin formation is absent, whereas in type 2 DM, insulin resistance is present, so that the insulin produced cannot be used effectively.

Oral Problems Associated With Diabetes.—When their disease is uncontrolled, oral infections can develop in type 1 diabetic patients more easily and can become more severe than those in type 2 diabetic patients, although age, duration of DM, and degree of metabolic control can be contributing factors. Oral complaints include xerostomia with enlarged parotid glands and decreased salivary flow rate, altered taste sensations, increased caries development, and periodontal disease. Small blood vessel changes occur in the gingiva of patients with diabetes and produce thickened vessel walls and narrowed lumens. Periapical lesions are more prevalent among type 1 diabetic patients, along with a high rate of asymptomatic tooth infections.

Case Report.—Woman, 32, reported mild, constant, gnawing toothache bilaterally. Her medical history was unrevealing, and her oral and radiographic evaluation showed minimal caries, several shallow fillings, and a few small periapical lesions. Her condition remained undiagnosed until 6 weeks later, when she had unilateral pain, and her physician reported that she had a high blood sugar that required insulin therapy. Seven teeth that had not responded to the initial pulp testing demonstrated periapical radiolucencies. The patient was diagnosed with previously undetected DM, for which endodontic treatment proved successful.

Conclusions.—Diabetic states are linked to higher susceptibility to inflammatory reactions; increased local inflammation can intensify the diabetes and potentially allow the diabetic state to become uncontrolled. Thus, infection of the dental pulp should be removed, thereby preventing future episodes. Pain may be present, referred to as dental odontalgia, even when there is no pulp response during pulp testing, and the teeth are noncarious. Evidence of bacterial leakage may also be lacking. Histologic evaluation can reveal diabetic circulatory impairment characteristic of uncontrolled DM conditions. When DM is controlled, healing of periapical lesions is normal.

▶ This is a very good review article on diabetes and its effects on the dental pulp and other oral tissues. With an aging population and an increasing life span, increasing numbers of patients who exhibit various chronic diseases and complex pharmacologic regimens will be seen by practitioners. Diabetes is certainly one of those long-term chronic diseases that compromises a patient's health and about which dental practitioners must be knowledgeable. This article will be very helpful to practitioners in that regard. As we focus on evidence-based dentistry, it would be very helpful to have these types of clearly written articles available on a host of chronic diseases that can complicate oral diseases and the delivery of dental care.

K. L. Zakariasen, DDS, MS, MS(ODA), PhD

Reliability of the Dye Penetration Studies

Camps J, Pashley D (Faculté d'Odontologie, Marseille, France; Med College of Georgia, Augusta)
J Endodont 29:592-594, 2003   5–21

Background.—It is not possible to completely eliminate bacteria in the root canal by any technique; thus, some bacteria are entrapped in dentinal tubules. Infection or reinfection of the periapical zone by these bacteria can be prevented by a hermetic apical seal. Numerous studies have addressed evaluation of the sealing efficiency of a variety of filling techniques or endodontic sealers. Recently, the filtration technique was introduced in endodontics. However, the dye penetration technique has remained the most commonly used technique for evaluation of the sealing efficiency of endodon-

TABLE 1.—Evaluation of the Apical Leakage of 4 Endodontic Sealers by 3 Methods

	Filtration Technique $(L\,s^{-1}\,Kpa^{-1})$ ANOVA $(p < 0.01)$	Dye Penetration (mm) ANOVA (NS)	Dye Extraction (Absorbance) ANOVA $(p < 0.01)$
Pulp Canal sealer	$0.17 \pm 0.09\ 10^{-11}\ L\,s^{-1}\,Kpa^{-1}$ [a]	2.2 ± 1.4 mm	268 ± 235 [a]
Sealapex	$8.42 \pm 4.2\ 10^{-11}\ L\,s^{-1}\,Kpa^{-1}$ [b]	2.1 ± 2.4 mm	567 ± 257 [b]
AH Plus	$2.10 \pm 1.39\ 10^{-11}\ L\,s^{-1}\,Kpa^{-1}$ [a]	1.8 ± 0.8 mm	376 ± 120 [a]
Ketac-Endo	$0.32 \pm 0.24\ 10^{-11}\ L\,s^{-1}\,Kpa^{-1}$ [a]	3.6 ± 2.3 mm	316 ± 168 [a]

The groups identified with the same superscript letter were not statistically significant.
Abbreviations: NS, Not significant; ANOVA, analysis of variance.
(Courtesy of Camps J, Pashley D: Reliability of the dye penetration studies. *J Endodont* 29[9]:592-594, 2003.)

tic sealers. The classic dye penetration method was compared with novel dye extraction technique, using a fluid-filtration method as a control.

Methods.—Forty teeth were prepared with a ProFile device and then divided into 4 groups according to the sealer (Pulp Canal Sealer, Sealapex, AH Plus, and Ketac-Endo) used for the lateral condensation. The apical seal was evaluated on the same teeth with all 3 methods in succession: a fluid-filtration method, a dye penetration method with 2% methylene blue, and a new method in which the roots were dissolved in 65% nitric acid so that methylene blue could be extracted before reading of the absorbance of the solution.

Results.—No difference among the sealers was demonstrated with the classical dye penetration technique, and there were no correlations among the classical technique and the other 2 techniques. The fluid filtration and dye extraction techniques showed that Sealapex had the highest apical leakage. There was a significant degree of correlation between the results of the fluid filtration and dye extraction techniques (Table 1).

Conclusion.—The limitations of the classic dye penetration studies were manifest in this study, which also showed that the dye extraction method provided the same results as fluid filtration, but in much less laboratory time.

▶ In my comments for some of the previous endodontic articles, I discussed the importance of sealing the root canal from fluid exchange between the root canal space and the periapical tissues and, of course, also from the oral environment. Many different methods have been utilized to measure root canal leakage. This research compares 3 different techniques for measuring root canal leakage and illustrates one of the problems with in vitro research and generalizing the results to the real clinical situation. The traditional dye penetration method indicated no differences among 4 different sealers, while the 2 fluid volume–oriented studies indicated, with agreement, that 1 of the sealers was less effective than the other 3.

Of course, as I have discussed previously, we still don't know from such research how much leakage is clinically significant. As we continually move toward more evidence-based practice, we will require increasingly sophisticated research, as seen with these volume-oriented leakage study methods, upon which to draw more valid conclusions. However, the real "acid test" will always be well controlled clinical trials.

As a final note, I would like to point out that my colleague and I published 2 research abstracts on a dye extraction method for measuring root canal leakage in 1981.[1] I certainly agree with these authors regarding the advantages of the dye extraction method.

K. L. Zakariasen, DDS, MS, MS(ODA), PhD

Reference

1. Program and Abstracts of Papers. *J Dent Res* 60(special issue A). March 1981.

6 Implant Surgery

Introduction

This year's chapter on Implant Surgery presents a potpourri of topics relating to specific clinical issues ranging from ways to make the implant delivery protocol more efficient to histomorphometric analysis of the effect of location of the microgap on the adjacent tissue. While implant therapy has an overall success rate that is impressive, we must remember that in most studies success is defined by the implant remaining in function with minimal morbidity. In recent years, we have seen our patients increase their esthetic demands, and this forces us as a profession to learn more and more about what it takes to have an inflammation-free implant in the correct position, and then to monitor the health of that implant so that inflammation, bone resorption, and the subsequent recession can be held at bay. It also motivates us to keep up with exciting new areas of potential, such as laser-decontamination of diseased implant surfaces. This diverse selection of articles is intended to help the reader stay abreast of some new knowledge in these areas that has presented in the last year.

Douglas N. Dederich, DDS, MSc, PhD

Effects of Implant Healing Time on Crestal Bone Loss of a Controlled-load Dental Implant
Ko CC, Douglas WH, DeLong R, et al (Univ of Minnesota, Minneapolis; Mayo Clinic, Rochester, Minn; Mayo Med School, Rochester, Minn)
J Dent Res 82:585-591, 2003   6–1

Introduction.—The universally accepted concept of strategic early loaded dental implants is presently under debate. An intraoral hydraulic device was used to control in vivo load and healing quantitatively in 17 pigs to determine whether an early application of a mechanical stimulus (reduced implant-healing time) leads to increased bone formation.

Methods.—Mini-pigs were placed in either an experimental or an internal or external control group. Each group was separated into subgroups for nonloaded implant-healing times of 1, 2, or 4 months (Fig 1). The right and left fourth premolars were extracted from each animal. Dental implants were placed in the healed extraction sites 2 months later. The timing of the extraction was dependent on group assignment. Radiographic and histo-

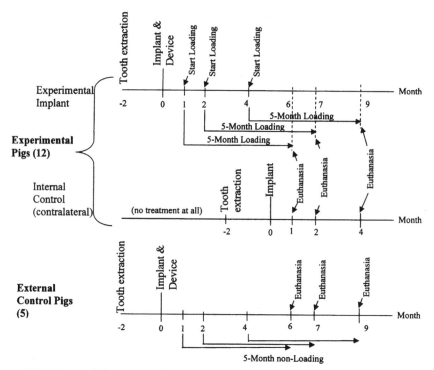

FIGURE 1.—Study design: surgical schedules, healing, and loading times of the implants. The experimental group included 12 pigs; for each pig, 1 implant was used as the experimental implant, and the implant in the contralateral side was used as an internal control. The experimental animals were divided into 3 equal subgroups with 1-, 2-, and 4-month implant healing periods. The daily load was applied for 5 months for all experimental implants. For the internal control on the contralateral side, the implant was allowed to heal for 1, 2, or 4 months, the same as the experimental implant in the same pig. Since both the internal control and experimental implants were recovered at the same time, control implants were placed at appropriate times before the animal's death. Five animals with 2 bilateral implants were used as external controls to provide a baseline of bone loss. These were also divided into 3 groups with the same healing periods as the experimental implants. The external control implants stayed in the jaw for the appropriate healing period plus an additional 5 months with no loading. (Courtesy of Ko CC, Douglas WH, DeLong R, et al: Effects of implant healing time on crestal bone loss of a controlled-load dental implant. *J Dent Res* 82:585-591, 2003.)

logic evaluations were made of the osseointegrated bone changes for 3 healing times (between implant insertion and loading) after 5 months of loading.

Results.—The effect of loading on crestal bone loss was dependent on healing time. Delayed loading was linked with significantly more crestal bone loss versus that of nonload control subjects (2.4 mm vs 0.64 mm; $P < .05$) (Fig 2).

Conclusion.—Histologic evaluation and biomechanical analyses of the healing bone indicate that loading and bioactivities of osteoblasts exert a synergistic effect on osseointegration, supporting the theory that early loading provides more favorable osseointegration.

▶ There has been a debate for some time now regarding the advantages and disadvantages of early loading. This in vivo pig study looks at very low level

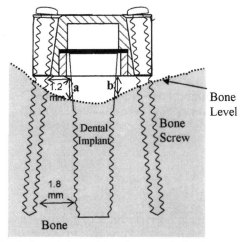

A. Schematics of implant and device

	Healing Time (mo.)	CBL (mm)	n
Experiment	1	0.84±0.54	8
(Load)	2	1.20±0.66	8
	4	2.40±0.53*	6
Control	1	0.72±0.15	4
(Non-load)	2	0.58±0.12	2
	4	0.64±0.30*	6

B. Averaged crestal bone loss

FIGURE 2.—(A), Diagram for measurements showing mesial-distal cross-section of the implant-bone and hydraulic device. Two crestal bone loss measurements per implant (*a* and *b*, in mm) were taken along the implant surface from the subtracted radiographic images. (B), Averaged crestal bone loss for experimental and external control groups. The symbol *n* represents number of measurements obtained, 2 from each implant. The data (*CBL*, in mm) were averaged for the 3 healing-time subgroups. The loading effect on crestal bone loss significantly depends on healing time (loading-by-month interaction, $P = .03$), increasing as time proceeds. *Asterisk* indicates a significant difference between the experimental and the control groups. (Courtesy of Ko CC, Douglas WH, DeLong R, et al: Effects of implant healing time on crestal bone loss of a controlled-load dental implant. *J Dent Res* 82:585-591, 2003.)

forces (6.5N and 1 Hz) applied axially with an ingenious intraoral hydraulic device for 10 minutes a day for up to 4 months. The authors noticed that at 1 month, the bone density was greater than at the start, while at 2 and 4 months it was less. The authors also noted that delayed loading (positive controls) resulted in twice the crestal bone loss. This might suggest that light loading for short periods after placement may result in less loss of the alveolar ridge, but that you don't want to load it for more than 1 month at these light levels.

The primary intent of this study was to test the hypothesis that an early application of a mechanical stimulus (ie, a decreased implant-healing time) leads to increased bone formation. The answer is that it does, at least initially, in pigs, which heal slightly faster than humans. The time-dependency of the bone loss also offers insight into what mechanisms may be in play. It is important to remember that the forces used here were very small, so this study does not really address the situation where excessive forces are present.

D. N. Dederich, DDS, MSc, PhD

Masticatory Function and Patient Satisfaction With Implant-Supported Mandibular Overdentures: A Prospective 5-Year Study
Bakke M, Holm B, Gotfredsen K (Univ of Copenhagen)
Int J Prosthodont 15:575-581, 2002   6–2

Introduction.—Good long-term outcomes with implant-supported mandibular overdenture (ISO) treatment have been reported, even in patients with severely resorbed mandibular ridges. Outcome has been described primarily in terms of implant survival rates and durability of implant superstructures. The outcome of treatment with ISO with 2 implants was examined in a longitudinal, prospective, controlled clinical trial to determine (1) patient satisfaction with the ability to chew and bite and (2) chewing efficiency, bite force, and electromyographic (EMG) recordings.

Methods.—Twelve edentulous patients who had worn dentures for a minimum of 5 years were evaluated. All patients were in good health. They had retention problems with their mandibular dentures. The mean participant age was 63 years. Before placement of implants, the conditions for complete dentures were optimized by using prosthetic surgery. Three months after fabrication of new dentures, 2 Astra Tech implants were placed in the anterior portion of the mandible (right and left canine regions). Abutments were connected 6 months later. Patient satisfaction was determined by questionnaire. Functional recordings of chewing ability, bite force, and EMG activity were performed at the time of placement of the new dentures and at 3 months, 1 year, and 5 years after overdenture treatment.

Results.—No implants were lost at 5-year follow-up. All patients required a minimum of 1 small correction or repair of the mandibular overdenture. The maxillary denture needed to be relined or remade in 7 patients. All patients reported improved ability to chew and bite after ISO. Only 5 patients reported that they were entirely satisfied with their denture function after ISO in all recording series. The 7 patients not fully satisfied with the function of the ISO had lower muscle activity, even before implant placement, compared to patients who reported satisfaction. Patients were able to chew hard and tough food.

The chewing inefficiency index was significantly decreased at 1 year. The type and texture of food significantly influenced muscle activity. Generally, the harder the food item, the shorter the chewing cycle and the higher the EMG amplitude.

Conclusion.—Implant-supported mandibular overdenture treatment provides better biting and chewing function, compared to conventional complete dentures.

▶ ISOs have become exceedingly popular because they offer a vast improvement in function and stability for our patients with complete lower dentures. While this is most probably clinically obvious to anyone who has utilized this modality, it is nevertheless reassuring to know that the clinical data also support this therapy. This simple but relevant clinical study does just that, looking at both function and patient satisfaction.

D. N. Dederich, DDS, MSc, PhD

Temperature Changes at the Implant-Bone Interface During Simulated Surface Decontamination With an Er:YAG Laser

Kreisler M, Haj HA, d'Hoedt B (Johannes Gutenberg-Univ Mainz, Germany)
Int J Prosthodont 15:582-587, 2002   6–3

Introduction.—Most titanium implants have a rough surface to enhance implant-bone contact and anchorage force in the alveolar bone. The surface roughness makes elimination of bacteria from implants challenging. Sterilization and cleaning of implants using lasers has been suggested. Yet some lasers are not suitable for decontamination of implant surfaces since they can also damage the surfaces. Temperature elevations were examined at the implant-bone interface during simulated surface decontamination with a 2940-nm Er:YAG laser.

Methods.—Stepped cylinder implants with 3 different surfaces (titanium plasma–sprayed, sandblasted and acid etched, and hydroxyapatite-coated) were positioned in bone blocks excised from freshly resected pig femurs. An artificial peri-implant bone defect (size, 6 mm²) allowed access for laser irra-

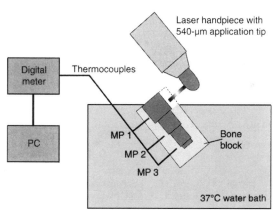

FIGURE 1.—Bone block is placed in a 37°C water bath. The optic fiber is positioned perpendicular to the implant surface at a distance of 0.5 mm. Thermocouples connected to a digital meter are positioned at 3 measuring points (*MP*) at the implant (*MP 1* is directly opposite the spot of irradiation at 3 mm below the artificial alveolar crest; *MP 2* is the most inferior part of the second cylinder step; and *MP 3* is the most inferior part of the third cylinder step). (Courtesy of Kreisler M, Haj HA, d'Hoedt B: Temperature changes at the implant-bone interface during simulated surface decontamination with an Er:YAG laser. *Int J Prosthodont* 15:582-587, 2002.)

diation in the coronal third of the implant. A 540-μm peri-implantitis application tip was used at 0.5 mm from the implant surface.

The pulse energy varied between 60 and 120 mJ at 10 pps. The bone block was submerged into a 37°C water bath to simulate in vivo thermal conductivity and diffusivity of heat (Fig 1). Temperature changes were registered at 3 levels of the peri-implant bone via K-type thermocouples connected to a digital meter.

Results.—The temperature at the implant-bone interface did not surpass 47°C after 120 seconds of continuing laser irradiation. Temperature elevations were significantly higher with the hydroxyapatite-coated implants, compared to the 2 titanium surface groups ($P < .001$).

Conclusion.—Decontamination of implant surface using the Er:YAG laser did not excessively heat the peri-implant bone in the energy range used in this series. This approach appeared to be clinically safe with the surfaces studied.

▶ Too often, when new devices are introduced into our profession, having been cleared or approved by the US Food and Drug Administration for specific applications, the technology is used outside the indications for other creative purposes that do not yet enjoy adequate scientific support. Some of these novel uses eventually gain the data to validate their use, and some fall by the wayside. While it is our hope that both cause no harm to the patient, we all know that, unfortunately, that hope is not always fulfilled.

One example of an apparently successful innovation is illustrated by this article. The Er:YAG laser came into dentistry with some fanfare as a novel way to remove enamel and dentin. It had the advantage of being very kind to the dental pulp due to its wavelength of light being highly absorbed on the surface of the target material. It became known that this laser could also detoxify surfaces, and this led to the use of this laser in the detoxification of ailing implants during surgery.

One question that needed answering, however, was whether the energy that was deposited on the contaminated implant surface would heat the implant to any clinically significant degree, placing the peri-implant tissues at risk. This in vitro study creates a thermal model and then, using this model, generates temperature data which suggest that the thermal risk to the peri-implant tissues is very low. This positive result paves the way to test this hypothesis in an in vivo model.

D. N. Dederich, DDS, MSc, PhD

Treatment Planning for Success: Wise Choices for Maxillary Single-Tooth Implants

Gregory-Head BL, McDonald A, Labarre E (Univ of the Pacific, Calif)
Calif Dent Assoc J 29:766-771, 2001   6–4

Introduction.—When a patient is intent on having a missing anterior tooth replaced with an implant, there is an expectation for something that looks good, feels good, and works like a real tooth. It is challenging to fulfill these treatment goals. The patient may consider treatment a failure if any of these criteria cannot be satisfied. The esthetic limitations of dental implant treatment were discussed.

Limitations of Implants.—Nine issues must be addressed to determine whether a patient is likely to experience an esthetically successful outcome.

Assessment of Patient Expectations.—Unreasonable demands from the patient and unrealistic promises by the practitioner can lead to an unsatisfactory experience for all involved. It is crucial that the patient be involved and educated concerning risks, esthetic or otherwise, that might occur, along with the need for rigorous dental hygiene.

Assessment of Gingival Display.—The patient's ability to display gingiva is paramount. The most important element in esthetic success is the anterior smile line. It is strongly recommended that the first few patients treated in a practice have a lower lip line.

Gingival Thickness.—An ideal first implant for a dentist would have an abundance of thick, flat, fibrous gingival tissue and thus be resistant to gingival recession around the restoration.

Papillary Presence or Absence.—The greater the distance from the free gingival margin to the osseous crest, the higher the esthetic risk. An esthetic risk would be a sounding depth of over 3 mm at the midface aspect or 4 mm at the interproximal position.

Morphology of Adjacent Teeth (Crown-to-Root Ratio).—If the apical limit of the contact area is 5 mm or less from the osseous crest, a papilla will be present nearly 100% of the time in the natural dentition. An additional 1-mm distance diminishes the likelihood of a papilla being present to 56%. The position of the osseous crest may be challenging to adjust, but the restorative dentist may change the position of the contact areas.

Available Bone Height.—The ideal patient would have sufficient bone height to house a long implant (13 mm or more) with the crest of the residual ridge 2 mm below the cementoenamel junction of the adjacent teeth.

Available Bone Width.—A minimum of 1.5 mm of healthy bone is needed between the implant and neighboring root surfaces. The standard implant is about 4 mm in diameter. The smallest mesiodistal space that can accommodate an implant between 2 teeth is 7 mm.

Determining Available Bone.—Evaluating available bone in the mesiodistal and buccolingual dimensions can be accomplished by thorough clinical evaluation or measuring directly from casts. The CT scan is the most accurate diagnostic tool.

Conclusion.—When the 9 factors to consider for single-tooth implants are carefully evaluated, patients with significant esthetic risks will be screened out and those with predictably good prognoses will be chosen.

▶ A very common application of dental implants is for single-tooth replacement in the esthetic zone, ie, the maxillary anterior area. With increasing use in this area, our patients are becoming much more aware of the benefits that implants have to offer and are escalating their esthetic demands even further. This article is a good place for those who wish to embark on restoring anterior implants to begin. It addresses many of the most pertinent issues in a short and digestible form.

D. N. Dederich, DDS, MSc, PhD

The Use of Small Titanium Screws for Orthodontic Anchorage
Deguchi T, Takano-Yamamoto T, Kanomi R, et al (Okayama Univ, Japan; Kanomi Dental Clinic, Japan; Indiana Univ, Indianapolis; et al)
J Dent Res 82:377-381, 2003   6–5

Introduction.—Anchorage control is essential to the success of orthodontic treatment. The potential advantage of a miniature implant is that it increases the number of sites where anchorage implants can be placed. The bone healing reaction and response to applied load for the miniature implants were examined in canines.

Methods.—Ninety-six small titanium screws (5.0 mm × 1.0 mm) were equally placed in 8 eight-month-old male dogs. Within each jaw, both force-applied and healing control implants were further separated into 3 groups (3-, 6-, and 12-week). There were 8 implants per group. The healing control implants were placed in the jaw for 3, 6, or 12 weeks before the experiment ended so that bone could be evaluated at the initiation of loading.

A force of 200 to 300 g was applied for 12 weeks with the use of an elastomeric chain attached from the implant to a hook on the crowns of the premolars. The force was evaluated and adjusted every 4 weeks with a force gauge to maintain the 200- to 300-g range. Histomorphometric analysis was performed for all teeth to determine the effects of healing and application of force on the histomorphometric indexes of the maxilla and mandible.

Results.—Successful rigid osseous fixation was observed in 97% of the 96 implants placed in the 8 dogs and 100% of the elastomere chain-loaded implants. All of the loading implants stayed integrated. Mandibular implants had significantly higher bone-implant contact, compared with maxillary implants. Within each arch, the significant histomorphometric indexes seen in the "3-week unloaded" healing group were increased labeling rate, higher woven-to-lamellar-bone ratio, and increased osseous contact.

Conclusion.—Titanium screws were able to function as rigid osseous anchorage against orthodontic load for 3 months with a minimal (under 3 weeks) healing period in young canine jaws.

▶ This article furthers our knowledge of an innovative use of dental implants, that of using small titanium implants to provide orthodontic anchorage. Traditional implants used to replace teeth are often too large to be practical in this application, so the authors have focused their attention on small titanium screws and attachment plates to provide this capability. This dog study provides a histologic assessment of the integration of these small screw implants after having various times to heal subsequent to placement and then also functioning for 3 months.

The results were very encouraging: a 97% success rate when they were allowed to heal for only 3 weeks. It is important to keep in mind, however, that orthodontic therapy usually lasts much longer than 3 months and that humans heal slower than dogs.

D. N. Dederich, DDS, MSc, PhD

Role of the Microgap Between Implant and Abutment: A Retrospective Histologic Evaluation in Monkeys
Piattelli A, Vrespa G, Petrone G, et al (Univ of Chieti, Italy; Univ of Milano, Italy; Univ of Rome "La Sapienza")
J Periodontol 74:346-352, 2003   6–6

Introduction.—Most trials have focused on bone reactions to bone implants. Little attention has been directed to the dimensions and relationships of the soft tissues around implants. It has been suggested that a certain width of the peri-implant mucosa is needed to enable an adequate epithelial–connective tissue attachment; otherwise bone resorption will occur to ensure the establishment of attachment with an appropriate biological width. The reason for the accelerated bone loss around submerged 2-piece implants in the first year after restoration has not been determined. It may be that the gap between the components has a role in this process.

Recent trials have indicated that for all 2-part implants, the bone crest level changes seem to be dependent on the location of the microgap. A retrospective histological evaluation of the bone response to implants inserted 1 to 2 mm above the alveolar crest (group 1; 15 implants), at the level alveolar crest (group 2; 12 implants), or 1 to 1.5 mm below the alveolar crest (group 3; 13 implants) was performed.

Methods.—The bone response to early loaded implants, immediately loaded implants, and implants inserted immediately postextraction was evaluated. One hundred eight implants inserted, retrieved, and histologically examined in 10 monkeys from 3 trials were compared with those of the implants in the current trial.

Results.—A mean 0.13-mm increase, a mean 2.1-mm vertical bone loss, and a mean 3.6-mm vertical bone loss extending in an apical direction were identified in groups 1, 2, and 3, respectively. Statistically significant differences were seen among all 3 groups.

Conclusion.—These data support earlier findings that if the microgap is moved coronally away from the alveolar crest, less bone loss will occur and if the microgap is moved apically to the alveolar crest, greater amounts of bone resorption will occur. The observed remodeling was not dependent on early or immediate loading of the implants or on immediate postextraction insertion.

▶ One decision that faces every implant surgeon in every 2-stage implant placement surgery is that of where to place the implant in the vertical dimension. Several considerations go into this decision, one of which is the long-term effect on the peri-implant tissues. The idea here is that the microgap that exists between the implant table and the abutment provides space for microorganisms to collect and create an inflammatory response, and the vertical location of this gap influences the amount of bone loss down the road.

This was an in vivo study done in monkeys, which provided the opportunity for histologic analysis. The results suggested that the closer the microgap is to the bone crest the greater the amount of subsequent bone loss will be. Contrarily, when the microgap was positioned 1 to 2 mm coronal to the bone level, there was no bone loss, and in some cases there was actually a slight increase in bone height. This corroborates several other studies and much of our own anecdotal clinical experience. If you choose to use a 2-stage implant system, periodontal health appears to be generally better if you can position the microgap at or near the gingival margin, at least on the lingual in cases where esthetic demands require placement within the sulcus on the facial.

D. N. Dederich, DDS, MSc, PhD

Persistent Acute Inflammation at the Implant-Abutment Interface
Broggini N, McManus LM, Hermann JS, et al (Univ of Texas, San Antonio; Univ of Zürich, Switzerland; Univ of Bern, Switzerland; et al)
J Dent Res 82:232-237, 2003   6–7

Introduction.—The inflammatory response adjacent to implants has not been well examined and may influence peri-implant tissue levels. How changes in abutment connection timing (submerged vs nonsubmerged 2-piece implants) or the presence of a microgap (2-piece, nonsubmerged implants vs 1-piece, nonsubmerged implants) influences the composition of inflammatory cells immediately adjacent to the implant was evaluated in dog mandibles.

Methods.—The 3 implant designs were placed in the edentulous mandibular regions of 5 foxhound dogs. Every implant type was included in duplicate in each animal, with random placement in both the left and right mandibles. Abutment connection was done at the time of initial surgery for the 2-piece, nonsubmerged implants and at 3 months after initial placement for the 2-piece, submerged implants.

At 4, 8, and 10 weeks after second-stage surgery of submerged implants, abutments were loosened, then immediately tightened in all of the 2-piece implants to imitate clinical restorative methods. The remaining implant was 1-piece. At 6 months after initial placement, tissues were prepared and histologic and histomorphometric analyses were performed.

Results.—Both of the 2-piece implants had a peak of inflammatory cells about 0.50 mm coronal to the microgap that consisted primarily of neutrophilic polymorphonuclear leukocytes. No such peak was seen with the 1-piece implants. Significantly greater bone loss was seen in both 2-piece implants, compared to the 1-piece implant.

Conclusion.—The absence of an implant-abutment interface (microgap) at the bone crest was linked to decreased peri-implant inflammatory cell accumulation and minimal bone loss.

▶ The previous study by Piattelli et al (Abstract 6–6) looked at the position of the microgap and its histologic effect on the tissue. This study histomorphometrically compares a microgap at the osseous crest with no microgap in a 1-stage implant system. It appears that the absence of the microgap in 1-stage systems is associated with substantially less inflammation and bone loss than the 2-stage systems with a microgap. This result is not surprising and supports the hypothesis that the microorganisms harbored in the gap have a potentially negative effect on the adjacent soft tissues.

While this inflammation may not directly affect the overall success/failure rate of the implant, it does have clinical importance in that it can cause recession and crestal bone loss in addition to edematous-looking tissue. These results also argue in favor of using 1-stage systems for posterior applications where esthetics is not as great a concern.

D. N. Dederich, DDS, MSc, PhD

Some Soft Tissue Characteristics at Implant Abutments With Different Surface Topography: A Study in Humans
Wennerberg A, Sennerby L, Kultje C, et al (Göteborg Univ, Sweden; MediTeam Dentalutveckling AB, Sävedalen, Sweden)
J Clin Periodontol 30:88-94, 2003   6–8

Introduction.—When an implant with a rough surface is exposed to the oral cavity, it may accumulate higher amounts of plaque, compared to a smooth surface. This can lead to severe problems with mucositis and peri-implantitis. The early inflammatory response to mucosa-penetrating abutments prepared with varying surface roughness was examined in abutments created with topographies similar to commercially available fixtures.

Methods.—Nine patients willing to participate had all 5 of their original abutments exchanged to evaluate titanium test abutments for a 4-week period. The test abutments were prepared with 5 different degrees of roughness. The surface roughness was determined with the use of an optical profilometer.

At completion of the test period, the test abutments were examined. The health of the surrounding mucosa, the amount of accumulated plaque, and marginal bleeding were documented. One biopsy specimen was obtained from each test abutment. Qualitative and quantitative histologic assessments were conducted.

Results.—There was a statistically significant difference between patients concerning the amount of accumulated plaque on the abutment surfaces and inflammatory cells. The morphology of the abutment contact zone varied greatly between specimens. The histologic appearance was similar among the 5 different titanium surface modifications. The thickness and appearance of the epithelium ranged from a relatively thick one with retepegs to a thin structure more like contact epithelium with a diminishing number of cell layers in the apical direction. There was no difference between the surface modifications in relation to plaque accumulation or number of inflammatory cells.

Conclusion.—There was no relationship between inflammatory response and abutment surface roughness after an evaluation period of 4 weeks in a human test model.

▶ This was a 1-month human clinical study that looked at the relationship between the roughness of implant surfaces and the degree of inflammatory soft tissue response in adjacent soft tissues. The authors' initial expectation was that the rougher surfaces would collect more plaque and elicit more inflammation. As commonly occurs in research, however, their expectations were not supported. They found no relation between surface roughness and inflammation either histologically or clinically.

While this result may seem surprising, it should be mentioned that the study was done on 10 patients with no natural teeth. All had multi-implant–supported prostheses. We know that the microbiology of the edentulous patient is typically different than that of those with natural teeth remaining. It is a reasonable hypothesis to suggest that these results may have been different had patients with natural teeth been the subjects of this investigation.

D. N. Dederich, DDS, MSc, PhD

Immediate Functional and Non-functional Loading of Dental Implants: A 2- to 60-Month Follow-up Study of 646 Titanium Implants
Degidi M, Piattelli A (Univ of Chieti, Italy)
J Periodontol 74:225-241, 2003   6–9

Introduction.—A healing time of about 4 to 6 months without loading is needed to obtain mineralized bone tissue at the dental implant interface. These time periods have been set up empirically and have never been confirmed experimentally. A large number of implants subjected to immediate functional loading (IFL) and to immediate nonfunctioning loading (INFL) (Table 1) in various anatomical configurations were evaluated clinically.

Methods.—One hundred fifty-two patients underwent placement of 646 implants inserted into 39 totally edentulous mandibles, 14 edentulous maxillae, 23 edentulous posterior mandibles, 16 edentulous anterior maxillae, and 15 edentulous posterior maxillae. Of these, 58 implants were used to replace single missing teeth. In 65 cases, IFL was performed for 422 implants and INFL was performed in 116 cases (224 implants).

Results.—Six of the 422 (1.4%) implants in the IFL group failed and 2 of the 224 (0.9%) implants in the INFL group failed (Tables 2 and 3). From clinical and radiographic observations, all other implants seemed to have successfully osseointegrated and were functioning satisfactorily from the

TABLE 1.—Loading Mode Definitions

Loading Mode	Definition
Submerged	Flush with bone level, covered by the gingiva
Nonsubmerged	Nonsubmerged, flush or within 1 to 2 mm of gingival level
Immediate functional loading	Temporaries same day of the surgery; in occlusion
Immediate non-functional loading	Temporaries same day of the surgery; not in occlusion
Early loading	Final crowns within 3 weeks from surgery; in occlusion
Anticipated loading	Temporaries within 8 to 10 weeks from surgery

(Courtesy of Degidi M, Piattelli A: Immediate functional and non-functional loading of dental implants: A 2- to 60-month follow-up study of 646 titanium implants. *J Periodontol* 74:225-241, 2003.)

TABLE 2.—Immediate Functional Loading Implants

Implant	N Implants	N Failures	% Implant Survival	% Prostheses Survival
Frialit 2*	82	6	94.7	93.7
IMZ*	44	0	100	100
Frialoc*	37	0	100	100
Brånemark†	63	0	100	100
Restore‡	70	0	100	100
Maestro§	126	0	100	100
Total	422	6	98.6	98.5

*Friadent, Mannheim, Germany.
†Nobel Biocare, Göteborg, Sweden.
‡ LifeCore Biomedical, Chaska, Minn.
§Biohorizons, Birmingham, Ala.
(Courtesy of Degidi M, Piattelli A: Immediate functional and non-functional loading of dental implants: A 2- to 60-month follow-up study of 646 titanium implants. *J Periodontol* 74:225-241, 2003.)

TABLE 3.—Immediate Nonfunctional Loading Implants

Implant	N Implants	N Failures	% Implant Survival	% Prostheses Survival
Frialit 2*	62	2	96.6	95
IMZ*	7	0	100	100
Restore†	27	0	100	100
Maestro‡	116	0	100	100
Brånemark§	10	0	100	100
3 I‖	2	0	100	100
Total	224	2	99.1	98.3

*Friadent, Mannheim, Germany.
†LifeCore, Biomedical, Chaska, Minn.
‡Biohorizons, Birmingham, Ala.
§Nobel Biocare, Göteborg, Sweden.
‖Implant Innovations, Inc, West Palm Beach, Fla.
(Courtesy of Degidi M, Piattelli A: Immediate functional and non-functional loading of dental implants: A 2- to 60-month follow-up study of 646 titanium implants. *J Periodontol* 74:225-241, 2003.)

time of insertion. All failures occurred in the first few months after implant loading.

Conclusion.—IFL and INFL appear to be a technique that provides satisfactory results in selected cases.

▶ Many of the protocols we use in dentistry are based on historic experience that can, in some cases, date back to a time when the technology we were using was not nearly as advanced as it is today. This makes it necessary to periodically reassess our paradigms in light of new developments.

This is exactly what this article does. It looks at the 4- to 6-month healing criteria that so many of us use and asks whether immediately loaded implants are a viable option. The authors make an important distinction between implants restored and placed in occlusion at the time of surgery and those restored at the time of surgery kept out of occlusion. The success rate demonstrated by this study was very high and similar to other reports from longer healing times, and the failures—when they did occur—seemed to occur within the first few months after placement and loading. The final message is that IFL and INFL may provide satisfactory results in selected cases.

While these results are not corroborated by some of the other published work in this area, the authors do a good job in their discussion of the opposing views. This article does not by itself settle this issue of whether and when immediate loading is appropriate, but it does a service to us all by the analysis that it offers.

D. N. Dederich, DDS, MSc, PhD

Periimplant Probing: Positives and Negatives
Atassi F (Univ King Saud, Riyadh, Saudi Arabia)
Implant Dent 11:356-362, 2002   6–10

Introduction.—Periodontium in normal dentition is different from the periodontium surrounding an implant area. Peri-implant probing cannot be performed the same way as periodontal probing in normal dentition due to inherent anatomical differences. The issues concerning peri-implant probing were reviewed to develop a peri-implant probing protocol.

Peri-Implant Probing.—Data should be documented within the first week after the suprastructure has been seated, every 3 months for 1 year, then every 6 months thereafter. This timing allows evaluation of the stability of the supracrestal connective tissue over time. It is not as good an indicator as clinical attachment level measurements. Clinicians should not be concerned about absolute measurements; rather, they should focus on progressive attachment level assessment. Various probing depth values may be considered as normal in different implant systems. The probing depth may not be meaningful unless these points are considered:

• There needs to be a consistent and repeatable reference point on the implant or its suprastructure. For every probing, the same reference should be used.

- Peri-implant probing does not cause irreversible damage on the soft tissue seal.
- Probe penetration tends to be deeper at implant sites, compared to teeth.
- Peri-implant probing may cause bleeding during probing that is not associated with the amount of inflammation.
- Peri-implant probing is more sensitive to force variation, compared to periodontal probing.
- The soft tissue seal inhibits probe tip penetration in healthy and slightly inflamed peri-implant soft tissues. Tissue around peri-implantitis is sensitive and does not resist probing. This is a reliable finding.
- Relying on this 1 clinical parameter is not enough; the entire clinical picture must be considered before making treatment decisions.

Conclusion.—Probing is important in determining the health status of implants, yet it is only 1 clinical parameter and the entire clinical picture must be appraised before making treatment decisions.

▶ I've included this article because it provides an excellent summary of the issues related to whether or not to probe dental implants. Probing remains an important activity in assessing the health status of implants, but because of the anatomical differences between the natural tooth/tissue and implant/tissue interfaces, several points that should be taken into consideration when probing dental implants are listed as follows: (1) Use a repeatable reference point on the implant; (2) peri-implant probing does not irreversibly damage the soft tissue seal; (3) implants usually probe deeper than natural teeth; (4) it's likely that you will get more bleeding on probing with implants than natural teeth; (5) peri-implant probing is more sensitive for force variation than periodontal probing; (6) healthy peri-implant tissue resists probing, and tissues in cases of peri-implantitis do not; therefore, probing around implants should be considered a valid and reliable thing to do; and (7) one should not rely only on probing; the clinician should assess the whole clinical picture before making clinical decisions.

D. N. Dederich, DDS, MSc, PhD

7 Implant Restorative Dentistry

Introduction

If you are not restoring dental implants in your practice, it is time to incorporate the procedure into your practice. Numerous implant systems and courses on how to use them are now on the market. The risk of placing implants in simple locations is less than extracting impacted third molars. Implant dentistry is an important part of today's dental practice. The dental practitioner should incorporate the concept into their practice as their personal comfort allows.

This year's literature focused on the implant-abutment interface. Research and clinical studies are included in this chapter to better help your understanding of the dynamics of the implant-abutment interface.

Frederick M. McIntyre, DDS, MS

Technical

Cyclic Loading of Implant-Supported Prostheses: Changes in Component Fit Over Time

Hecker DM, Eckert SE (Univ of Minnesota, Minneapolis; Mayo Clinic, Rochester, Minn)
J Prosthet Dent 89:346-351, 2003   7–1

Background.—Osseointegration has provided new treatment options for the edentulous and partially edentulous patient. The bone-to-implant interface may be reliable, but clinical complications can occur at the prosthetic level, and technical problems continue to challenge clinicians. The literature suggests that an implant-supported prosthesis must demonstrate a passive fit to prevent implant fracture, component breakage, and screw loosening. However, passive fit is impossible to attain from a practical standpoint, and minimal misfit may instead be the clinical goal. No specific range of acceptable misfit has been established. The purpose of this study was to determine whether the fit of an implant-supported prosthesis is altered in response to cyclic loading and to quantify the amount of change between the gold cylinder and implant abutment over time.

TABLE 1.—Summary of the Distributions of Gap Measurements (Averaged Over Reference Points, Implant Positions, and Frames) by Load Location and Cycling Interval

Load Location	Cycle	Geometric Mean	Median	Mean (std)	Minimum	Maximum	25th Percentile	75th Percentile
Unilateral Posterior	Pre-load	0.067	0.076	0.108 (0.092)	0.009	0.334	0.038	0.142
Unilateral Posterior	50,000	0.062	0.068	0.105 (0.095)	0.007	0.334	0.033	0.150
Unilateral Posterior	200,000	0.066	0.069	0.104 (0.091)	0.010	0.325	0.038	0.131
Anterior	Pre-load	0.054	0.047	0.082 (0.077)	0.014	0.346	0.039	0.115
Anterior	50,000	0.052	0.049	0.082 (0.082)	0.013	0.378	0.035	0.110
Anterior	200,000	0.049	0.048	0.075 (0.070)	0.014	0.299	0.025	0.123
Bilateral Posterior	Pre-load	0.047	0.052	0.078 (0.060)	0.005	0.199	0.034	0.124
Bilateral Posterior	50,000	0.042	0.050	0.075 (0.059)	0.007	0.212	0.034	0.122
Bilateral Posterior	200,000	0.041	0.055	0.071 (0.058)	0.006	0.209	0.027	0.116

(Reprinted by permission of the publisher from Hecker DM, Eckert SE: Cyclic loading of implant-supported prostheses: Changes in component fit over time. J Prosthet Dent 89:346-351, 2003. Copyright 2003 by Elsevier.)

Methods.—A total of 15 implant-supported frameworks were fabricated with conventional casting techniques and cyclically loaded under 3 different loading conditions. Five frameworks were loaded on the anterior portion, 5 on the left unilateral posterior cantilever, and 5 bilaterally on the posterior cantilevers with a servohydraulic testing machine. Each framework received a cyclic load of 200 N for up to 200,000 cycles. Linear measurements were made in micrometers of the gap between the prosthetic cylinder and the implant-supported abutment at 4 predetermined reference points.

Results.—A significant decrease in gap dimensions was noted at specific reference points, and a significant decrease in the average gap was observed when the load was applied to the anterior portion of the framework (Table 1). However, significant gap closure was not observed when the load was applied unilaterally or bilaterally on the posterior cantilever.

Conclusion.—This study found changes in the fit between the prosthetic superstructure and the implant-supported abutment when simulated functional loading was performed at the anterior portion of the prosthesis. Simulated functional loading applied unilaterally or bilaterally to the posterior cantilever portion of the prosthesis did not alter the measured gap sizes.

▶ It is the goal in implant restorative dentistry to achieve a passive fit between the implant and its restorative components. Many factors can make it difficult to achieve passive fit. Manufacturing tolerance alone can limit our abilities to achieve passive fit. Manufacturers have made great strides in materials and implant interface design, but forces applied to the interface are multidirectional and of different loads, making it difficult to predict passive fit under function. This article studied the fit of an implant-supported prosthesis under various directional forces during cyclic loading.

F. M. McIntyre, DDS, MS

Fatigue Resistance of Two Implant/Abutment Joint Designs
Khraisat A, Stegaroiu R, Nomura S, et al (Niigata Univ, Japan)
J Prosthet Dent 88:604-610, 2002   7–2

Introduction.—A commonly reported mechanical problem with osseointegrated single-tooth implant replacements is screw joint instability. A simulation trial was designed to evaluate the effect of joint design on the fatigue strength and failure mode of 2 single-tooth implant systems: Brånemark and ITI.

Methods.—Seven 10-mm implants from the Brånemark and 7 from the ITI implant system were embedded to a depth of 7 mm in cylindrical acrylic resin blocks. CeraOne and solid abutments with cement-retained castings were assembled to both implant systems. The assembled units were mounted in a lever-type testing machine that was outfitted with an automatic counting device and shutoff sensors. This enabled recording of the number of cycles until failure. Each specimen was firmly mounted and a cyclic load of 100 N was used perpendicular to the long axis of the assemblies at a rate of 75

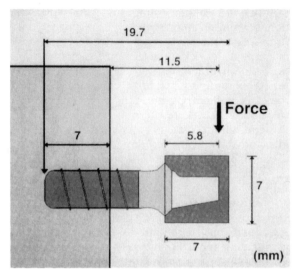

FIGURE 3.—Schematic illustration of tested specimen. (Reprinted by permission of the publisher from Khraisat A, Stegaroiu R, Nomura S, et al: Fatigue resistance of two implant/abutment joint designs. *J Prosthet Dent* 88:604-610, 2002. Copyright 2002 by Elsevier.)

cycles/min (Fig 3). To determine specimen resistance to fatigue during 6 years of simulated function, a target of 1,800,000 cycles was defined. Specimen preparation and testing were conducted by the same operator.

Results.—In the Brånemark group, the gold alloy abutment screw in all specimens fractured between 1,178,023 and 1,733,526 cycles (standard deviation, 224,477 cycles). In the ITI group, no specimens had failure until 1,800,000 cycles. A highly significant difference was observed between the 2 groups ($P = .000582$).

Conclusion.—A significant difference in fatigue resistance was observed between the Brånemark and ITI single-tooth implant systems. Failure of the abutment screw in the Brånemark system may act as a safety mechanism in securing the implant and the surrounding structure from bending overload.

▶ Great strides have been made to perfect the junction of the abutment to the implant. Screw failure or loosening were often common failures early in implant restorative dentistry. Often implants were splinted to adjacent implants or natural teeth to prevent rotation and loosening at the implant/abutment interface. Today, the interface has been improved with new screw designs, hex designs, taper, thread design, and specific torque loads. This article compares the fatigue resistance of 2 implant/abutment joint designs.

F. M. McIntyre, DDS, MS

Fracture Strength and Failure Mode of Five Different Single-Tooth Implant-Abutment Combinations

Strub JR, Gerds T (Albert-Ludwigs Univ, Freiburg, Germany)
Int J Prosthodont 16:167-171, 2003   7–3

Purpose.—The replacement of anterior single teeth continues to pose clinical challenges. Osseointegrated implants offer high cumulative implant and crown success rates. An "artificial mouth" setup was used to study fracture strength and failure modes with various implant-abutment combinations for single-tooth replacement.

Methods.—Standardized maxillary central incisor specimens were prepared with the use of 5 different implant-abutment combinations as follows: group 1, Steri-Oss/Novostil; group 2, Steri-Oss/Anatomic abutment; group 3, Steri-Oss/straight HL; group 4, IMZ Twin +/Esthetic abutment; and group 5, Steatite/gold UCLA. Each group included 16 specimens; all were luted with Panavia 21 (Kuraray). Half of the specimens in each group were aged in an artificial mouth, with simulated chewing and thermocycling. Compressive fracture strength testing was then performed on the aged and unaged specimens.

Results.—In all 5 groups, at least half of the specimens survived exposure to the artificial oral environment. Fracture strengths were similar before and after artificial aging, with median values of 537 N in group 1, 817 N in group 2, 893 N in group 3, 473 N in group 4, and 743 N in group 5. After static loading, abutment-screw bending and abutment fractures were consistent findings across groups. Group 4 specimens showed distortion of the implant neck.

Conclusion.—In this artificial mouth study, 3 of the 5 combinations for single-tooth replacement (Steri-Oss/Anatomic abutment, Steri-Oss/straight HL, and Osseotite/gold UCLA) appear to have the properties needed to withstand physiologic biting forces. In contrast, improvement is needed in the physical properties of the screws and screw joints used in the Steri-Oss/Novostil and IMZ Twin +/Esthetic abutment combinations. The findings support the use of the artificial mouth setup for assessing the stability of implant-abutment-screw interfaces.

▶ The present study investigates 5 different single-tooth implant-abutment combinations from 3 different manufacturers. The single-tooth implant is a difficult restorative challenge. Early in implant system development, the implant-abutment interface was unpredictable. Abutment rotation or loss from screw flexure or fracture was a common problem. The present implant-abutment designs provide for much more predictable results. In this study, an artificial mouth model was used to evaluate the implant-abutment-screw interface stability. With the present implant-abutment interface designs, the clinical efficacy of osseointegrated implants for single-tooth replacement has become an acceptable alternative to conventional fixed or removable partial dentures.

F. M. McIntyre, DDS, MS

Osseointegration Under Immediate Loading: Biomechanical Stress–Strain and Bone Formation–Resorption

Kawahara H, Kawahara D, Hayakawa M, et al (Osaka Dental Univ, Japan; Inst of Clinical Materials, Osaka, Japan; Ehime Univ, Japan)
Implant Dent 12:61-68, 2003   7–4

Objective.—Over the past decade, many clinicians have used immediate loading of 2-piece dental implants to promote early recovery of function and esthetics. The biomechanical and bone formation responses to immediate implant loading were assessed in a series of experiments in dogs.

Methods and Results.—Four separate experiments were designed to evaluate the effects of immediate implant loading on biomechanical stress-strain and bone formation-resorption in beagle dogs. Histologic examination several weeks after implant placement and loading showed that at least 80% of the implant surface showed fibrous encapsulation, often with osteogenesis originating centripetally from the implant surface. New bone developed centrifugally from the implant surface. By 24 weeks, the implant surface was covered with mature bone. The extent of bone resorption and remodeling depended on the characteristics of stress-strain in the implant-sheath bone. Histometric studies performed 6 to 24 weeks after implant loading showed similar bone contact areas with titanium, Co-Cr-Mo alloy, and sapphire endodontic pin stabilizers.

Under horizontal loading conditions of 8 N and 10 seconds, there was a direct, proportional relationship between the amount of micromotion displacement and the measured Periotest values. The Periotest records allowed assessment of the maximum micromotion of implants in response to biting stress. For implants and abutment teeth, Periotest values increased for the first 6 weeks after loading, then decreased significantly from 6 to 24 weeks. Insertion of a pin stabilizer led to significantly reduced Periotest values.

Conclusion.—The experimental results lend new insights into the biomechanical effects of immediate loading of dental implants. As long as it is under 30 μm, micromotion at the implant-bone interface doses not appear to interfere with osteogenesis and new bone growth. Periotest values appear to provide a useful indicator of micromotion of implants and natural teeth. When implants are placed in poor bone density, splinting to a healthy proximal tooth appears to optimize the implant's status.

▶ Two-piece implants have been mainstream because osteogenesis and osseointegration can be disturbed by micromotion at the implant-bone interface. However, the duration of healing can be a problem for many patients. During the past 10 years, many clinicians have used 2-piece implants as 1-piece systems for immediate loading to accomplish early recovery of function and esthetics. This present study evaluates micromotion of implants using Periotest values. Periotest values have become useful parameters to predict micromotion of implants and predictability of their success.

F. M. McIntyre, DDS, MS

Photoelastic Stress Analysis of Implant-Tooth Connected Prostheses With Segmented and Nonsegmented Abutments

Ochiai KT, Ozawa S, Caputo AA, et al (Univ of California, Los Angeles)

J Prosthet Dent 89:495-502, 2003   7–5

Background.—Implant restoration and the treatment of partial edentulism has a history of success. However, a number of clinical concerns have been raised regarding the dentition and possible connection to osseointegrated implants. A point of controversy is the connection of implants to natural teeth. The use of implants in partially edentulous patients requires enough implant support to render the restoration independent of tooth connection. In situations in which increased implant support is untenable, there is the option of implant-tooth connection. However, there is some question as to whether implant abutment selection affects the transfer of load between connected implants and natural teeth. Stress transfer patterns with either 1 or 2 posterior implants connected to a single anteriorly located simulated natural tooth were compared with either 1 or 2 segmented and nonsegmented implant abutments under relevant functional loads by use of the photoelastic stress analysis technique.

Methods.—A model of a human left mandible was fabricated from photoelastic materials. The model was edentulous posterior to the first premolar and had 2 screw-type implants embedded within the edentulous area in the first and second molar positions. Two fixed partial denture prosthetic restorations were fabricated with either segmented conical abutments or nonsegmented UCLA abutments. Vertical occlusal loads were applied at fixed locations on the restorations.

Photoelastic stress fringes that developed in the supporting mandible were monitored visually and recorded photographically. Subjective comparisons were made of the number of fringes (stress intensity), the closeness of fringes (stress concentrations), and their location.

Results.—Apical stresses of similar intensity at the tooth and the first molar implant were generated with loading on the restoration over the simulated tooth for both abutment types. Low-level stress was transferred to the second molar implant. Loading directed on the implant-supported region of the restoration showed low transfer of stress to the simulated tooth. The nonsegmented abutment showed nonvertical stress transfer with slightly higher intensity.

Conclusion.—This study found similar degrees of stress distribution and intensity for either 1 or 2 posterior implants with segmented or nonsegmented abutment designs. The magnitude of stresses observed for both abutment designs was similar for the single implant condition. Vertical loading resulted in more nonaxial stresses away from the force applied for the single-implant condition with the nonsegmented abutment. Both abutment designs produced similar direct loading results. Clinical criteria should be the basis of specific recommendations for selection of implant abutment and application.

▶ There is controversy related to implant restorations utilizing adjacent natural tooth abutments. Several complications have been noted in the literature pertaining to implant-tooth–connected prostheses. Many designs and materials have been used over the years to facilitate restoration of implant–natural tooth connections. This article evaluates the stress transfer between implants connected to stimulated natural teeth. Stress distribution appears to be similar for segmented and nonsegmented abutment designs.

F. M. McIntyre, DDS, MS

Clinical Studies

Residual Ridge Resorption in the Edentulous Maxilla in Patients With Implant-Supported Mandibular Overdentures: An 8-Year Retrospective Study
Kreisler M, Behneke N, Behneke A, et al (Johannes Gutenberg Univ Mainz, Germany)
Int J Prosthodont 16:295-300, 2003   7–6

Introduction.—The rate of residual ridge resorption after tooth loss varies significantly among patients and is probably affected by various anatomical, metabolic, psychosocial, and mechanical factors. The effects of an implant-retained mandibular overdenture on the rate of alveolar bone resorption in the edentulous maxilla were evaluated.

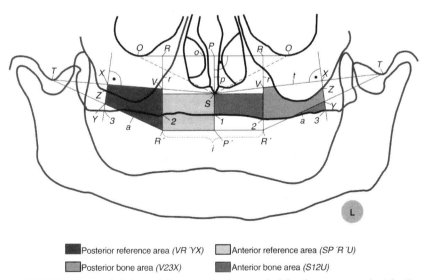

■Posterior reference area *(VR ′YX)*   □Anterior reference area *(SP ′R ′U)*
■Posterior bone area *(V23X)*   ■Anterior bone area *(S12U)*

FIGURE 2.—Geometric design used. Bone areas are shown on the left, reference areas on the right. (See Materials and Methods in original article for the definition of reference points.) (Courtesy of Kreisler M, Behneke N, Behneke A, et al: Residual ridge resorption in the edentulous maxilla in patients with implant-supported mandibular overdentures: An 8-year retrospective study. *Int J Prosthodont* 16:295-300, 2003.)

Methods.—The radiographic study included 25 edentulous patients undergoing placement of implants between the mental foramina, followed by fabrication of bar-retained mandibular overdentures and maxillary complete dentures. Before initial loading, standardized panoramic radiographs were obtained from each patient. These films were repeated every year for up to 8 years to assess maxillary alveolar bone loss. Resorption rates were compared for the anterior versus posterior parts of the maxilla (Fig 2).

Results.—It was highly variable among patients, but residual ridge resorption continued throughout the follow-up period. As a percentage of original bone height, median bone resorption ranged from 5% to 11%. Bone loss was greater in the anterior maxilla (5% to 12%) than in the posterior maxilla (2% to 7%). Two patients had extreme ridge resorption, probably related to osteoporosis.

Conclusion.—In edentulous patients, the presence of implant-supported mandibular overdentures is associated with continued residual ridge resorption in the maxilla. Resorption varies widely among patients and occurs significantly faster in the anterior than in the posterior maxilla.

▶ There have been several studies in the literature regarding combination syndrome. "Combination syndrome" is a term used to identify maxillary anterior ridge resorption in edentulous patients who have their remaining mandibular anterior teeth. It has been reported that retention of mandibular anterior teeth may create accelerated maxillary ridge resorption in some maxillary edentulous patients. The present study found similar results with a mandibular implant–supported bar overdenture, a situation that mimics mandibular anterior teeth against a maxillary edentulous ridge. I question whether a ball-retained mandibular overdenture might be less traumatic to the maxillary ridge. Is the implant-supported bar overdenture really more advantageous for our patients? Are we over-engineering the restoration as we have done for years with cast-post cores in endodontically treated teeth?

F. M. McIntyre, DDS, MS

Evaluation of Distraction Implants for Prosthetic Treatment After Vertical Alveolar Ridge Distraction: A Clinical Investigation

Feichtinger M, Gaggl A, Schultes G, et al (Univ Hosp of Graz, Austria)
Int J Prosthodont 16:19-24, 2003   7–7

Background.—Initial techniques for distraction osteogenesis in the edentulous mandible required a second operation to remove the distraction devices before implants could be placed. More recently, a distraction system that remains in the alveolar ridge after distraction has been used; in this system, the device head is changed to transform it from a distraction to a permanent implant. The results of distraction implant placement for prosthetic treatment are presented.

Methods.—The experience included 35 patients undergoing placement of a total of 62 distraction implants for vertical distraction of the alveolar ridge.

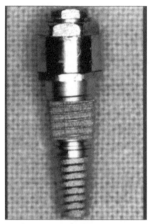
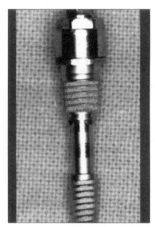

FIGURE 2.—Distraction implant in the nonactivated position (*left*) and acitivated position (*right*). (Courtesy Feichtinger M, Gaggl A, Schultes G, et al: Evaluation of distraction implants for prosthetic treatment after vertical alveolar ridge distraction: A clinical investigation. *Int J Prosthodont* 16:19-24, 2003.)

Sixteen had severe posttraumatic alveolar ridge defects, 9 had localized defects after single tooth loss, and the rest had severe mandibular or maxillary atrophy. The DISSIS distraction implant was used in each case (Fig 2). Implants were loaded with prosthetic superstructures 4 to 6 months after alveolar ridge distraction was complete. Metal-ceramic fixed partial dentures were placed in 16 patients, removable overdentures in 10, and single-crown restorations in 9 (Fig 3). Clinical and radiographic outcomes and complications were assessed at 9 months after implant loading.

Results.—Two implants were removed because of failed osseointegration. All remaining implants were successfully loaded after fabrication and placement of abutments. At follow-up, all superstructures were in place and functional, with good occlusion and healthy peri-implant mucosa. Periotest val-

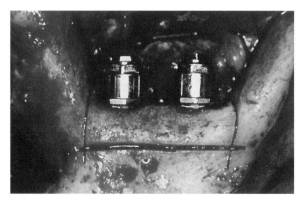

FIGURE 3.—Intraoperative situation after placement of 2 distraction implants in anterior mandibular area after performing a segment osteotomy. (Courtesy Feichtinger M, Gaggl A, Schultes G, et al: Evaluation of distraction implants for prosthetic treatment after vertical alveolar ridge distraction: A clinical investigation. *Int J Prosthodont* 16:19-24, 2003.)

ues and probing depths decreased within the first 9 months after implant loading.

Conclusions.—Distraction implants provide important advantages for alveolar ridge distraction and prosthetic restoration. Both distractor and implant can be placed in a single surgical procedure, with low rates of complications and implant loss. Gentle distraction and the use of individual abutments lead to good functional and aesthetic results.

▶ Distraction osteogenesis was first used in 1996. It is a technique that can be used to augment alveolar ridges for implant placement. Its advantages over bone grafting procedures relate to faster healing and better predictability. A disadvantage is the second operation usually needed to remove the distraction device. This article evaluates a distraction system that remains in the alveolar ridge after distraction and can be used as a permanent implant for prosthetic reconstruction.

F. M. McIntyre, DDS, MS

A Dual-Purpose Guide for Optimum Placement of Dental Implants
Çehreli MC, Çalis AC, Şahin S (Hacettepe Univ, Ankara, Turkey)
J Prosthet Dent 88:640-643, 2002   7–8

Introduction.—Correct implant placement is crucial for patients undergoing implant treatment. It is important to obtain accurate radiographic images of the potential recipient sites, and proper surgical guides are needed to place implants in their predetermined position. CT has become part of the preoperative evaluation of the maxilla or mandible for implant treatment. The use of precise surgical guides may be useful in placing implants accurately in low-density bone in which there is an increased risk of malaligning implants, compared with dense bone. Described was the use of internally stacked prefabricated surgical guides in a dual-purpose guide to place implants in the anterior maxilla.

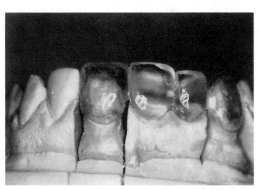

FIGURE 1.—Labial view of polished resin portion of guide on cast. (Reprinted by permission of the publisher from Çehreli MC, Çalis AC, Şahin S: A dual-purpose guide for optimum placement of dental implants. *J Prosthet Dent* 88:640-643, 2002. Copyright 2002 by Elsevier.)

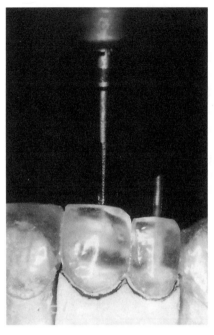

FIGURE 2.—Pins secured to guide on surveyor. Angulation of pins determined by assumptions made on possible angulation of bone. (Reprinted by permission of the publisher from Çehreli MC, Çalis AC, Şahin S: A dual-purpose guide for optimum placement of dental implants. *J Prosthet Dent* 88:640-643, 2002. Copyright 2002 by Elsevier.)

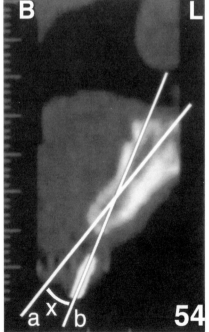

FIGURE 3.—Correction angulation of implants determined by angulation of bone. Line *a* is angulation of bone, line *b* is angulation of pin incorporated into guide, and *x* represents desired change in angle. The buccopalatal angle of the pin is used to determine correct implant alignment and to incorporate internally stacked stainless steel guide channels into the acrylic resin carrier. (Reprinted by permission of the publisher from Çehreli MC, Çalis AC, Şahin S: A dual-purpose guide for optimum placement of dental implants. *J Prosthet Dent* 88:640-643, 2002. Copyright 2002 by Elsevier.)

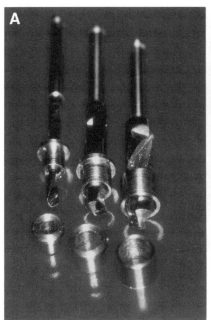
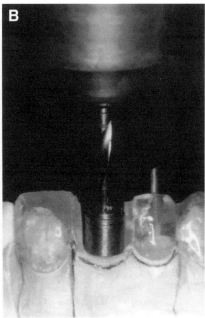

FIGURE 4.—A, Interplaced stainless steel surgical guides matching drills with diameters of 2 mm and 3.8 mm (from left to right). **B,** Two-millimeter surgical drills inserted into guides on surveyor. Tubes incorporated into guide according to CT data. (Reprinted by permission of the publisher from Çehreli MC, Çalis AC, Şahin S: A dual-purpose guide for optimum placement of dental implants. *J Prosthet Dent* 88:640-643, 2002. Copyright 2002 by Elsevier.)

Technique.—Impressions are made of both arches with the use of irreversible hydrocolloid impression material. Casts are poured in type III dental stone. Casts are mounted in a semiadjustable articulator. Dental implant recipient sites are determined. A single-mix condensation impression is made of artificial teeth. The impression and denture teeth are removed from the cast after being allowed to set. A mix of autopolymerized methyl methacrylate resin is placed in the impression where the artificial teeth were and the cast is reinserted into the impression. After polymerization, the resin guide is removed from the cast and the guide is finished and polished (Fig 1).

The cast and the acrylic resin guide are placed as an assembly on a surveying table and the table is tilted to ascertain the desired angulation of the proposed dental implants. A pinhole (1 mm in diameter) is prepared for each site at the anticipated central axis of the implant in the acrylic resin guide. A pin is secured in each hole (Fig 2). The guide is placed in the patient's mouth and 2-dimensional CT images are obtained. If a change is needed in implant angulation, it can be implemented by using the angulation of the radiographic pins as a reference.

The surveying table is retilted to obtain the correct implant angulation (Fig 3), then reoriented to remove the portion of the guide

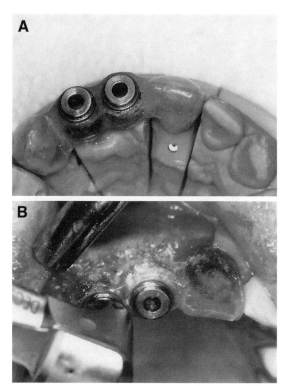

FIGURE 5.—A, Occlusal view of converted guide for surgery. B, Use of dual-purpose guide for surgery during site preparation with 2-mm drill. (Reprinted by permission of the publisher from Çehreli MC, Çalis AC, Şahin S: A dual-purpose guide for optimum placement of dental implants. *J Prosthet Dent* 88:640-643, 2002. Copyright 2002 by Elsevier.)

where the stainless steel surgical guides are incorporated. The drill is passed through the assembled prefabricated stainless steel surgical guides (Fig 4). The internally stacked guides are secured to the surgical guide with acrylic resin. The procedure is repeated for each implant site and the guide is ready to be used for surgery after sterilization (Fig 5).

Conclusion.—The technique of dual-purpose guide with interplaced stainless steel surgical guides can be used to assist the clinician during site preparation.

▶ Over the years, the philosophy for placement of implants has changed dramatically. Originally, implants were placed where the bone was available. Today, implant placement is restoratively driven, and bone grafting procedures are used to idealize the sites for implant placement. CT scans are used to measure the quality and quantity of bone available. However, the accurate placement of implants is not possible without an accurate surgical template.

This article describes a dual purpose guide for optimum placement of dental implants.

F. M. McIntyre, DDS, MS

Split-Frame Implant Prosthesis Designed to Compensate for Mandibular Flexure: A Clinical Report
Paez CY, Barco T, Roushdy S, et al (Indiana Univ, Indianapolis; Heleopolis, Cairo, Egypt)
J Prosthet Dent 89:341-343, 2003   7–9

Background.—It has been shown in several reports that the lateral pterygoid muscles contract in an almost frontal plane during opening and protrusion of the mandible, pulling the condyles together. The result of this contraction is flexure of the mandible around the mental symphysis, with resultant sagittal movement of the posterior segments. Flexure of the mandible during opening and protrusion may alter the position of the structures located inside of it. Mandibular flexure in an edentulous mandible restored with 4 or more implants connected by a metal bar and retained with screws may cause screw loosening and unnecessary stresses and strains on the prosthesis and implants. This case report demonstrates that separation of the prosthesis at the midline may relieve these stresses and strains.

> *Case Report.*—Man, 57, was seen with complete dentures as a result of loss of natural dentition to decay. The patient was dissatisfied with the mandibular denture and requested a fixed prosthesis for the mandible. A split-frame, implant-supported prosthesis was designed for this patient to compensate for mandibular flexure.
> The separation at the mandibular midline was evaluated with shim stock to ensure that the 2 framework pieces did not contact during opening and protrusive movements of the mandible. The internal medial surfaces of the metal frameworks were airborne-particle abraded, and after 2 weeks, the frameworks were removed from the mouth to determine whether there had been any contact during function. There was no evidence of contact. At 2 years after placement, the patient had reported no complaints and no screw loosening.

Conclusion.—This report describes the midline separation of a hybrid mandibular denture. Such a split-frame, implant-supported prosthesis is designed to minimize the adverse effects of mandibular flexure, which reduces unnecessary stress and strain on the metal substructure and retaining screws and may increase the longevity of the prosthesis.

▶ It has been known for years that the mandible flexes upon opening, especially in a protrusive movement. This is the first article that I have read that questions the possible effects flexure of the mandible may have on an edentulous mandibular fixed-implant prosthesis. The article reviews literature pertaining to mandibular flexure and presents a case report that describes the design of a hybrid mandibular denture that is designed to compensate for mandibular flexure.

F. M. McIntyre, DDS, MS

8 Oral and Maxillofacial Surgery

Introduction

The section of Oral and Maxillofacial Surgery continues to include relevant issues of current anesthesia practice and dentoalveolar surgery. Two areas that have expanded recently are pediatric maxillofacial surgery and reconstruction. These are fast becoming subspecialty areas of expertise and focus as technology and our understanding of bone and tissue repair drive management of maxillofacial disorders in these patients.

Bruce B. Horswell, MD, DDS, MS

Dentoalveolar Surgery/Anesthesia

Adverse Events With Outpatient Anesthesia in Massachusetts

D'Eramo EM, Bookless SJ, Howard JB (Boston Univ; Tufts School of Dental Medicine, Boston; Massachusetts Society of Oral and Maxillofacial Surgeons, Norwell, Mass)

J Oral Maxillofac Surg 61:793-800, 2003   8–1

Introduction.—Data are sparse regarding national morbidity and mortality statistics on office anesthesia as practiced by qualified oral and maxillary surgeons. The incidence of various complications associated with outpatient anesthesia was examined retrospectively.

Methods.—As part of a long-term survey of ambulatory oral surgical office deaths in Massachusetts since 1984, a questionnaire was mailed to the 157 active members of the Massachusetts Society of Oral and Maxillary Surgeons. The response rate was 100%. Morbidity data were obtained for 1999 and the preceding 4 years. Data included anesthesia-associated complications and all office deaths of patients treated by this cohort of oral and maxillary surgeons.

Results.—Syncope remains the most common complication. Of 178,647 patients who received local anesthesia alone, 1119 experienced syncope (1/160 patients). Laryngospasm (1/345) was about 9 times more common than bronchospasm in patients who received office general anesthesia. Dysrhythmia necessitating drug therapy occurred in 43 of 80,323 patients (1/1868).

One episode of neck injury or nerve injury associated with positional changes during general anesthesia was reported.

Aspiration of a tooth or foreign body was rare (2 patients aspirated, 1 during parenteral sedation and 1 during local anesthesia). During 1999, 13 patients were sent to a hospital from the oral and maxillofacial surgeon's office (1/47,692 patient visits). There were 2 treatment-associated deaths among 1,706,100 patients treated during the 5-year period 1995 through 1999 (mortality rate, 1/853,050).

Conclusion.—Data from this retrospective practitioner survey showed a mortality rate consistent with those of the 6 similar mortality reports since 1980. These 7 retrospective reviews reported 34 deaths during 28,399,193 office visits involving anesthesia, for an overall dental anesthesia rate of 1/835,000 patients.

▶ These reviews are always of interest to those of us who utilize outpatient general anesthesia or IV sedation in our daily practices. As this article suggests, outpatient general anesthesia continues to be a safe and predictable mode of anxiety and pain control for the well-trained surgeon. As correctly suggested in the discussion that follows, proper patient evaluation and selection and increased technology with the advent of pulse oximetry and constant cardiovascular monitoring have contributed to this increased margin of safety over the last decades.

B. B. Horswell, MD, DDS, MS

Panoramic Radiographic Risk Factors for Inferior Alveolar Nerve Injury After Third Molar Extraction
Blaeser BF, August MA, Donoff RB, et al (Massachusetts Gen Hosp, Boston)
J Oral Maxillofac Surg 61:417-421, 2003   8–2

Introduction.—Inferior alveolar nerve (IAN) injury after third molar extraction is a well-recognized complication with a reported incidence of 0.5% to 5%. Contributing factors include age, history of infection, use of rotary instruments, use of concomitant general anesthesia, and level of impaction. The most important component contributing to IAN injury may be the anatomical proximity of the IAN to the third molar root. The relationship between specific panoramic radiographic signs and the IAN during mandibular third molar removal was examined with the use of a case-control design.

Methods.—The study included 8 cases and 17 control subjects. Cases were considered to be those patients with verified IAN injury after third molar extraction. Control subjects were patients with no nerve injury. Five oral surgeons blinded to injury status independently analyzed the preoperative panoramic radiographs for the presence of high-risk radiographic signs. Bivariate analyses were performed to evaluate the association between radiographic findings and IAN injury. The sensitivity, specificity, and positive and negative predictive values were determined for each radiographic sign.

Results.—Positive radiographic signs were significantly linked with an IAN injury ($P < .0001$). The presence of radiographic signs had positive predictive values that ranged between 1.4% and 2.7%; this represented a 40% or greater increase over the baseline likelihood of injury (1%) for each patient. The absence of radiographic risk factors had a strong negative (>99%) predictive value.

Conclusion.—Panoramic findings of diversion of the inferior alveolar canal, darkening of the third molar root, and interruption of the cortical white line are statistically correlated with IAN injury. On the basis of the estimated predictive values, the absence of positive radiographic findings was linked with a minimal risk of nerve injury. The presence of 1 or more risk factors was associated with an increased risk of nerve injury.

Litigation and the Lingual Nerve

Lydiatt DD (Univ of Nebraska, Omaha)
J Oral Maxillofac Surg 61:197-200, 2003   8–3

Introduction.—Injury of nerves during oral surgery can be due to anatomical variations. The oral surgeon must be aware of these variations and the regions in which injury may occur. Good communication with the patient regarding the possibility of injury before surgery is crucial. Injury to the lingual nerve causes considerable morbidity. Litigation analysis is useful in understanding and preventing lingual nerve injuries and resultant litigation suits.

Methods.—Jury verdict reports were obtained from a computerized legal database for the period of 1987 through 2000. All state and federal civil trials in the United States were reviewed. Data included information concerning plaintiffs and defendants, allegations of wrongdoing, reasons for litigation, anatomical sites of injuries, specialties of expert witnesses, verdict results, and awards received.

Results.—Thirty-three suits from 12 states were identified. Dentists or oral surgeons were involved in 87% and otolaryngologists were involved in 13% of lawsuits. Tooth extractions were involved in 79% of cases; 50% resulted in financial awards. Lack of informed consent was alleged in 52% of cases overall and in 46% of tooth extraction suits. Expert witnesses were of the same specialties for both plaintiffs and defendants in 81% of suits. Inadequate education and selection of the wrong surgical approach were cited in 18% and 15% of the suits, respectively. Anatomical variation was considered to be present in 15%.

Conclusion.—Surgeons must be aware of anatomical variations and regions in which injury to the lingual nerve is likely to occur. Written informed consent may help reduce litigation in known risk regions.

▶ I have placed both of these articles (Abstracts 8–2 and 8–3) together as they relate to a problem that many of us see in our offices, which is nerve injury after treatment—most often after removal of the lower third molar. The first article by Blaeser et al (Abstract 8–2) looks at the use of the Panorex to determine the degree of risk of surgery to contents of the neurovascular canal. They nicely outline these risk factors in Table 1 of the original article.

The second article (Abstract 8–3) is authored by Professor Lydiatt, who is both an oral surgeon and an ENT surgeon. He highlights that the lingual nerve will more often result in litigation because of the difficulty of the patient in accommodating to perceived taste and sensory disruption. The article also confirms that dentists are more often involved in lingual nerve injuries, and this comes after tooth extraction. He also highlights the anatomical variations in the lingual nerve as it approaches the lingual aspect in the third molar region in some patients, necessitating care in surgical technique. For both of these nerve entities, I do not think we will be seeing any decrease in the challenges, both in avoiding injury or the litigious tendencies of our patients regarding nerve injury. Nevertheless, we need to remain informed, careful, and vigilant.

B. B. Horswell, MD, DDS, MS

Office-Based Ambulatory Anesthesia: Outcomes of Clinical Practice of Oral and Maxillofacial Surgeons

Perrott DH, Yuen JP, Andresen RV, et al (American Assoc of Oral and Maxillofacial Surgeons, Rosemont, Ill; Harvard School of Dental Medicine, Boston; Massachusetts Gen Hosp, Boston)
J Oral Maxillofac Surg 61:983-995, 2003   8–4

Background.—Delivery of ambulatory anesthesia services in an office setting is an essential part of the daily practice of oral and maxillofacial surgeons. Retrospective studies and data sources that include surveys or analyses of malpractice claims have been used to document the quality and safety of office-based ambulatory anesthesia care in oral and maxillofacial practices, and these studies have found an improvement in associated mortality with the introduction of modern anesthetic agents and techniques. However, these types of studies introduce biases that cannot be eliminated or controlled. Prospective studies have supported the efficacy and safety of office-based anesthesia services, but these studies have generally had small study populations.

There is a need for a system for collection of prospective data from a large patient population undergoing office-based ambulatory anesthesia. This report provided an overview of current anesthetic practices of oral and maxillofacial surgeons in an office-based ambulatory setting.

Methods.—A prospective cohort study was conducted using patients undergoing oral and maxillofacial procedures in an office setting. Patients were included if they received local anesthesia, conscious sedation, or deep sedation/general anesthesia. Predictor variables were classified as demographic, anesthetic technique, staffing, adverse events, and patient-oriented outcomes.

Results.—A total of 34,191 patients were enrolled. Deep sedation/general anesthesia was the most commonly used technique (71.9%), followed by conscious sedation (15.5%) and local anesthesia (12.6%). Only 2 patients experienced complications that required hospitalization. The majority of patients (80.3%) reported some anxiety before the procedure. However, after the procedure, 61.2% of patients reported having no anxiety about future operations. Overall, 94.3% of patients reported satisfaction with the anesthetic, and more than 94% of all patients would recommend the anesthetic technique to a loved one.

Conclusion.—The use of local anesthesia, conscious sedation, or deep sedation/general anesthesia delivered in an oral and maxillofacial surgery office setting is safe and can provide a high degree of patient satisfaction.

Patient Safety in Anesthesia Practice: Partnerships That Make the Impossible Routine
Assael LA
J Oral Maxillofac Surg 61:981-982, 2003   8–5

Background.—Patient safety in anesthesia practice is a primary concern of every oral and maxillofacial surgeon. Safety has been enhanced by technological advances such as pulse oximetry and capnography, but the effectiveness of these technologies is dependent on the presence of a skilled clinician who can immediately interpret findings and act to ensure an uneventful outcome. A recent publication by Perrott et al in the *Journal of Oral and Maxillofacial Surgery* highlighted the essential partnership necessary among oral and maxillofacial surgeons and their staff, the American Association of Oral and Maxillofacial Surgeons, educators, researchers, and the patients. Highlights of that Perrott et al report were presented.

Overview.—A great majority of patients in the study experienced significant anxiety before ambulatory oral and maxillofacial surgery but after their procedure, the majority of patients said they would have no anxiety about a future procedure, and nearly all of the patients indicated that they would recommend a similar technique to a loved one. Fear and anxiety are among the main reasons that patients delay and refuse necessary health care, and these emotions amplify the experience of pain. A comfortable anesthesia/oral and maxillofacial surgery experience can prevent future fear and anxiety and thus promote improved health. Insurance company denials of coverage for these services are hard to understand and run contrary to the goal of improving the health of the insured.

The study found that compliance with the American Association of Oral and Maxillofacial Surgeons Parameters of Care was excellent but not universal. Operating room staffing and the use of pulse oximetry were areas in which compliance was over 90%, but this would appear to be an area in which 100% compliance is required. The most critical outcome of the Perrott et al study is anesthesia safety, and the study findings support the view that ambulatory anesthesia in the office setting provides the safest possible care for oral and maxillofacial surgery patients.

Conclusion.—Ambulatory anesthesia in the oral and maxillofacial surgery setting is extremely safe and provides a valuable service to the public.

Office-Based Ambulatory Anesthesia: Outcomes of Clinical Practice of Oral and Maxillofacial Surgeons
Windell HC (Gresham, Ore)
J Oral Maxillofac Surg 61:995-996, 2003   8–6

Background.—This discussion described the valuable contribution to oral and maxillofacial surgery provided by an evidence-based outcomes investigation that presented the first and most complete prospective study of outpatient anesthesia in the practice setting.

Overview.—The delivery of anesthesia has been a fundamental component of oral and maxillofacial surgery practice. Over the years, there has been much progress in ensuring the safe delivery of anesthesia, in part through the publication of studies and the establishment of programs for improvement of the delivery of anesthesia.

Previous articles have addressed mortality and morbidity studies on a retrospective basis and have included small numbers of study participants. Unlike these previous articles, the present study of office-based ambulatory anesthesia utilized a large number of patients and generated a much greater volume of useful data. The patient satisfaction portion of the study was the most difficult aspect, as having patients come back to the office to complete a survey or contacting the patients by telephone would result in a low return.

To address these problems, patients recovering at the office were kept somewhat longer so that the surveys could be completed immediately. The increased scrutiny that the dental profession has experienced in the past several years and the regulations promulgated by individual state dental boards provide strong incentives to continue this study to obtain additional data from both participant oral and maxillofacial surgeons and patients to further demonstrate the efficacy and safety of the delivery systems used for ambulatory anesthesia in the office setting.

Conclusion.—This discussion piece represents the concern that oral and maxillofacial surgeons have for ensuring the safety and reducing the anxiety of their patients. The continuing development of evidence-based outcomes in regard to ambulatory anesthesia is important in maintaining the excellent safety record of the profession in regard to outpatient anesthesia.

▶ Due to the increasing medical complexity of our patients and the increased need for safe outpatient or ambulatory anesthesia, these articles (Abstracts 8–4 and 8–5) and the editorial discussion that follows (Abstract 8–6) help us to clarify and focus in regard to delivering that care in the oral and maxillofacial surgical setting. Like the previous article by D'Eramo (Abstract 8–1) in regard to outpatient anesthesia in Massachusetts, this article demonstrates the high level of safety of outpatient anesthesia as practiced in contemporary oral and maxillofacial surgery. It is very important to develop evidence-based outcomes in regard to ambulatory general anesthesia or sedation in our practices, as this will no doubt help to direct future public health delivery, insurance coverage, and (the bottom line) our patients' expectations for safe and predictable pain and anxiety control, which, as noted in these articles, is reasonably and confidently assured as currently practiced.

B. B. Horswell, MD, DDS, MS

Sevoflurane General Anesthesia: An Alternative Technique in the Pediatric Oral and Maxillofacial Surgery Patient
Lee M, Bennett HE, Gordon N (Univ of California, San Francisco)
J Oral Maxillofac Surg 61:1249-1252, 2003   8–7

Background.—Sevoflurane was used successfully in Japan for many years before it was approved for use in the United States. Numerous publications over the past decade have described the safety and efficacy of this potent inhalational anesthetic agent with rapid onset and recovery for use in both the adult and pediatric populations. The traditional method of obtaining IV access before induction is not a viable option for many pediatric patients in the oral and maxillofacial surgery clinical setting because of their uncooperative behavior. Administration of an inhalational anesthetic agent makes it possible to obtain IV access. An acceptable and effective technique for administration of outpatient sevoflurane anesthesia without preoperative sedatives in pediatric patients was described.

Methods.—This prospective study involved 20 pediatric patients over a period of 4 months at a large urban hospital. Mask induction of general anesthesia with sevoflurane and maintenance with a nasal trumpet as airway was used throughout the surgical procedure. A standard anesthesia and recovery record was made for each patient and included observations for untoward effects and complications.

Results.—The average time for induction of anesthesia was 95 seconds, and the time from termination of sevoflurane to eye opening was 8 minutes. The duration of recovery was 30 minutes. No procedure time for any patient exceeded 10 minutes. Transient tachycardia developed in 2 patients.

Conclusion.—The indication is that this alternative general anesthetic technique, using mask induction and maintenance with sevoflurane, is an effective approach for the control of fear and anxiety in the pediatric patient undergoing an outpatient oral or maxillofacial surgical procedure.

▶ Sevoflurane is a rapid onset, well tolerated, and safe inhalational anesthetic agent which has been utilized with great success in operating room general anesthesia and now has found its way into the ambulatory setting in oral and maxillofacial surgical practices. This does require a general anesthetic machine for the precise and safe delivery of anesthetic gases, but when this is in place then Sevoflurane can be safely administered with predictability. Obviously, monitoring of partial pressure of arterial oxygen and end-tidal carbon dioxide is important when delivering general anesthetic inhalational agents. I am sure, as anesthetic machines become more affordable for the office-based surgical practice, that this procedure will become more widespread, particularly its use in children.

B. B. Horswell, MD, DDS, MS

Medicine

Maxillofacial Surgery in World War I: The Role of the Dentists and Surgeons

Strother EA (Louisiana State Univ, New Orleans)
J Oral Maxillofac Surg 61:943-950, 2003   8–8

Introduction.—Because trench warfare dominated World War I (WWI), soldiers' most serious injuries were to the head and neck. Steel helmets saved lives, yet increased the number of facial injuries from shells, bullets, and other projectile fragments. Of 8607 total facial injuries (32% cheek, 25% eye, and 13% mandible [about 11% of mandibular fractures resulted in nonunion and necessitated bone grafting]), there were 316 deaths (3.67%), a lower rate than the average of deaths for all types of injuries (7.73%). The roles of dentists and surgeons in treating maxillofacial injuries during WWI were discussed.

Treatment of Maxillofacial Injuries.—Before WWI, there were no formal educational programs for the treatment of maxillofacial injuries. British and French soldiers injured early in the war wore masks to hide their deformities. The Surgeon General's Office for the American Expeditionary Forces (AEF) named surgeon Vilray P. Blair to organize the effort to treat maxillofacial injuries in the AEF and Robert H. Ivy, a dentist, as his assistant.

Short, intensive courses ranging from 3 to 6 weeks were conducted from October 1917 through March 1918 in St Louis, Philadelphia, and Chicago. About 86% of 164 medical officers and 123 dental officers completed the course and were assigned in teams of 1 surgeon and 1 dentist to each unit overseas. By the time the United States entered WWI, the allies had already gained significant experience in the surgery and reconstruction of maxillofacial patients.

Teams of US surgeons/dentists were sent to France to observe the work of prominent practitioners until they were needed in their own hospitals. Special reports created during treatment of maxillofacial injuries included photographs, drawings, plaster and wax models, and plaster masks. The Surgeon General's Office had detailed plans for treatment of maxillofacial patients, yet the realities of war resulted in inadequate personnel and equipment for the AEF. Surgeons and dentists were often sent to the front lines to perform emergency surgery. Specialized equipment for the maxillofacial unit was sent, but it was not received until after the war.

Dentists on the maxillofacial team became adept at improvising appliances for their patients, often creating splints from coins, telephone wire, or meat tins. Results were often less satisfactory than anticipated due to inadequate numbers of trained army surgeons and dentists and lack of adequate supplies. The general principle of thorough debridement of gunshot wounds was discouraged in maxillofacial wounds to save as much tissue as possible. Lack of proper drainage, tissue debridement, and removal of foreign bodies were the primary causes of infection.

Early restoration of tissues to their normal position was effective in preventing infection; immediate fixation of jaw fractures was critical. Innovations during WWI included bone grafting and pedicle flaps.

Conclusion.—Many dentists and surgeons who innovated the treatment of maxillofacial injuries during WWI also had a significant role in the development of their profession following the war. Oral surgery was relatively unformed as a dental specialty before WWI. The need for treatment of maxillofacial trauma led to an understanding of the unique skills of oral surgeons.

▶ This is a historical review of the role of dentists and maxillofacial surgeons who were primarily dental surgeons or physicians interested in facial injuries during WWI. This is an important review as it accurately describes the history of the dental profession's involvement regarding trauma. WWI marked the birth of maxillofacial surgery as a specialty and area of interest both in medicine and dentistry due to the large number of maxillofacial injuries which were seen during the long and destructive global conflict. Enjoy the article!

B. B. Horswell, MD, DDS, MS

Allergic Rhinitis: Broader Disease Effects and Implications for Management
Baroody FM (Univ of Chicago)
Otolaryngol Head Neck Surg 128:616-631, 2003   8–9

Introduction.—Allergic rhinitis (AR) is a benign, yet burdensome disease for a significant proportion of both adults and children. The broader disease effects of AR and implications for management were discussed.

Managing Allergic Rhinitis.—AR increases medical costs, decreases patients' productivity and quality of life, and impairs learning and socialization skills. Poorly controlled AR can trigger exacerbations of asthma, sinusitis, and otitis media since it shares pathophysiologic elements with these diseases. Early diagnosis and treatment needs to be a priority for both patients and physicians, both to control the symptoms of AR and to improve the management of associated diseases.

Several pharmacologic treatments are available for AR and include antihistamines (intranasal and systemic); intranasal cromolyn; intranasal anticholinergic agents; intranasal steroids; systemic steroids; immunotherapy; and, most recently, leukotriene receptor antagonists. Frequently, combinations of these treatments are used to maximize control of refractory symptoms.

Conclusion.—Early diagnosis and treatment of AR needs to be a priority for both patients and physicians to control the condition and to improve the management of other related comorbid diseases.

▶ I wanted to include this article for review as all of us will be treating patients with significant AR and upper respiratory airway issues in our practices. This is an entity which is also increasing in this country for unknown reasons, and it behooves us to be well aware of the pathophysiology and management for our patients who are afflicted with AR. I therefore highly recommend this reading, which is a nice review of AR, its basic science, associated diseases, and appropriate treatment.

B. B. Horswell, MD, DDS, MS

Xerostomia: Etiology, Recognition and Treatment
Guggenheimer J, Moore PA (Univ of Pittsburgh, Pa)
J Am Dent Assoc 134:61-69, 2003   8–10

Introduction.—The presence of saliva is usually assumed and is not necessary for any life-sustaining functions. Yet, its diminution or absence may cause significant morbidity and a decrease in a patient's quality of life. The etiology, recognition, and treatment of xerostomia, commonly called "dry mouth," were evaluated retrospectively.

Methods.—Clinical and scientific reports of xerostomia published in the last 20 years of dental and medical literature were obtained using the Index Medicus.

Results.—Xerostomia often occurs when the amount of saliva that bathes the oral mucous membranes is diminished. Symptoms may ensue without a measurable decrease in salivary gland output. The most common cause of xerostomia is the use of xerostomic medications. Several frequently prescribed drugs with a variety of pharmacologic actions produce xerostomia as a side effect. Xerostomia often occurs in Sjögren's syndrome, a condition that involves both dry mouth and dry eyes and may be associated with rheumatoid arthritis or a related connective tissue disease. Xerostomia is also common in patients who have undergone radiotherapy to the head/neck region.

Conclusion.—Xerostomia is an uncomfortable and common oral complaint for which patients may seek relief from dental practitioners. Its complications can include dental caries, periodontitis, mucositis, candidiasis, or difficulty with the use of dentures. Practitioners need to identify the possible cause(s) and treat patients accordingly. Treatment of xerostomia is usually palliative, yet may offer protection from its complications.

▶ Xerostomia is a common malady affecting primarily the elderly population. This is a nice review of the etiology of xerostomia and its treatment. I can certainly confirm that the patients I see that have xerostomia are patients who are on certain antihypertensive agents as listed in the Table (see original article), patients with certain rheumatologic diseases and obviously, patients who have undergone radiation for head and neck cancer. This is an article to keep in one's file cabinet for ready reference.

B. B. Horswell, MD, DDS, MS

Trauma Reconstruction

Non-Surgical Treatment of Condylar Fractures in Adults: A Retrospective Analysis

Smets LMH, Van Damme PA, Stoelinga PJW (Univ Medical Centre, Nijmegen, The Netherlands)
J Craniomaxillofac Surg 31:162-167, 2003　　　　　　　　　8–11

Introduction.—Although the consensus for some time has been to treat condylar mandibular fractures in a nonsurgical fashion, there has been recent uncertainty that this is the ideal approach. The results of nonsurgical condylar fracture were examined in 60 patients with 71 condylar fractures to establish a protocol for selecting patients for surgical treatment of condylar fractures.

Methods.—A retrospective review of patients treated for unilateral or bilateral fractures on the condyle between 1995 to 1999 was performed. Data were obtained regarding the clinical assessment of occlusion, asymmetry at rest and during mouth opening, maximum interincisal distance, signs of TMJ dysfunction, and analysis of radiographic data (ie, shortening of the ascending ramus as measured on sequential orthopantomograms).

Results.—Five patients (8%) had an unacceptable malocclusion; 1 of these patients had considerably limited mouth opening. Fifty-five patients (92%) had no or only minor signs of TMJ dysfunction that did not need further treatment.

Conclusion.—Surgical repositioning and rigid internal fixation are recommended only in selected patients with shortening of the ascending ramus of 8 mm or more or considerable displacement of the condylar fragment.

▶ One of the most challenging entities in facial trauma is that of the condylar fracture in the adult patient for reasons relating to treatment and recovery. The nondisplaced or minimally displaced condylar fracture is adequately treated with a combination of intermaxillary fixation for a period of 10 to 14 days with training elastics and/or physical therapy modalities with close surveillance. The difficult entity is the displaced condylar fracture which may result in condylar ramal shortening on the affected side.

As this study points out, this is the fracture that will result in malocclusion and/or dysfunction for the patient once healing has ensued. Therefore, these adult patients may benefit from open reduction internal fixation with a view toward thorough physical therapy modalities in order to recover pretraumatic condylar ramal height and achieve acceptable masticatory function. I would refer the reader to the OMS Knowledge Update[1] referenced below in regard to condylar fractures.

B. B. Horswell, MD, DDS, MS

Reference

1. Condylar fractures, in Trauma, OMS *Knowledge Update*. Kelly JP (ed). AAOMS, 1995, p Tra 83.

Referral Patterns for the Treatment of Facial Trauma in Teaching Hospitals in the United States

Le BT, Holmgren EP, Holmes JD, et al (Univ of Southern California, Los Angeles; Oregon Health Sciences Univ, Portland; Univ of Alabama, Birmingham)
J Oral Maxillofac Surg 61:557-560, 2003   8–12

Introduction.—The management of facial trauma is considered a necessary component in the education of several specialties, including general plastic surgery, otolaryngology (ENT), and oral and maxillofacial surgery. The referral patterns for patients with facial trauma to the various specialty areas differ institutionally according to physician preferences and protocols. The referral patterns for facial trauma at teaching hospitals in the United States were examined.

Methods.—One hundred questionnaires were sent by facsimile to physician-chiefs of emergency or trauma services at teaching hospitals in the United States. Surveyed hospitals were limited to those for whom appropriate consultation services were available. Scenarios involving a variety of facial injury patterns were presented and respondents were asked to make a hypothetical referral. Questions concerning preferences and opinions about the various services were included.

Results.—Most teaching hospitals had a formal protocol for the referral of patients with facial injuries that were even across 3 specialties (ENT, oral and maxillofacial surgery, and general plastic surgery). Only 56% of respondents would seek the same referral for themselves or their relatives in the same manner in which they would refer a patient, based on their in-house protocol. Regarding timeliness, efficiency, and perceived competency in handling facial trauma, oral and maxillary surgery had statistically significantly higher scores, compared to ENT and plastic surgery, which were not statistically distinguishable from each other.

Conclusion.—All 3 specialties seem to be involved in the management of facial trauma at teaching institutions in the United States. It appears unlikely that any one specialty will be singled out as the sole provider of these services at all teaching institutions.

▶ This is a short study which surveyed emergency and trauma services at major teaching hospitals in the United States. Due to the overlap of specialty interests in the head and neck region, it is no surprise that 3 specialties—oral and maxillofacial surgery, ENT, and plastic surgery—vie for position on the traumatized face. In some major institutions where requirements for training are high and numbers of patients are lower, this may result in competition between specialties. To be sure, there are regional differences, and for my practice in

Appalachia and southern West Virginia, my two oral and maxillofacial surgery partners and myself are the sole providers of facial trauma for our level I trauma center in this area. There is essentially no competition for patients among providers.

B. B. Horswell, MD, DDS, MS

Cranio-Maxillofacial Trauma: A 10 Year Review of 9543 Cases With 21 067 Injuries

Gassner R, Tuli T, Hächl O, et al (Univ of Innsbruck, Austria; Univ of Pittsburgh, Pa)
J Craniomaxillofac Surg 13:51-61, 2003   8–13

Introduction.—An understanding of the cause, severity, and temporal distribution of maxillofacial trauma can help institute clinical and research priorities for effective treatment and injury prevention. Data regarding patients with facial bone fractures, dentoalveolar trauma, and soft tissue injuries were examined. The impact of the 5 main causes of facial injury was assessed, along with the statistical patterns of cranio-maxillofacial trauma in relation to accident causes.

Methods.—Between 1991 and 2000, 9543 patients were treated for maxillofacial trauma. Data were prospectively documented concerning cause of injury, age and gender, type of injury, injury mechanisms, location and frequency of soft tissue injuries, dentoalveolar trauma, facial bone fractures, and concomitant injuries.

Results.—Of 5 major categories/mechanisms of injury, the causes were as follows: activity of daily living in 3613 patients (38%), sports in 2991 (31%), violence in 1170 (12%), traffic accidents in 504 (5%), and other causes in 149 (2%). A total of 3578 patients (37.5%) had 7061 facial bone fractures, 4763 patients (49.9%) had 6237 dentoalveolar injuries, and 5968 patients (62.5%) had 7769 soft tissue injuries.

There was an overall male-to-females ratio of 2.1:1 and the mean patient age was 25.8 years, but both varied depending on the mechanism of injury. Mechanisms were as follows: facial bone fractures, 35.4 years, high risk for males; soft tissue injuries, 28.7 years, no gender preference; dentoalveolar trauma, 18 years, elevated risk for females. Patients with facial trauma were at increased risk for facial bone fractures (225%).

Soft tissue lesions were observed in 58% of patients involved in traffic accidents. Dental trauma was present in 49% of activities of daily living and play accidents. When compared with other causes, the probability of experiencing soft tissue injuries and dental trauma, but not facial bone fractures, is higher in sports-associated accidents.

Conclusion.—Surgeons treating cranio-maxillofacial trauma are the main source of information for the public and legislators regarding implementing preventive measures concerning high-risk activities. In facial trauma, older patients are prone to bone fractures (increase of 4.4%/y of age) and soft tissue injuries (increase of 2%/y of age). Children are more susceptible to dentoalveolar trauma (decrease of 4.5%/y of age).

▶ This is a very nice review from a busy trauma center in Austria where the authors have looked at approximately 10,000 cases of maxillofacial trauma over a 10-year period. The epidemiology is interesting in that the majority of facial injuries are due to what were termed "activities of daily living" and play accidents, whereas in the American trauma literature, motor vehicle crashes are responsible for most of our facial injuries. Sport is a larger category of trauma in Austria as opposed to violence in the American trauma experience. The patients more susceptible are younger, which would agree with our experience here in the United States.

B. B. Horswell, MD, DDS, MS

The Buccinator Musculomucosal Island Flap for Partial Tongue Reconstruction

Zhao Z, Zhang Z, Li Y, et al (Chongqing Med Univ, China)
J Am Coll Surg 196:753-760, 2003   8–14

Introduction.—The ideal tongue reconstruction after partial or total glossectomy should be performed using similar tissue. The buccinator musculomucosal island flap consists of thin, pliable mucosa, with a high cell renewal rate and minimal scar formation, good color, contour, texture match, and buccinator muscle fibers over the flap's entire length to provide acceptable tongue reconstruction without conspicuous donor site defect. An application of the buccinator myomucosal island flap for partial tongue reconstruction after cancer ablation is discussed.

Methods.—The buccinator musculomucosal flap is designed in a shuttle or in a fish-mouth fashion, approaching the oral commissure anteriorly. If the flap design is contoured in a 3-leaf shape, a larger flap will be obtained without oral corner deformity or mouth opening difficulty. The flap is safe and easy to raise on the facial musculature. The pedicle of the flap is longer and reliable and has a wide range of applicability. The flap may be used for reconstruction of a partial glossectomy defect (defect not more than half a tongue). The surgeon must be knowledgeable concerning possible anatomic variations, particularly in the venous system, and should plan to raise a contralateral buccinator musculomucosal island flap when homolateral facial vascular variation compromises the flap's survival.

Results.—The flap was successfully used for partial tongue reconstruction in 16 patients. All flaps survived without any complications. Results were satisfactory (including configuration and function of the reconstructed tongue). Electromyography performed in 1 patient with half glossectomy demonstrated reinnervation of the muscle in the flap with active motion of the reconstructed tongue.

Conclusion.—The buccal musculomucosal island flap, which is based on the facial artery and vein, is a good local flap option for reconstruction of the tongue. Reinnervation of the flap offers the potential for improved physiologic motion.

▶ The buccal mucosal and fat pad flaps are some of my favorite local flaps for reconstructing small defects in the oral region. These authors disclose their experience using the buccal island flap that is based upon the buccal branches of the facial artery in lining lateral tongue and floor of mouth defects. This is a nice review of a predictable and easy flap for intraoral reconstruction with minimal complications.

B. B. Horswell, MD, DDS, MS

TGF-β3 Decreases Type I Collagen and Scarring After Labioplasty
Hosokawa R, Nonaka K, Morifuji M, et al (Kyushu Univ, Fukuoka, Japan; Natl Inst of Health, Bethesda, Md)
J Dent Res 82:558-564, 2003   8–15

Background.—Cleft lip (with or without cleft palate) is one of the most common congenital malformations and represents a unique clinical management challenge in facial surgery. Labioplasty performed on infants for repair of cleft lip often results in severe scar formation. Transforming growth factor-beta (TGF-β) has been implicated in regulating the rate and extent of wound healing and tissue repair. The hypothesis that TGF-β is a contributor to reduced scar formation after labioplasty for cleft lip was tested with the use of sutured mouse lip in both in vivo and in vitro experiments.

Methods.—The mice were divided into 4 groups as follows: (1) unoperated control animals; (2) sutured only; (3) sutured with phosphate-buffered saline (PBS) injection; and (4) sutured with 100 μL of TGF-β3 injection at 0.1 ng/μL. A like volume of PBS was used in the third group. Injections were repeated every 12 hours for 3 days.

Results.—In the in-vivo experiments, scar formation was reduced by exogenous TGF-β. Endogenous TGF-β expression was also increased during labioplasty. In the in vitro experiments, accumulation of type I collagen was reduced by exogenous TGF-β3, which also inhibited alpha-smooth-muscle actin expression. Alpha-smooth-muscle actin is a marker for myofibroblasts. In tandem, TGF-β3 induced the expression and activity of matrix metalloproteinase (MMP)-9.

Conclusions.—TGF-β3 is normally secreted after labioplastic wound healing. An increase of TGF-β3 reduces the deposition of type I collagen by restricting myofibroblast differentiation and collagen synthesis and promoting collagen degradation by MMP-9. The combination of these events results in mediation of reduced scar formation by TGF-β3.

▶ It is noteworthy and exciting to see the elaboration of tissue growth factors that not only accelerate and optimize wound healing, but also harness those that may decrease a certain amount of scarring after procedures. This is most true in cleft lip surgery, which, although successful, still leaves a noticeable scar and reminds the patient and those around him of his condition. I am sure that in the next several years, we will, in fact, be developing growth factors and determining proper dosages and timing in regard to administration of these growth factors to augment, facilitate, and modify wound healing after surgery. Although this article describes the successful administration in an animal model, the human studies are in the not too distant future. Keep posted!

Bruce B. Horswell, MD, DDS, MS

Temporospatial Expression of Vascular Endothelial Growth Factor and Basic Fibroblast Growth Factor During Mandibular Distraction Osteogenesis
Hu J, Zou S, Li J, et al (Sichuan Univ, Chengdu, China)
J Craniomaxillofac Surg 31:238-243, 2003   8–16

Background.—Distraction osteogenesis has become a safe and effective approach to the treatment of select congenital craniofacial deformities or acquired skeletal defects. Studies have suggested that osteogenesis is a vascular-dependent process, and angiogenesis is associated closely with distraction osteogenesis in mandible or limb lengthening. Neovascularization is an essential component of bone formation and remodeling, and osteogenesis may be amplified by endogenous production of angiogenic mediators. The expression patterns of vascular endothelial growth factor (VEGF) and basic fibroblast growth factor (bFGF) in the distracted calluses were investigated after mandibular lengthening in an animal model.

Methods.—Bilateral mandibular osteotomies were performed in 15 young adult goats. After 7 days, the mandibles were elongated by means of custom-made distractors at a rate of 1 mm per day for 10 days. Three animals were distracted at the end of the latency period and at 0, 7, 14, and 28 days after completion of distraction. The lengthened mandibles were then harvested and processed for histologic and immunohistochemical examinations.

Results.—Elevated cellular expression of VEGF and bFGF was observed after mandibular lengthening, along with neovascularization in the distraction gap. VEGF staining was observed in the endothelial cells and osteoblasts, and bFGF staining was observed in the fibroblast-like cells, osteoblasts, and immature osteocytes. The expression of these angiogenic factors was strongest in the first 7 days after the end of distraction and declined with maturation of the newly formed bone.

Conclusion.—This study found a temporal and spatial pattern of VEGF and bFGF expression during distraction osteogenesis in goat mandibles. The findings suggest that distraction forces can stimulate the production of VEGF and bFGF, which contribute to the formation of new bone during gradual distraction of the mandible. Thus it appears that the application of angiogenic factors is a potential method for enhancement of angiogenesis and osteogenesis in osteodistraction, particularly at sites with insufficient vascularization.

▶ Other studies have reported on the elaboration of important growth factors such as VEGF and bFGF during active bone healing and, in particular, distraction osteogenesis. This article goes on to identify the temporal and spatial association of the production of these growth factors during distraction. This is important as it may clue us into when we might harvest these growth factors for their administration, not only during distraction but during any phase of bony healing. I believe that in the next 3 to 5 years many of these growth factors will find their place in our medical armamentarium for rapid predictable and satisfactory wound healing results.

B. B. Horswell, MD, DDS, MS

Pathology

Dedifferentiation of Odontogenic Keratocyst Epithelium After Cyst Decompression
August M, Faquin WC, Troulis MJ, et al (Massachusetts Gen Hosp, Boston; Harvard School of Dental Medicine, Boston; Harvard Med School, Boston)
J Oral Maxillofac Surg 61:678-683, 2003   8–17

Introduction.—Cytokeratin-10 expression by cystic epithelium has been observed in the suprabasilar layers of odontogenic keratocytes (OKCs) but not in dentigerous cysts. Cyst decompression and irrigation produce loss of keratinization. Cytokeratin-10 antibody staining was used to assess changes in OKC epithelium to ascertain whether decompression/irrigation treatment produces an epithelial modulation that may be linked with lower long-term recurrence.

Methods.—Fourteen consecutive patients with biopsy-confirmed OKCs have been treated by compression and longitudinal irrigation between 1997 and the present. The OKCs underwent exteriorization via removal of mucosa and bone. An irrigation port was positioned in the cyst for twice-daily irrigations. At 3-month intervals, panoramic radiographs were taken and cyst-lining cells were obtained and stained for cytokeratin-10. Residual cystectomy was performed when needed, based on clinical and radiographic criteria. The lining was assessed by histologic and immunohistochemical evaluations.

Results.—The mean age of 6 men and 8 women was 32 years. There were 10 mandibular and 4 maxillary cysts. The average irrigation lasted 8.4 months (range, 6-12 months). The mean shrinkage of the radiolucency was 65% (range, 5% to 91%). Cytokeratin-10–positive epithelial cells were detected in all cytologic samples obtained at 3 and 6 months. At the time of cystectomy, 9 of 14 cases were cytokeratin-10–negative and no longer showed histologic characteristics of OKCs. Specimens from the other 5 patients were histologically consistent with OKCs and were cytokeratin-10–positive. The mean treatment times were 7 and 9 months, respectively, for the cytokeratin-10 positive and cytokeratin-10 negative groups.

Conclusion.—Epithelial dedifferentiation and loss of cytokeratin-10 production were seen in 64% of patients treated by cyst decompression/irrigation after an average treatment time of 9 months. Longitudinal follow-up of these patients will ascertain whether this change is linked to lower rates of recurrence versus alternative OKC therapy.

▶ There is some controversy regarding the treatment of OKCs among surgeons. This has to do with the perception that OKCs are both aggressive and tend to recur. The controversy exists regarding radical excision of cysts versus more conservative therapy with either enucleation or marsupialization of the cyst. Both camps are well versed and have produced studies to confirm their perceptions and treatment protocols. This study seeks to identify the pathologic behavior of the OKC by identifying the diminution of cytokeratin-10 in OKCs which have been decompressed or marsupialized. The authors go on to conclude that perhaps this decrease in cytokeratin-10 elaboration results in a more clinically less aggressive OKC, therefore more amenable to conservative modes of treatment. My feeling is that the study will need to be reproduced in other centers with a larger group of patients. Also, we need to identify which OKCs may be "responders" and thus be treated more conservatively.

B. B. Horswell, MD, DDS, MS

The Prognostic Implications of the Surgical Margin in Oral Squamous Cell Carcinoma
Sutton DN, Brown JS, Rogers SN, et al (Univ Hosp Aintree, Liverpool, England)
Int J Oral Maxillofac Surg 32:30-34, 2003   8–18

Introduction.—In the surgical treatment of oral squamous cell carcinoma (OSCC), the primary objective is adequate tumor clearance with a margin of normal tissue. There is a lack of consistency in the literature concerning what constitutes tumor involvement at the resection margin. The factors associated with close and involved surgical margins in the management of OSCC were examined.

Methods.—Two hundred consecutive patients undergoing primary surgery for previously untreated OSCC between 1990 and 1996 provided material for the investigation. All patients underwent clinical examination and either CT or MRI. All patients underwent neck dissection, usually by a "staging" selective procedure; more extensive neck surgery was performed in patients with clinically node-positive necks. Various clinical, operative, and pathologic parameters were related to the status of the surgical margin, along with time to recurrence and survival.

Results.—Of 200 patients evaluated, 107 (53.5%) had clear margins, 84 (42%) had close margins, and 9 (4.5%) were involved. There was a poor correlation between the status of the surgical margins and clinical factors and a high correlation between histologic indicators of aggressive disease and close or involved surgical margins.

Conclusion.—Close margins were strongly correlated with histologic indicators of aggressive disease behavior. Clinical management should reflect these findings.

▶ This is a very nice review article by a well-established head and neck clinic in Liverpool, United Kingdom. The authors are known to be fastidious in their evaluation processes and outcome-based studies. As they correctly point out, those oral cancers that approach the margin on histology (ie, those within 0.5 cm) should be regarded as high indications for aggressive disease which will recur. For these reasons, OSCC continues to require wide margins in those areas where disease is more aggressive, for example, in the base of the tongue, palate, pharynx, etc, and in areas that require close surveillance.

B. B. Horswell, MD, DDS, MS

Is Detection of Oral and Oropharyngeal Squamous Cancer by a Dental Health Care Provider Associated With a Lower Stage at Diagnosis?

Holmes JD, Dierks EJ, Homer LD, et al (Legacy Hosp System, Portland, Ore; Oregon Health Science Univ, Portland)
J Oral Maxillofac Surg 61:285-291, 2003   8–19

Introduction.—Stage at diagnosis is the most critical prognostic indicator for oral and oropharyngeal squamous cell cancers (SCCs). Yet, about 50% of these cancers are detected at stage III or IV. The detection patterns of oral and oropharyngeal SCCs were examined. Detection of SCCs by various health care providers was also assessed to ascertain whether there was an association with a lower stage.

Methods.—Data were obtained by patient interview and medical record audit of 51 consecutive patients with newly diagnosed oral or oropharyngeal SCCs. Patients were queried regarding demographic information and the circumstances surrounding the identification of the lesion. The primary outcome measure was tumor stage grouping, based on detection source.

Results.—The health care providers who detected oral and oropharyngeal SCCs during non–symptom-driven (screening) examinations were dentists, hygienists, oral and maxillofacial surgeons, and a denturist in 1 case. All lesions detected by physicians occurred during a symptom-driven evaluation. Lesions detected during a non–symptom-driven examination were of a statistically significant lower average clinical and pathologic stage (1.7 and 1.6, respectively), compared to lesions during a symptom-directed evaluation (2.6 and 2.5, respectively). A dental office was the most likely source of detection of a lesion during a screening examination ($P = .0006$).

Overall, patients referred from a dental office had a significantly lower stage, compared to those referred from a medical office. Patients who were initially evaluated by a regional specialist (dentist, oral and maxillofacial surgeon, or otolaryngologist) with symptoms related to their lesions were more likely to receive appropriate treatment, compared to those who initially sought care from their primary care provider.

Conclusion.—Overall, the detection of oral and oropharyngeal SCCs during a non–symptom-driven evaluation is correlated with a lower stage at diagnosis and is most likely to occur in a dental office. A regional specialist was more likely than a primary care provider to identify an oral or oropharyngeal SCC and initiate appropriate treatment during the first visit for symptoms associated with the lesion.

▶ The authors have conducted a small study reviewing referral patterns from head and neck cancer seen in their clinic. It was noted—and on a broader scale, this has been confirmed—that dentists who provide good head and neck screen exams as a routine in their offices are those who are primarily the first screeners and detectors of oral cancer. Oral cancer, like colon cancer, has a high survival rate when caught at an early stage. It is unfortunate that oral cancer has not received the press notoriety of colon cancer, with a view toward public education and an increased media profile to encourage thorough oral screening by a dental health provider. Perhaps, as articles like this become more confirmatory and widespread, the message will come across, not only to other dental health professionals but also to our medical colleagues and, in a larger sense, the medical community and public.

B. B. Horswell, MD, DDS, MS

Tongue Piercing and Its Adverse Effects
Shacham R, Zaguri A, Librus HZ, et al (Barzilai Med Ctr, Ashkelon, Israel; Hebrew Univ, Jerusalem)
Oral Surg Oral Med Oral Pathol Oral Radiol Endod 95:274-276, 2003   8–20

Introduction.—Oral piercing is usually performed with no anesthesia or infection control. Piercers are often unlicensed and self-educated and have little clinical or anatomical knowledge. Presented were 3 cases that highlight complications caused by tongue piercing.

Case 1.—Woman, 20, was seen in the emergency department (ED) with pain and swelling in the submental area of 4 days duration. A tongue ornament was in the middle of the anterior third of the tongue, which was swollen, firm, and erythematous, accompanied by elevation of the floor of the mouth. IV Augmentin 1 g × 3/d was administered and the ornament was removed. The infection was completely resolved in 1 week and the patient did not replace the ornament.

Case 2.—Man, 18, was seen in the ED with bleeding from the tongue. He had had his tongue pierced the day before and had experienced slow, active bleeding from the ventral side of the pierced side. The ornament was removed in surgery and coagulation was obtained by electrocautery. The patient was discharged after 2 days of observation.

Case Report 3.—Girl, 16 years, was seen in the ED with tongue pain. She had attempted to remove a barbell-shaped ornament placed 2 years previously. Physical examination revealed a palpable hard swelling mid tongue, and a lateral encephalometric radiograph identified the ornament embedded in the tongue. The ornament was removed and the patient was discharged the next day.

Conclusion.—For patients with an inflamed tongue caused by piercing, the clinician should remove the jewelry, perform a local debridement, institute antibiotic therapy, and administer chlorhexidine mouthwash. Patients need to be monitored closely for infection. The opening in the tongue will spontaneously close.

▶ I have submitted this article because of its obvious interest in our younger population, and I am sure many of us have treated patients with either tongue posts in place or ones that have been removed with the telltale puncture dents in the tongue. Though I have not seen an acute infectious process relating to a tongue post, I have seen significant scarring in the floor of the mouth that resulted in stenosis of the salivary gland ducts and chronic sialadenitis. The involved glands were subsequently removed.

B. B. Horswell, MD, DDS, MS

Juvenile Mandibular Chronic Osteomyelitis: A Distinct Clinical Entity
Heggie AA, Shand JM, Aldred MJ, et al (Royal Children's Hosp of Melbourne, Australia; Univ of Melbourne, Australia; Dorevitch Pathology, Heidelberg, Victoria, Australia)
Int J Oral Maxillofac Surg 32:459-468, 2003   8–21

Introduction.—Sclerosing osteomyelitis of the mandible is a rare disease with unknown cause. Among the recorded cases of sclerosing osteomyelitis in the literature, children have been described in isolated case reports, incorporated within series of adult cases, or included in association with other osteomyelitic syndromes. To date, a specific analysis of a series of pediatric cases has not been reported. Eight females with a distinct mandibular inflammatory disease were evaluated (Table 1).

Methods.—The study included patients from 6 to 12 years old. On initial history and physical examination, all patients reported pain and had recurrent soft-tissue swelling overlying a predominantly unilateral mandibular enlargement (Fig 1). Imaging revealed the deformity was a mixture of patchy sclerosis and radiolucency (Fig 2). An increased erythrocyte sedimentation count was the only consistent serologic finding. Treatment ranged from symptomatic control with nonsteroidal anti-inflammatory medication to surgical management with decortication and contouring; 1 patient underwent resection with reconstruction.

Conclusion.—The early age of onset of the disease process and the uniformity of the features separate this condition from other groups of disorders that, previously, have been collectively designated as chronic diffuse sclerosing osteomyelitis. It is proposed that this inflammatory disease of mandibular bone in the pediatric patient be named as a separate clinical entity: juvenile mandibular chronic osteomyelitis.

TABLE 1.—Presentation and Management of Patients with Juvenile Mandibular Chronic Osteomyelitis

Age at Diagnosis and Sex	History	Presentation	ESR	Management
Case 1 11 yrs F	• Delay of 2 yrs from onset of disease to diagnosis • Courses of antibiotics • Seen by many practitioners	• Intermittent painful right facial swelling / erythema • Right hemi-mandibular involvement • Strongly positive bone scan • Mild to moderate trismus	24	• Decortication, debulking and masseteric myomectomies • Indomethacin 25mg TDS • Right hemimandibulectomy, free flap reconstruction
Case 2 12 yrs F	• Delay of 1 yr from onset of disease to diagnosis • Two courses of A/B • Treated for parotitis	• Intermittent 2 weekly right facial swelling • Right hemi-mandibular involvement • Strongly positive bone scan • Mild trismus	70	• Decortication and debulking • Indomethacin 25mg TDS daily • Episodes of swelling less frequent / reducing in severity
Case 3 12 yrs F	• Onset of symptoms age 9 yrs • Several courses of A/B	• Intermittent 2 monthly episodes left facial swelling • Left hemi-mandibular involvement • Mild trismus	12	• Bone biopsy • Indomethacin 25mg TDS PRN • Regular follow-up
Case 4 9 yrs F	• One month to diagnosis • One course of A/B	• 2 episodes of right facial pain and swelling • Right hemi-mandibular involvement • Moderate trismus	92	• Bone biopsy • Indomethacin 25mg TDS PRN • Regular follow-up
Case 5 11 yrs F	• Facial swelling commenced age 6 yrs • 5 years until diagnosis • Multiple courses A/B including IV, treated for parotitis	• Intermittent right facial swelling and pain • Right hemi-mandibular involvement • Mild trismus • No polyarthralgia or isolated joint involvement	61	• Previous bony biopsy reported as 'fibrous dysplasia' • Indomethacin 25 mg TDS daily • Episodes reducing, mouth opening improving with NSAID therapy
Case 6 7 yrs F	• Facial swelling and pain commenced age 5 yrs • Multiple courses A/B, including IV • Seen by many practitioners	• Intermittent right facial swelling and pain • Right hemi-mandibular involvement • Reviewed by orthopaedic surgeon, no other areas of bony involvement	85	• Two bone biopsies reported as 'low grade chronic osteomyelitis' • Commenced on indomethacin with improvement in symptoms
Case 7 10 yrs F	• Progressive facial swelling and pain • 6 months to diagnosis	• Bony expansion of left hemi-mandible • Trismus, opening 10 mm • Strongly positive bone scan	64	• Initial biopsy reported as fibrous dysplasia • Debulking procedure 6 months after presentation, histology reviewed • Commenced on indomethacin with improvement
Case 8 12 yrs F	• 10 month history of nonresolution of right facial swelling • Course of A/B	• 4 episodes of exacerbation of swelling • Mild pain • Right hemi-mandibular enlargement • Strongly positive bone scan	65	• Bone biopsy • Commenced on indomethacin 25 mg TDS

Abbreviations: ESR, Erythrocyte sedimentation rate mm/h; *A/B,* antibiotic therapy; *NSAID,* nonsteroidal anti-inflammatory drug; *PRN,* as required.
(Courtesy of Heggie AA, Shand JM, Aldred MJ, et al: Juvenile mandibular chronic osteomyelitis: A distinct clinical entity. *Int J Oral Maxillofac Surg* 32:459-468, 2003. Reprinted by permission of Blackwell Publishing.)

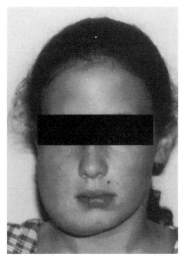

FIGURE 1.—Case 1, frontal view with swelling right facial region. (Courtesy of Heggie AA, Shand JM, Aldred MJ, et al: Juvenile mandibular chronic osteomyelitis: A distinct clinical entity. *Int J Oral Maxillofac Surg* 32:459-468, 2003. Reprinted by permission of Blackwell Publishing.)

▶ This is a review article written by authors with whom I am familiar and from a well-renowned institution. This describes an entity that is not commonly seen nor clearly delineated as to its diagnosis and treatment. For this reason, I believe that dentists and surgeons would be well served in having some familiarity with juvenile mandibular chronic osteomyelitis. I have had 2 female children in my clinical experience who have had similar entities, and whom I felt had this disease process. Indeed, it is a chronic and frustrating lesion to bring

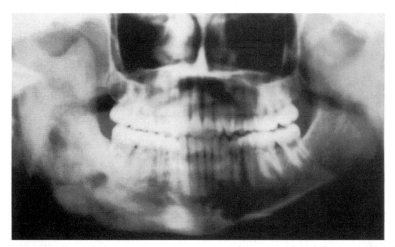

FIGURE 2.—Case 1, Orthopantomogram demonstrating enlargement of the right hemi-mandible, with patchy radiolucency and radiopacity. (Courtesy of Heggie AA, Shand JM, Aldred MJ, et al: Juvenile mandibular chronic osteomyelitis: A distinct clinical entity. *Int J Oral Maxillofac Surg* 32:459-468, 2003. Reprinted by permission of Blackwell Publishing.)

under control, both in alleviating symptoms and in achieving resolution of the deforming process. I agree that oftentimes the less-involved lesion will respond to conservative medical management with NSAIDs after ruling out other pathologic processes through biopsy, as indicated. For those patients with more deforming and symptomatic lesions, early resection with a view toward limited reconstruction will provide a "cure" in the child patient. I refer the reader to Table 1 for the review of this study's patient log, as well as to Figs 1 and 2, which demonstrate the clinical entity.

B. B. Horswell, MD, DDS, MS

Extent of Extracapsular Spread: A Critical Prognosticator in Oral Tongue Cancer

Greenberg JS, Fowler R, Gomez J, et al (Baylor College of Medicine, Houston; Univ of Texas, Houston)
Cancer 97:1464-1470, 2003   8–22

Background.—Patients with squamous cell carcinoma of the oral tongue (SCCOT) have a high rate of occult nodal metastases, ranging from 20% to 40%, without clinical or radiographic evidence of regional spreading. Evidence indicating regional nodal metastases shows a relationship with a marked decrease in both overall and disease-specific survival rates; further decreases of survival occur if extracapsular spreading (ECS) is also present, and ECS has been linked to an increased incidence of regional recurrence and distant metastases. In one investigation, a high percentage of patients who had ECS and who had received adjuvant radiotherapy still had a regional recurrence rate exceeding 33%, which suggests that more intense adjuvant therapy may be in order, including systemic chemotherapy, biological therapy plus irradiation, or both. The outcomes of patients with ECS, in terms of overall and disease-specific survival and whether distant metastases occurred, were assessed to determine whether the degree of ECS affects distant metastasis rates and survival.

Methods.—The 266 patients underwent treatment of SCCOT involving surgery with or without adjuvant radiotherapy in a tertiary care center. Histopathologic evaluation determined the extent of ECS in involved lymph nodes, as determined by measurement from the capsular margin to the farthest perinodal extension. Results in terms of the extent of ECS and the number of lymph nodes exhibiting pathologic characteristics with or without ECS were assessed for disease-free interval, survival rates, and presence of distant metastases.

Results.—Patients were divided into those whose ECS was 2 mm or less and those whose ECS was more than 2 mm; no difference in survival rates was noted between the 2 groups. A significantly poorer prognosis was obtained for patients who had more than 1 ECS-positive node; most patients died within 1 year of treatment. The disease-specific and overall survival rates were markedly worse for patients who had multiple nodes that were ECS positive: these patients had an extremely brief disease-free interval and a median time to recurrence of 6 months. Regardless of ECS status, the outcomes for patients with 2 or more positive lymph nodes were worse in terms of disease-specific and overall survival rates. Patients who had multiple positive nodes had more ECS than did patients who had a solitary positive node. Patients with multiple nodes that were ECS positive had the worst prognosis and lowest survival rates.

Conclusions.—Patients with SCCOT who had ECS and multiple nodes with or without ECS had both poor survival and early recurrence rates for their disease. Treatment failure rates are high; therefore, therapy intensification may be warranted.

▶ Head and neck cancer has met with very little improvement in terms of survival over the last decades. This has to do with late detection of disease and the sometimes difficulty in control of local aggressive disease. This article nicely demonstrates that the presence of extracapsular spread or involvement in multiple lymph nodes portends a poor prognostic indicator for the patient. Patients who present with oral squamous cell carcinoma where metastatic disease has spread outside of the capsular node or in multiple lymph nodes require initial aggressive adjuvant therapy. As suggested, this may qualify these patients for clinical trials that intensify and redirect adjuvant therapy as indicated.

B. B. Horswell, MD, DDS, MS

Oral Cancer: Material Deprivation, Unemployment and Risk Factor Behaviour—An Initial Study
Greenwood M, Thomson PJ, Lowry RJ, et al (Univ of Newcastle upon Tyne, England)
Int J Oral Maxillofac Surg 32:74-77, 2003   8–23

Background.—Regional variations in the incidence of oral cancer may be associated with material deprivation, or lower socioeconomic status. In England and Wales a distinct North-South gradient is discernible in the incidence of oral cancer, with higher rates observed in the North. It has been suggested that this difference may be due in part to material deprivation. Consumption of both tobacco and alcohol has been shown to increase with deprivation, and both are risk factors for oral cancer. However, it is not known whether material deprivation is itself a risk factor for oral cancer or whether it reflects lifestyles that involve greater exposure to risk factors for oral cancer. The purpose of this study was to identify an index of material deprivation, employment history, smoking, and alcohol consumption among a population of patients with oral cancer.

Methods.—This prospective case-control study included 100 consecutive patients with oral cancer of various stages and grades. These patients were matched by age and sex with control subjects with no history of oral cancer. Patients and control subjects were asked to complete a questionnaire regarding prediagnosis smoking and alcohol consumption. Patients were assigned to a Carstairs Deprivation category ranging from 1 (least deprived) to 5 (most deprived), with categories derived from census data regarding occupational social class, car ownership, home overcrowding, and the proportion of residents unemployed.

Results.—There was a statistically significant trend for patients to come from the most materially deprived groups. Two thirds of the patients (66%) had experienced long-term unemployment. However, the high proportion of patients with long-term unemployment was not statistically significant when multivariate analysis adjusted for the confounding effects of smoking and alcohol use.

Conclusion.—There was a distinct trend toward patients with oral cancer coming from the most materially deprived segments of society. However, after adjustment for the confounding effects of alcohol and tobacco use, it was not possible to determine the strength of the association between oral cancer and each risk factor. These findings suggest that high alcohol consumption and smoking are the most important risk factors for oral cancer, but the possible association with long-term unemployment requires further investigation.

▶ This is a most interesting survey questionnaire study conducted by a head and neck surgical unit in the United Kingdom which sought to identify risk factors in terms of socioeconomic status and the incidence of oral cancer. The long-established association of smoking and alcohol is well known for oropharyngeal cancer, but this study also investigates duration of unemployment and low socioeconomic status.

It was interesting to note that when the confounding factors of smoking and alcohol were removed, the incidence of cancer was still higher amongst the lower economic classes. This most likely relates to a combination of seeking health care at a later stage of signs or symptoms, poor health habits as relates to diet and exercise, and inconsistent presentation for management once a diagnosis is made. Although no studies have been done in the Appalachian region where I practice, I would not be surprised if the same factors and challenges faced our population in regard to development of head and neck cancer.

B. B. Horswell, MD, DDS, MS

Pediatric

Stability Consideration for Internal Maxillary Distractors
Cheung LK, Zhang Q, Wong MCM, et al (Univ of Hong Kong; Polytechnic Univ of Hong Kong; Queen Mary Hosp, Hong Kong)
J Craniomaxillofac Surg 31:142-148, 2003   8–24

Introduction.—To secure sound fixation for distraction osteogenesis, it is crucial to carefully evaluate both the implants and the implant sites. For bone-bone distractors applied to the maxilla, anatomical considerations need to be taken in order to optimize favorable fixation. The holding strengths of various fixation systems for maxillary distraction in various locations in the midfacial skeleton were studied.

Methods.—Cross-sectional images of 10 dry human skulls were obtained by CT. Bone thickness of the maxillae was measured in 5 anatomical regions: paranasal, infra-orbital, posterior sinus wall, zygomatic, and alveolar. Screws of 1.5 and 2 mm diameter and 3-screw mini-plates in triangular and straight configurations were assessed for holding strength by pull-out tests on fresh animal bone cortices of defined thickness.

Results.—The thickest cortical bone was observed in the paranasal and zygomatic regions. The next thickest was the alveolar region (2 mm). In bones of 2 mm and 4 mm thickness, the 2-mm screws were stronger than the 1.5-mm screws in pull-out tests. The pull-out behavior of screws of various diameters in 1-mm–thick bones and both configurations of mini-plates showed no significant differences.

Conclusion.—The paranasal and zygomatic bones are the thickest for fixation of internal maxillary distractors. Fixation screws of 2-mm diameter in either triangular or straight mini-plates can provide good stabilization for distractors.

▶ For those of us who have been utilizing distraction osteogenesis for correction of maxillomandibular defects and asymmetries, we have long been challenged with finding adequate fixation bone for the placement of distractors, particularly in the maxilla. This is a small but nice study which correctly confirms that the locations in the mid face for placement of fixation foot plates are the zygomatic buttress regions, paranasal rims, and infraorbital rims. This agrees with my experience in placement of internal maxillary distractors. The challenge arises when placing these in children, who have various degrees of mid face hypoplasia such as in the cleft lip and palate deformity, where thin bone around the paranasal region or missing bone may be the situation.

B. B. Horswell, MD, DDS, MS

Dento-Alveolar Development in Unilateral Cleft Lip, Alveolus and Palate
Noguchi M, Suda Y, Ito S, et al (Sapporo Med Univ, Japan)
J Craniomaxillofac Surg 31:137-141, 2003   8–25

Introduction.—Surgical intervention in the maxilla, especially the alveolar process, has an important role in growth inhibition of the maxilla in patients with cleft palate. Dentoalveolar development of the permanent dentition and morphology of the palate after 2 types of palatoplasty (supraperiosteal [SP] flap vs mucoperiosteal [MP] flap) was examined in patients with unilateral, cleft of the lip, alveolus, and palate in a cross-sectional investigation.

Methods.—Of 38 patients born between 1976 and 1983 with a complete cleft lip, alveolus, and palate, 15 were treated with SP flaps and 23 were treated with MP flaps. Dental casts of Hellman's dental stage IV A (14-18 years of age) were used for each participant. Distances measured were transverse distance C-C', transverse distance M-M', palatal length, and palatal height.

Results.—No statistically significant differences were observed between the SP and MP groups in measures of C-C' or M-M'. Palatal length ($P < .017$) and palatal height ($P < .001$) were significantly greater in the SP group than in the MP group.

Conclusion.—It is premature to consider this data definitive. It appears that less invasive surgical intervention in the area of the alveolar crest is advantageous for palatal development.

▶ The cleft mid face deformity is felt to be due to extensive palatal periosteal elevation and denudation of the palate during initial repair. As this article suggests, complete elevation of the mucoperiosteum with exposure of the palatal bone predisposes the palate to significant scarring, with decreased development in the anteroposterior and horizontal dimensions. The article suggests that leaving some of the periosteum attached will result in more normal development of the dentoalveolar complex and transverse dimension of the maxillary arch. This has also been established in some animal studies and is nicely confirmed in this small cleft palate unit in Japan. The challenge is to achieve adequate palatal closure of the cleft defect while also maintaining a well-vascularized periosteum.

B. B. Horswell, MD, DDS, MS

Preliminary Results of Standardized Occipital Advancement in the Treatment of Lambdoid Synostosis
Zöller JE, Mischkowski RA, Speder B (Univ of Cologne, Köln, Germany)
J Craniomaxillofac Surg 30:343-348, 2002   8–26

Introduction.—Lambdoid suture synostosis is seen occurring unilaterally, bilaterally, or in combination with other forms of craniosynostosis. A method of occipital advancement for correcting lambdoid suture synostosis is discussed.

Methods.—The technique of occipital advancement consists of osteotomy, removal, and reshaping of the calvarial bone segments, which are then replaced to achieve an "advancement" of the occipital region. Artificial sutures are constructed as a result of the osteotomy. Intraoperative remodeling provides a well-proportioned skull shape, and advancement provides an increase in intracranial volume for brain growth.

Results.—Standardized occipital advancement was performed in 21 patients treated in a multidisciplinary center. Patients were from 5 to 28 months old at the time of surgery. An esthetically satisfactory skull shape and normalization of the intracranial pressure was achieved. One patient experienced a life-threatening intraoperative hemorrhage.

Conclusion.—Standardized occipital advancement allows precise, reproducible and predictable positioning of the calvarial bone segments. Remodeling through brain growth produces a well-proportioned skull shape. Posterior advancement produces an increase in intracranial volume.

▶ As a craniofacial surgeon, I am always interested in any new techniques regarding surgical correction of craniofacial deformities. Unilateral lambdoidal synostosis, which results in unilateral flattening of the back of the head, is usually well tolerated as other than a mild deformity. It is noted more in infancy and oftentimes is not seen as an entity necessary for surgical treatment here in the United States. Where there is bilateral involvement, then this will adversely impact the developing calvarial vault with perhaps increased intracranial pressures. One must be sure that they are, indeed, dealing with synostosis where the sutures have fused prematurely and not deformational plagiocephaly, which results from supine positioning and *not* synostosis. Synostosis will usually be manifest on a CT scan. Deformational plagiocephaly will usually correct itself with physical therapy modalities and/or cranial remodeling devices.

B. B. Horswell, MD, DDS, MS

Le Fort III Osteotomy: A New Internal Positioned Distractor
Riediger D, Poukens JMN (Univ Hosp Maastricht, The Netherlands)
J Oral Maxillofac Surg 61:882-889, 2003   8–27

Background.—The treatment of patients with severe midfacial hypoplasia is a continuing problem in craniomaxillofacial surgery. The Le Fort III osteotomy and other surgical procedures may provide a solution for these patients, but antero-inferior displacement may be restricted because of anatomical limitations and retromaxillary scar formation in conventional Le Fort III surgery. Distraction osteogenesis has become an accepted, and in many cases, a preferred technique for the treatment of severe midfacial hy-

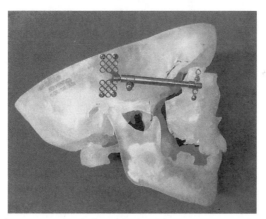

FIGURE 5.—The osteotomy and distraction procedure is preoperatively simulated on the stereolithographic model. The translation of the osteotomized bone segment and the resulting occlusion can be evaluated. (Courtesy of Riediger D, Poukens JMN: Le Fort III osteotomy: A new internal positioned distractor. *J Oral Maxillofac Surg* 61:882-889, 2003.)

poplasia; however the distraction devices currently available have several disadvantages. To address these issues, a new internal and temporal positioned distraction device has been developed. The initial findings with use of this new distractor device for patients undergoing Le Fort III osteotomy are presented.

Methods.—This new internal position distractor device was used in 5 patients, 8 to 15 years old, who were undergoing Le Fort III osteotomy (Fig 5). Nine distractors were used in 4 patients with midfacial retrusion and in 1 patient with hemifacial microsomia.

Results.—No complications were noted in obtaining the preoperative planned position of the osteotomized Le Fort III segment. The distractor was activated by rotation of a small lateral activation rod (Fig 9). Midface advancement, which was measured as anterior displacement of the infraorbital rim, ranged from 14 to 20 mm (Fig 11). The distractor was nearly invisible, and the daily activities of the patients were not disrupted by the presence of the distractor.

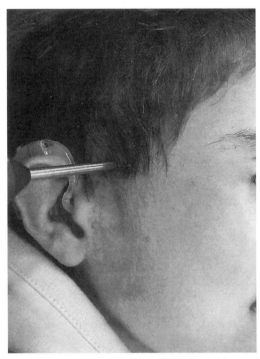

FIGURE 9.—Activation at the right side with the mounted screwdriver in the preauricular region. (Courtesy of Riediger D, Poukens JMN: Le Fort III osteotomy: A new internal positioned distractor. *J Oral Maxillofac Surg* 61:882-889, 2003.)

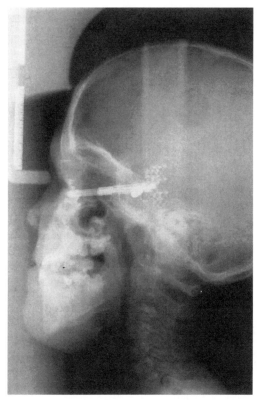

FIGURE 11.—Lateral cephalogram at the end of the distraction procedure. The teeth show an almost end-to-end bite in the front region. The distractor devices have almost reached their maximal distraction capacity. (Courtesy of Riediger D, Poukens JMN: Le Fort III osteotomy: A new internal positioned distractor. *J Oral Maxillofac Surg* 61:882-889, 2003.)

Conclusions.—This new internal distractor device is a promising development in the treatment of patients with midfacial retrusion. Further studies in a larger series of patients are warranted.

▶ As a craniofacial surgeon, I am very interested in those procedures that can effectively advance the midface in children. Internal distraction is a key component in management of these children, particularly those with severe craniofacial midface hypoplasia and/or cleft lip and palate deformities. Although the external distraction devices are very effective, easy to place, and easy to care for, their one major drawback is the wearing of a large obvious external apparatus, which is cumbersome for the child and somewhat of a social inhibitor, particularly for those children in school. For this reason, internal distractors, such as illustrated in this article (note Figs 5, 9, and 11) are placed via a craniofacial approach under the scalp and facial soft tissues. The devices are easily distracted at home by caregivers as the ports are external, are hidden in the hairline most of the time, and are more hygienic, as they can be cared for with local cleansing techniques.

B. B. Horswell, MD, DDS, MS

Complications in Bilateral Mandibular Distraction Osteogenesis Using Internal Devices
van Strijen PJ, Breuning KH, Becking AG, et al (Gelderse Vallei Hosp, Ede, The Netherlands; Tiel, The Netherlands; VU Med Centre/ACTA, Amsterdam)
Oral Surg Oral Med Oral Pathol Oral Radiol Endod 96:392-397, 2003   8–28

Background.—The use of distraction osteogenesis as an alternative to conventional surgery has resulted in the publication of several reports on the biology of the distraction process, its technical aspects, and indications and costs. There is ongoing controversy regarding the viability of distraction osteogenesis as a justifiable alternative to bilateral sagittal split osteotomy. The potential for distraction osteogenesis was explored as an alternative to conventional bilateral sagittal split osteotomy through a retrospective evaluation of complications encountered with this procedure.

Methods.—A total of 70 consecutive patients, including 40 males and 30 females, aged 11 to 37 years (mean, 14 years) underwent distraction osteogenesis for lengthening of the mandible. Surgery was performed with the patient under general anesthesia. After the osteotomy was performed, 2 intraoral monodirectional distraction devices were positioned on the mandibular cortex in the third molar region. The rate of distraction was 1 mm per day. The various complications that developed during all phases of the distraction procedure were recorded.

Results.—There were 28 instances of complications in the 70 procedures performed (40%). The complications were both technique- and device-related, and all occurred early in the learning period. Infection developed in 5 patients (7.1%), and prolonged sensory loss in the distribution of the alveolar nerve occurred in 3 patients (4.3%). Severe complications occurred in 6 patients (8.6%), and rehospitalization was necessary for 5 patients (7.1%), of whom 4 (5.7% of the series) required additional surgery.

Conclusion.—Distraction osteogenesis is a safe and predictable procedure for lengthening of the mandible, with a low incidence of major complications. The rate of infection and incidence of damage to the inferior alveolar nerve are low. The success of this procedure depends in large measure on the compliance of both patients and parents throughout the entire treatment period.

▶ With the advent of distraction osteogenesis for the facial skeleton, and particularly the mandible, many of us have discovered challenges and complications regarding its application. This article reviews the authors' experience in a busy maxillofacial unit in Europe. I have had similar experiences in regard to placement of internal mandibular distractors regarding incomplete fracture of the segments, which may result in return to the operating room to more completely obtain an osteotomy in order for the device to begin distraction.

I have not had any observed infections as compared to the authors' experience where 7% of the patients had infections requiring antibiotics. The greatest number of complications seem to be related to a technique or the devices utilized, and this speaks to the learning curve that we all have experienced in utilizing distraction devices, particularly the internal distractors which require more precise surgical technique and placement of the devices. As mentioned in other reviews, distractors are here to stay, and therefore we need to be aware of their indications, application, and perioperative challenges.

B. B. Horswell, MD, DDS, MS

Analysis of Bone Resorption After Secondary Alveolar Cleft Bone Grafts Before and After Canine Eruption in Connection With Orthodontic Gap Closure or Prosthodontic Treatment
Schultze-Mosgau S, Nkenke E, Schlegel AK, et al (Univ of Erlangen-Nuremberg, Germany)
J Oral Maxillofac Surg 61:1245-1248, 2003   8–29

Background.—The treatment of patients with clefts of the lip, alveolus, or palate requires a multimodal approach involving surgery, orthodontia, audiology, and dental care. The timing for secondary bone grafts/osteoplasties is often dependent on the stage of canine eruption. However, the optimal timing of the secondary grafts in relation to the eruption of canine teeth has not been resolved, and previous studies have not taken into account the influence of orthodontic gap closures or openings. The success rate of secondary alveolar cleft lip bone grafts before and after canine eruption was evaluated in connection with orthodontic gap closure and gap opening.

Methods.—Sixty-eight secondary alveolar cleft defects grafted with iliac crest marrow were performed in 57 patients with 11 bilateral and 46 unilateral clefts of the lip, alveolus, or palate. The mean age of the patients was 9 years, with an age range of 8 to 11 years. Gap closures were carried out after 53 bone grafts (78%), and gap openings with subsequent dental implants were performed with 15 bone grafts (22%). The parameters for success are determined by orthopantomograms at surgery and at follow-up examination were bone resorption in relation to the interdental height of the alveolar process in the vicinity of the cleft and root growth of the teeth in the vicinity of the cleft. Resorption grades I and II were considered successful.

Results.—The overall success rate was 88%, with resorption at grade I in 69% of patients, grade II in 19%, grade III in 10%, and grade IV in 1%. At osteoplasty, the root growth of the tooth in the immediate vicinity of the cleft was fully complete in 27 teeth (39%), 75% complete in 23 teeth (26.5%), and semicomplete in 18 teeth (33.8%). Twelve teeth (18%) in the vicinity of the cleft remained unerupted and displaced after the surgery. In these patients, the teeth were surgically exposed to reposition them orthodontically. Resorption losses were significantly lower with gap closures than with gap openings; however, bone grafts performed before eruption of the canine teeth were intended mainly to accomplish orthodontic gap closure, unlike those grafts performed after canine eruption.

Conclusion.—In this study of secondary alveolar cleft bone grafts, the exact timing of surgery in regard to canine eruption was a secondary consideration. It was found that gap closures provide more favorable results than do gap openings in terms of resorption and that graft resorption is reduced by controlled dental eruptions or orthodontic gap closures.

▶ As a cleft surgeon, I am often confronted with the problem of resorption after placement of a bone graft in an alveolar cleft defect, which this article addresses in a small and concise study. The authors discovered that bringing functional teeth or loading into the grafted defect or orthodontic closure is of benefit in order to maintain the grafted bone height in the long term. Other studies[1,2] have indicated that functional loading of a grafted defect does maintain satisfactory height, whereas if the grafted defect is not functionally loaded with either teeth or a prosthetic appliance (optimally an endosseous implant), then bone is gradually remodeled, particularly after 1 year. It is my aim to bring the grafted defect under function within 6 months after bone placement.

B. B. Horswell, MD, DDS, MS

References

1. Collins M, James DR, Mars M: Alveolar bone grafting: A review of 115 patients. *Eur J Orthod* 20:115-120, 1998.
2. Long RE Jr, Paterno M, Vinson B: Effect of cuspid positioning in the cleft at the time of secondary alveolar bone grafting. *Cleft Palate Craniofac J* 33:225-320, 1996.

Outcome of Bone Grafting in Relation to Cleft Width in Unilateral Cleft Lip and Palate Patients

van der Meij AJW, Baart JA, Prahl-Andersen B, et al (Vrije Universiteit, Amsterdam)
Oral Surg Oral Med Oral Pathol Oral Radiol Endod 96:19-25, 2003   8–30

Background.—There are a variety of treatment options for patients with cleft lip and palate. Closure of the lip and soft palate at a young age is recommended, but there is disagreement in the literature as to the optimal age of closure of the alveolar cleft and hard palate. For bone grafting, the symphyseal area of the mandible, the iliac crest, calvaria, or the tibia may function as the donor site. The outcome of the bone graft is dependent on many factors that may directly or indirectly influence the resorption of the transplanted bone. The relationship between the cleft width and the residual amount of bone after bone grafting was evaluated in 53 patients with unilateral cleft lip and palate.

Methods.—Early secondary bone grafting before the eruption of the permanent canine teeth was performed in 26 patients with a median age of 9 years 5 months. Late secondary bone grafting after the eruption of the permanent canine teeth was performed in 16 patients with a median age of 13 years 3 months. Bone grafting was performed at a later stage (tertiary bone grafting) in 11 patients with a median age of 20 years 2 months.

The fate of the grafts was determined by the residual amount of bone calculated from CT scans performed immediately after surgery and at 1 year postoperatively. The initial width of the cleft was measured on the CT scans obtained immediately after bone grafting.

Results.—The average width of the cleft was 6.4 mm, with a range of 3.0 to 12.2 mm. The average amount of residual bone in the cleft area after 1 year was 64% of the initial graft. Linear regression analysis showed that a significant correlation existed for cleft width in relation to the percentage of residual bone after 1 year.

Conclusion.—Regression analysis of the outcomes of bone grafting in relation to cleft width demonstrated that there is a relationship between cleft width and the fate of the bone graft. Grafts in wider clefts are more likely to resorb than bone grafts in narrower clefts.

▶ As many of us have observed in cleft defect reconstruction, this article substantiates the association between wide cleft defects and bone graft resorption. This resorption increases when examined 1 year after placement of bone graft, as suggested also by the previous article by Schultze-Mosgau et al (Abstract 8–29). These and other studies suggest that cleft defect preparation by creating a more narrow defect with placement at an earlier age (5-7 years of age, if possible) and functional loading of the defect within a year after placement are predictors for a successful and long-term bone graft.

B. B. Horswell, MD, DDS, MS

Secondary Osteoplasty of the Alveolar Cleft Defect
Horswell BB, Henderson JM (Charleston Area Med Ctr, WVa)
J Oral Maxillofac Surg 61:1082-1090, 2003   8–31

Background.—Reconstruction of the alveolar cleft defect (ACD) has been controversial since 1955, when the first bone graft series was reported. Hundreds of studies have addressed issues such as perioperative orthopedics, timing of osteoplasty (bone grafting), types of grafts, simultaneous procedures, and other issues involved in ACD reconstruction. The controversy that surrounds the timing of ACD repair was discussed, with commentary on various types of bone grafts.

Overview.—Early secondary osteoplasty, which involves bone repair of the ACD when the patient is approximately 5 to 8 years of age, is considered the optimal cleft management. While there was early enthusiasm for primary osteoplasty, the secondary osteoplasty for ACD repair is now considered the gold standard and has provided a foundational support for cleft management. Among the benefits of secondary osteoplasty are maxillary

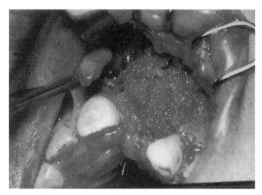

FIGURE 3.—Cleft defect filled with cancellous bone, condensed against repaired nasal floor. (Reprinted from Horswell BB, Henderson JM: Secondary osteoplasty of the alveolar cleft defect. *J Oral Maxillofac Surg* 61:1082-1090, 2003. Copyright 2003, with permission from the American Association of Oral and Maxillofacial Surgeons.)

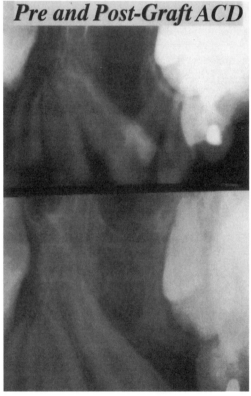

FIGURE 4.—Radiographs of alveolar cleft defect without preoperative orthodontic preparation. There is good bony fill and apparent osseous support for the teeth; however, postoperative arch expansion may result in some loss of alveolar height. (Reprinted from Horswell BB, Henderson JM: Secondary osteoplasty of the alveolar cleft defect. *J Oral Maxillofac Surg* 61:1082-1090, 2003. Copyright 2003, with permission from the American Association of Oral and Maxillofacial Surgeons.)

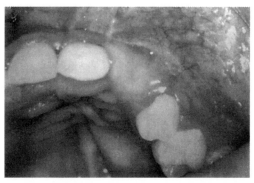

FIGURE 5.—Post graft alveolar cleft defect with good alveolar morphology and covered with healthy mucoperiosteum. This region should be functionally restored within 1 year to maintain alveolar bulk and height. (Reprinted from Horswell BB, Henderson JM: Secondary osteoplasty of the alveolar cleft defect. *J Oral Maxillofac Surg* 61:1082-1090, 2003. Copyright 2003, with permission from the American Association of Oral and Maxillofacial Surgeons.)

arch continuity, bone support for dentition, elimination of oronasal fistulas, ideal alveolar morphology, and facial growth (Figs 3 to 5).

Most bone grafts to the ACD have been particulate marrow harvested from the anterior iliac crest and represent the standard graft to which other materials are compared. Other sources have included the rib, tibia, calvarium, and mandible. New graft materials composed of resorbable and nonresorbable bone have been extensively studied. However, the unpredictability of resorption or the amount of bone formed has limited the use of the materials to late secondary osteoplasty or to adult patients with minor alveolar deficiency.

Recent animal studies have reported that bone defects can be reliably repaired with recombinant human bone morphogenetic protein. When appropriate dosing regimens are established, this material may replace autogenous bone as the ideal material. One of the most important factors in secondary osteoplasty is preparation of the recipient site. This requires the presence of sound dentition free of disease; healthy mucogingiva; a demonstrated ability of the patient (or parents) to maintain satisfactory oral hygiene; and control of nasal-sinus discharge through cleansing nasal sprays, decongestants, antihistamines, and aerosolized topical steroids, as indicated.

Conclusion.—This review of secondary osteoplasty addressed the indications for and benefits of autogenous bone repair. In the future, cleft reconstruction will focus on the development of graft substitutes that contain bone morphogenetic protein and can be safely and easily introduced during primary cheilorhinoplasty.

▶ This third article in regard to bone grafting of the ACD is one written by myself, and this is a review article of the literature examining bone graft placement during the mixed dentition years. It has been my experience, as well as many others in the cleft management world, that placement of autogenous bone in the well-prepared ACD in the early mixed dentition years provides for a predictable and satisfying result. This is demonstrated in Figs 3, 4, and 5 of the article. As I mentioned at the end of the article, most likely in several years autogenous bone graft will not be utilized, but rather we will see the elaboration of important growth factors to be placed in the defect at the appropriate time.

B. B. Horswell, MD, DDS, MS

9 Oral Medicine and Oral Pathology

Introduction

Oral Medicine and Oral Pathology are 2 inexorably intertwined disciplines that complement each other and complete the spectrum of etiology, pathogenesis, diagnosis, therapy, and management of oral disease. As a new section that spans such a wide variety of topics, a number of areas have been addressed, including the future of oral and maxillofacial pathology as a specialty, head and neck malignancies and their relationship to various etiologic factors and conditions, oral complications of immune dysfunction from various causes, and other topics of current interest in the practice of dentistry.

The goal of this chapter is to provide a potpourri of current literature in the hope that the readers will not only encounter new literature regarding topics with which they are already familiar, but also manuscripts that redirect their interest to new and different areas of the profession with which they are less familiar.

Denis P. Lynch, DDS, PhD

The Future of Oral and Maxillofacial Pathology
Wrights JM, Vincent SD, Muller S, et al (Baylor College of Dentistry, Dallas; Univ of Iowa, Iowa City; Emory Univ, Atlanta, Ga; et al)
Oral Surg Oral Med Oral Pathol Oral Radiol Endod 96:176-186, 2003   9–1

Introduction.—Findings from a survey of residents and recent postgraduates of oral and maxillofacial pathology (OMP) programs and results from the Long-Range Planning Committee (LRPC) of the American Academy of Oral and Maxillofacial Pathology (AAOMP) were reported at the annual meeting of the AAOMP, April 20 to 24, 2002, in New Orleans, Louisiana. Survey results were reported to help guide recommendations of the LRPC in charting the future direction of the Academy.

Methods.—One survey was for OMP graduates who had finished academic education since 1992, and one was for presently enrolled residents. The first halves of both surveys were similar. Questions regarding employment were directed only to OMP graduates. Residents were asked to project what they considered themselves doing after graduation. Surveys were mailed on September 4, 2001; the deadline for inclusion was January 2, 2002. The resident survey was mailed directly to the resident director to be administered to current residents.

Results.—Of 65 surveys mailed to postgraduates, there were 49 responses (75% response rate). The resident survey response rate was 100%. Respondents from both surveys indicated an interest in programs that offer an MD option. Opportunities for head and neck pathology fellowships generated favorable responses from both groups. There was a tendency of current residents to delay entry into OMP education, compared with postgraduates. Most current residents began residency programs within 4 years after dental school education. Among postgraduates, 84% practiced OMP in a dental school, a hospital, or a private practice. Respondents who had an active private clinical oral pathology patient practice were the exception. More than 50% of respondents did not see patients; only 4 oral and maxillofacial pathologists saw more than 30 patients a month. It was not possible to ascertain from survey results why patient consultation was not more common. The primary hindrance to a career in OMP was lack of job opportunities and low salaries.

Conclusion.—These perceptions have affected recruitment of new residents and have contributed to a recent decrease in the number of advanced education programs. The AAOMP must address the dilemma of employment opportunities in order to recruit qualified residents and employ graduates of OMP programs.

▶ As one of the smaller recognized specialties in dentistry with a primarily academically based membership, OMP continues to grapple with its changing identity, its role in contemporary dental practice, and its relationship with medicine. This article represents the summary of a symposium held at the most recent annual meeting of the AAOMP.

Oral and maxillofacial pathologists are currently finding that traditional academic positions are becoming increasingly difficult to identify. Newer generations of oral and maxillofacial pathologists are expanding their repertoire of skills and abilities to include fundable research, clinical practice within the scope of OMP (oral medicine), and hospital-based clinical and laboratory practices. The majority of oral and maxillofacial pathologists do not feel that an MD degree is necessary for practicing OMP and that it might be detrimental to the long-term vitality of the specialty.

D. P. Lynch, DDS, PhD

Factors Affecting Survival in Maxillary Sinus Cancer

Bhattacharyya N (Harvard Med School, Boston)
J Oral Maxillofac Surg 61:1016-1021, 2003   9–2

Introduction.—Malignancies of the nasal cavity and paranasal sinuses comprise a small proportion of newly diagnosed cancers every year. The Surveillance, Epidemiology, and End Results (SEER) database, which is maintained and rigorously updated by the National Cancer Institute, was reviewed to better delineate clinical trends and prognostic variables in maxillary sinus cancer.

Methods.—Cases of maxillary sinus malignancy from the SEER database from 1988 to 1998 were examined. Cases with distant metastatic disease were not included. Clinical data including tumor histology, grade and stage, and extent of surgery and radiation therapy were recorded. Kaplan-Meier survival and Cox proportional hazards analyses were performed to ascertain the influence of these factors on overall survival.

Results.—A total of 650 patients with maxillary sinus cancer (mean age, 64 years; male-to-female ratio, 3:2) were evaluated. The most frequently identified histology was squamous cell carcinoma (61.7%), followed by adenoid cystic carcinoma (9.8%). The overall mean survival was 52 months. On initial examination, 77.5% of patients had advanced (T3/T4) disease, and 7.4% had cervical metastasis. A total of 441 patients (67.9%) underwent radiation therapy, which significantly improved survival in patients with T4 lesions. Multivariate analysis revealed that increasing age, T stage, N stage, and tumor grade independently predicted poor survival. Gender was not predictive of survival. Adenoid cystic carcinoma was linked with significantly improved overall survival ($P < .001$).

Conclusion.—Survival in patients with maxillary sinus cancer is ascertained by TNM staging, histology, and grade. TNM staging can effectively stratify patients according to survival.

▶ When most dental health care providers think about "oral cancer," they instinctively associate that entity with squamous cell carcinoma of the lower lip, ventral lateral tongue, and floor of the mouth. This article is included for review because it illustrates that other oral malignancies must be considered within the diagnostic, if not therapeutic, realm of dentistry. The author reviews a 10-year history of maxillary sinus cancer from the SEER database of the National Cancer Institute. While the most common maxillary sinus cancer is squamous cell carcinoma, various adenocarcinomas, sarcomas, and melanomas have been reported in the same anatomic sight.

The 5-year survival rate for maxillary sinus cancer is low (<50%), with patients exhibiting advanced disease at the time of their initial diagnosis. As with any other malignancy, early diagnosis translates into increased long-term survival. It is important for dentists to appreciate the possible ominous implications of persistent unilateral nasal obstruction, discharge, cheek pain, and radiographic changes in the maxillary sinus that may be initially attributable to odontogenic infection.

D. P. Lynch, DDS, PhD

Alcohol-Containing Mouthwash and Oropharyngeal Cancer: A Review of the Epidemiology

Cole P, Rodu B, Mathisen A (Univ of Alabama, Birmingham)
J Am Dent Assoc 134:1079-1087, 2003   9–3

Introduction.—There is concern that the use of alcohol-containing mouthwash may increase the risk of oropharyngeal cancer (OPC). The epidemiologic literature regarding the relationship between alcohol-containing mouthwash use and the risk of developing OPC was reviewed.

Findings.—During the past 25 years, 9 English-language epidemiologic investigations have made reference to alcohol-containing mouthwash use and OPC. Of these, 3 reported some positive findings, and 6 reported no positive findings and offered no support for a possible relationship between mouthwash use and increased risk of OPC. One of the 3 reports with positive findings was a case series and included a follow-up case-control investigation, the results of which were negative. A reanalysis of the trial with the most positive results showed that findings were just as positive for nonmucosal cancers developing in the mouth as they were for the usual type of OPC. It is likely that this trial's positive findings resulted from recall bias.

Conclusion.—The use of alcohol-containing mouthwashes increasing the risk of developing OPC is unlikely. Dentists may recommend that their patients may use the mouthwashes of their choice, including those that contain alcohol.

▶ The synergistic effects of alcohol-containing beverages and tobacco use on the initiation of oral squamous cell carcinomas have been known for many years and are undisputed in the scientific community. Ethanol use alone is not considered carcinogenic when used therapeutically or ingested socially in moderation. Over 20 years ago, the relationship between alcohol-containing mouthwashes and oral cancer was questioned. Since that time, an additional 8 epidemiologic studies of oral cancer have been published that investigate, at least in part, the relationship of alcohol-containing mouthwash to oral malignancies. While 2 of the studies suggest some positive findings, the majority of evidence suggests that there is no relationship between the use of alcohol-containing mouthwashes and oral squamous cell carcinoma.

This article illustrates how inappropriate analysis of scientific data can lead to misperceptions by the public regarding the safety of over-the-counter products. In all likelihood, all mouthwashes will eventually have an alcohol-free formulation, not because there is any scientific evidence that alcohol-based mouthwashes have any negative health effects, but because of residual fear on the part of the public, based on poor data analysis that survived the review process and was published.

D. P. Lynch, DDS, PhD

The Possible Premalignant Character of Oral Lichen Planus and Oral Lichenoid Lesions: A Prospective Study
van der Meij EH, Schepman K-P, van der Waal I (Amsterdam/Vrije Universiteit Med Ctr)
Oral Surg Oral Med Oral Pathol Oral Radiol Endod 96:164-171, 2003   9–4

Background.—The literature contains conflicting reports concerning the malignant transformation of oral lichen planus (OLP) (Table 1). Generally the data presented have been insufficient to support the initial diagnosis of OLP in cases that eventually developed into squamous cell carcinoma. A detailed presentation of the data obtained in evaluations of OLP and oral lichenoid lesions (OLL) described the possible premalignant character of these lesions.

Methods.—Sixty-two patients diagnosed with OLP and 111 patients with OLL (age range, 23.1 to 79.2 years; mean age, 52.2 years) participated. The revised, modified World Health Organization diagnostic criteria were used in determining the diagnoses. Follow-up extended for a mean of 31.9 months (range, 6.6 to 72.0 months). Estimates of the number of patients with oral cancer among the OLP and OLL patients were determined by using a comparison between the number of patients, their ages, gender, and length of follow-up and the annual incidence rates for oral cancer in the general Dutch population.

Results.—Squamous cell carcinoma developed in 2 men and 1 woman (1.7% of the sample), all of whom were in the OLL group. Based on a mean follow-up of 31.9 months, the annual malignant transformation was 0.65%. The mean length of follow-up before the malignant transformation developed was 33 months, with a range of 11 to 70 months. Patients with a diagnosis of OLL had a 219-fold increased chance of malignant transformation compared to the general population. Although this number was not statistically significant because of the small size of the population and the short length of follow-up, it indicates a trend among patients with OLL.

Discussion.—The data seemed to indicate that OLLs are premalignant in nature, while no increased risk of malignancy was found among patients diagnosed with OLP. More patients followed up for a longer period of time should be studied before final conclusions regarding the premalignant nature of OLL and OLP are formulated.

TABLE 1.—Studies of the Possible Malignant Transformation of Oral Lichen Planus (1972-2002)

Authors	Year	Country	No. of OLP Patients	No. of Cancer Patients	MTR (%)	Mean Follow-up (y)	MTR per y (%)
Shklar[2]	1972	USA	600	3	0.5	Unknown	Unknown
Fulling[3]	1973	Denmark	225	1	0.4	3.6	0.12
Kövesi and Banoczy[4]	1973	Hungary	274	1	0.4	Unknown	Unknown
Silverman et al[5]	1985	USA	570	7	1.2	5.6	0.22
Murti et al[6]	1986	India	702	3	0.4	5.1	0.08
Holmstrup et al[7]	1988	Denmark	611	9	1.5	7.5	0.20
Salem[8]	1989	Saudi Arabia	72	4	5.6	3.2	1.74
Silverman et al[9]	1991	USA	214	5	2.3	7.5	0.31
Sigurgeirsson and Lindelöf[10]	1991	Sweden	2071	8	0.4	9.9	0.04
Voûte et al[11]	1992	The Netherlands	113	3	2.7	7.8	0.34
Barnard et al[12]	1993	UK	241	8	3.3	Unknown	Unknown
Moncarz et al[13]	1993	Israel	280	6	2.1	Unknown	Unknown
Gorsky et al[14]	1996	Israel	157	2	1.3	1.5	0.85
Markopoulos et al[15]	1997	Greece	326	4	1.3	4.8	0.26
Silverman and Bahl[16]	1997	USA	95	3	3.2	6.1	0.52
Lo Muzio et al[17]	1998	Italy	263	13	4.9	5.7	0.86
Rajentheran et al[18]	1999	UK	832	7	0.8	11.0	0.07
Mignogna et al[19]	2001	Italy	502	18	3.6	Unknown	Unknown
Chainani-Wu et al[20]	2001	USA	229	4	1.7	Unknown	Unknown
Eisen[21]	2002	USA	723	6	0.8	4.5	0.18

Abbreviations: OLP, Oral lichen planus; MTR, malignant transformation rate.

▶ The issue of whether or not OLP represents a premalignant condition has been debated for nearly a century, with reports in the literature of nearly 2% malignant transformation per year. Confounding this issue is the fact that de novo premalignant lesions can have a lichenoid appearance and exhibit lichenoid displasia microscopically.

This article illustrates several important points. First, the diagnosis of OLP should be made on the basis of a biopsy, not clinical signs and symptoms. Second, the histopathologic diagnosis of OLP should be made by individuals who are familiar with the disease to avoid misdiagnosis as lichenoid displasia or other histomorphologically similar entities. Third, regular, periodic follow-up is appropriate in patients with OLP, especially those with atrophic or erosive lesions.

While it has been postulated that immunomodulating agents, eg, corticosteroids, may cause unwanted immunosuppression concomitantly with symptomatic relief, until more information is gathered, it does not appear appropriate to discontinue their use. Finally, it seems appropriate to inform patients that there may be an increased risk of malignant degeneration with OLP, especially the atrophic/erosive variant.

D. P. Lynch, DDS, PhD

Dental Management of Patients With Human Immunodeficiency Virus
Campo-Trapero J, Cano-Sánchez J, del Romero-Guerrero J, et al (Complutense Univ of Madrid; Madrid Regional Service of Health)
Quintessence Int 34:515-525, 2003   9–5

Background.—With the improved treatment regimens available to patients who are HIV-positive, HIV infection is now viewed as a chronic disease. Patients with HIV/AIDS are increasingly seeking routine health care, including dental care. In particular, HIV-positive patients require dental treatment for dental caries, which is highly prevalent because of deficient oral hygiene practices, reduced saliva flow, and periodontal disease prevalence in these patients.

Dental practitioners may be reluctant to perform treatments involving blood exposure because of the perceived risk of infection. However, specific guidelines for handling accidents involving contaminated material have been developed, as have guidelines for performing invasive dental treatments.

Determining Immunologic Category.—In evaluating the seropositive patient, required components include a full medical history; examination of the head, neck, and soft tissues of the oral cavity; and a complete dental and periodontal assessment. Total platelet count is critical when surgical procedures are considered, as are coagulation tests. Viral load, determined by the number of HIV-1 RNA copies and the number and percentage of CD4 and CD8 lymphocytes, reflects the ability to combat infectious agents, reveals the patient's virologic and immunologic status, and permits classification of

---

TABLE 4A.—Protocol for Management of HIV-Positive Patients

Asymptomatic or symptomatic patients (> 200/14% CD4) (clinical categories A and B)*

1. Periodic examination of patients: Annual
   • Bacterial plaque control and Phase 1 periodontal treatment every 6-12 months

2. Annual radiologic examination

3. Appropriate personalized treatment plan
   • Prophylaxis, root scraping and smoothing (irrigate with 0.1% clorhexidine gluconate) Periodontal surgery
   • Caries removal and restoration
   • Surgical treatments: simple and surgical tooth extractions (elevate hemostasis and administer antibiotic prophylaxis if appropriate)
   • Endodontic treatments (symptomatic periapical lesions: periapical surgery or tooth extraction)
   • Complex prosthetic treatment (mixed denture, fixed denture, removable partial denture, implants)
   • Regular fluoride applications
   • Control of xerostomia
   • Diagnosis and treatment of mycotic, viral, bacterial, or other oral lesions (take biopsy if appropriate)

4. Removal of septic foci in cases of acute and progressive infection
   • Consult with patient's physician
   • Evaluate the immunologic situation (counts of CD4, CD8, platelets, red blood cells, etc)
   • Prophylactic antibiotic therapy if appropriate: 2 g amoxicillin 1 hour before (1.5 g erythromycin) or 600 mg clindamycin 1 hour before the procedure
   • In recurrences: 500 mg metronidazol 1 hour before and three 500 mg doses at 8-hour intervals after

5. Abcesses, cellulitis, and osteomyelitis
   • Penicillin V 2 g per day for 5-10 days + metronidazol (above dose)

6. Pathologic state of mind (depression, anxiety, excitability)
   • Consult with the psychiatrist, psychologist, or social worker (especially in ex-IDUs or IDUs)
   • If behavioral changes are observed, refer the patient urgently to a neurologist

---

*Clinical categories of the consensus classification of the HIV-positive patient.
Abbreviation: IDU, intravenous drug user.
Modified from Malagón S, Chimenos E, López J, et al: Protocolo del manejo odontoestomatológico de pacientes infectados por el VIH(I). Publicación oficial de SEISIDA 8:21-24, 1997 and Malagón S, Chimenos E, López J, et al: Protocolo del manejo odontoestomatológico de pacientes infectados por el VIH(II). Publicación oficial de SEISIDA 8:63-66, 1997.
(Courtesy of Campo-Trapero J, Cano-Sánchez J, del Romero-Guerrero J, et al: Dental management of patients with human immunodeficiency virus. *Quintessence Int* 34:515-525, 2003.)

---

the disease stage. The guidelines for treatment of dental conditions depend on disease status (Table 4).

Invasive Dental Procedures.—HIV-positive patients have been viewed as highly prone to having complications develop postoperatively, but studies reveal similar rates of complications between HIV-positive and HIV-negative patients, and the complications that do develop are readily treated. The most common complications seen are alveolitis and delayed wound healing. Antibiotic prophylaxis before tooth extraction has been recommended for patients with AIDS, sometimes limited to those who have neutropenia of more than 500 cells/mL or CD4 counts exceeding 100 cells and who are not receiving prophylactic antibiotics against pneumonia or tuberculosis. Analytic and coagulation test results are obtained before undertaking surgical tooth extractions in HIV-positive patients. Rarely do patients whose platelet

TABLE 4B.—Protocol for Dental Treatment of HIV-Positive Patients

Patients with AIDS (< 200/14% CD4)* (clinical categories C1, C2, and C3)†

1. Periodic examination of patients:
   • Bacterial plaque control and Phase 1 periodontal treatment every 3-6 months

2. Dental treatment
   • Caries removal and restoration of caried surfaces
   • Regular fluoride applications
   • Simple prosthetic treatment (removable partial denture or complete denture)
   • Supra- and subgingival scraping Postpone complex periodontal treatment (bone regeneration)

3. Evaluate hemostasis status
   • If there is a history of thrombocytopenic purpura or hepatic problems, postpone oral surgery

4. Assess the risk of septicemia (antibiotic prophylaxis)

5. Removal of septic foci, abscesses, and cellulitis
   • Antibiotic prophylaxis
   • Consult with the patient's physician

6. Diagnosis and treatment of oral lesions (mycotic, bacterial, and viral infections)

7. Control of xerostomia and glosodynia
   • Dietary (greater liquid intake) and oral hygiene recommendations
   • Gentle manipulation of buccal tissues (lubricate lips, commissures) with damp rolls of cotton and gauze
   • Saliva stimulation with xylitol chewing gum; avoid tobacco and alcohol; fluoride applications

8. Ulcers of viral origin (CMV ro SHV)
   • If recurrences occur, consult with the patient's physician

9. Cleaning of removable dentures
   • Benzal chloride 1:7.5 + water + antiseptic soap + 1% hypochlorite
   • 0.1% chlorhexidine gluconate (never use with nistatine)

10. In terminal phases (< 50 CD4)
   • Pain control, limitation of infection, removal of bacterial plaque, and cleansing of oral cavity when the patient is unable to do so. Do not carry out surgical treatments in emergencies, treat in the hospital setting
   • Treat acute infections of buccal origin only using systemic antimicrobial and analgesic therapy
   • Consult with the patient's physician

11. Consult with a psychiatrist, psychologist, or nurses for episodes of depression or anxiety

---

*In patients receiving highly active antiretroviral therapy, if their immunologic and virologic status allows it, more complex treatments can be contemplated.

†Clinical categories of the HIV-positive patient consensus classification.

Abbreviations: CMV, cytomegalovirus; *SHV*, simple herpes virus.

(From Campo-Trapero J, Cano-Sánchez J, del Romero-Guerrero J, et al: Dental management of patients with human immunodeficiency virus. *Quintessence Int* 34:515-525, 2003. Courtesy of Malagón S, Chimenos E, López J, et al: Protocolo del manejo odontoestomatológico de pacientes infectados por el VIH(I). Publicación oficial de SEISIDA 8:21-24, 1997 and Malagón S, Chimenos E, López J, et al: Protocolo del manejo odontoestomatológico de pacientes infectados por el VIH(II). Publicación oficial de SEISIDA 8:63-66, 1997.

counts exceed 50,000/mm³ develop postoperative bleeding complications, but most surgical procedures are contraindicated in patients whose counts are under 20,000/mm³. Simple tooth extraction is generally performed as long as the HIV-infected patient has no coagulopathy. The use of mouthrinses or topical hemostatics is advised.

When hemoglobin values are less than 6 g/dL, treatment is offered cautiously because oxygen transport mechanisms are often compromised and red blood cell transfusions are usually required. Few studies address the response to implant treatments in HIV-positive patients, but those available seem to support the use of implant treatment or guided tissue regeneration procedures for immunologically stable HIV-positive patients. Further study is required.

Periodontal techniques in patients who are seropositive are designed to control pain and gingival bleeding during the acute disease state, eliminate causative microorganisms, and prevent tissue destruction while supporting gingival health. The local antimicrobial agent of choice for periodontal disease is povidone iodine. Transient bacteremia is produced, yet root scraping and smoothing, curettage, and periodontal surgery can be performed in seropositive patients, with antibiotic prophylaxis needed only when neutropenia is less than 500 cells or CD4 less than 100. When linear gingival erythema refractory to conventional plaque control and oral hygiene measures is present, with acute necrotizing gingivitis or acute necrotizing periodontitis, and when the patient has fever, intense pain, necrosis, and bone exposure, systemic antimicrobial therapy is required, usually metronidazole in 250-mg doses every 6 hours for 5 days unless the patient has hepatopathy, requiring amoxicillin or amoxicillin with clavulanic acid.

Generally only nonsteroidal anti-inflammatory drugs and antibiotics are needed to treat complications from endodontic therapy. Some HIV-positive patients have radiolucid periapical lesions that remain asymptomatic for ex-

TABLE 3.—Drug Interactions Between Commonly Used Drugs in Dentistry and Those Used Against HIV Infection

Drug	Use Caution With	Administration
Clindamycin	Ritonavir	Consult dose
Cotrimoxazol	AZT, Lamivudine	Consult dose
Eritromicina	Indinavir, ritonavir, saquinavir	Consult dose
Metronidazol*	Didanosine, nevirapine, ritonavir	2 hours before ddl; consult dose
Tetracycline	ddl	2 hours before ddl
Trimethoprim	Ritonavir, lamivudine, nevirapine	Consult dose
Acyclovir	Indinavir	Increase liquid intake
Fluconazole†	AZT, rifampicin, ddl, sulfonilureas	2 hours before ddl; consult dose
Codeine†§	AZT, ritonavir	Consult dose
Ibuprofen	AZT, ritonavir	Observation
Paracetamol	AZT, isoniazid	Avoid prolonged treatment; risk of hepatoxicity
Prednisone	Indinavir, ritonavir, saquinavir	Consult dose
Piroxicam‖	—	—
Tramadol§	Ritonavir	Consult dose
Carbamazepine	Ritonavir, nelfinavir, saquinavir, indinavir	Consult dose

*Never administer with zalcitabine or estavudine.
†Never administer with oral coagulants (increases the prothrombin time).
‡Never administer with efavirenz.
§Never administer with methadone.
‖Never administer with ritonavir.
Abbreviations: AZT, Zidovudine; *ddl,* didanosine.
(Courtesy of Campo-Trapero J, Cano-Sánchez J, del Romero-Guerrero J, et al: Dental management of patients with human immunodeficiency virus. *Quintessence Int* 34:515-525, 2003.)

tended periods after endodontic treatment. Conventional conservative techniques or antimicrobial substances are not used because of their immunogenic capacity and possible antigenic dissemination. The treatment of choice for these acute phases is periapical surgery; tooth extraction is chosen for symptomatic radiolucid apical lesions.

Conclusion.—Complication rates for HIV-positive patients after invasive dental procedures are similar to those for HIV-negative patients. Special care is required before undertaking any dental treatment of symptomatic patients whose CD4 lymphocyte counts are less than 200, along with careful assessment of concomitant disease, hemostasis status, and pharmacologic treatment (Table 3). The risks faced by the dental staff are extremely low, and refusal of treatment to these patients is not justified.

▶ It has now been over 20 years since the HIV epidemic was first recognized. Since that time, over 60 million people have been infected, with over 20 million deaths. Oral manifestations of HIV infection have been described from the outset, and dentistry has played a major role in the diagnosis of HIV/AIDS-related lesions, eg, oral hairy leukoplakia, intraoral Kaposi's sarcoma, non-Hodgkin's lymphoma, oral candidiasis, and other lesions. While the apparently intentional infection of Kimberly Bergalis by her dentist, Dr David Acer, highlighted the potential of transmission in a health care setting, it is now known that such transmission is highly unlikely and easily prevented by routine infection control measures.

This article illustrates not only the safety with which HIV-infected individuals can be treated, but also addresses the treatment alterations that must be done to accommodate their particular illness. Hopefully, this article and others like it will reassure reluctant health care providers that proper treatment and management of HIV-positive individuals is easily within the realm of general dentistry and that appropriate oral health care for HIV-infected patients can provide a significant positive aspect to the patient's quality of life.

D. P. Lynch, DDS, PhD

Antibiotic Prophylaxis for Dental Patients With Total Joint Replacements
American Dental Association, American Academy of Orthopaedic Surgeons (Chicago)
J Am Dent Assoc 134:895-899, 2003   9–6

Background and Overview.—In 1997, the American Dental Association (ADA) and the American Academy of Orthopaedic Surgeons (AAOS) assembled an expert panel of dentists, orthopedic surgeons, and infectious disease specialists. This panel published their first Advisory Statement for Dental Patients With Prosthetic Joints. This represented the first time that national health organizations had addressed this topic on record. In addition, the organizations created a new patient handout that dentists may give to their patients. The 1997 Advisory Statement has been well used by both dentists and orthopaedic surgeons. Following established protocols for periodic review of existing advisory statements, the ADA and AAOS and their expert consultants reviewed and modified the 1997 statement. The 2003 advisory statement is the first periodic update of the 1997 statement.

Conclusions and Clinical Implications.—The 2003 statement contains some modifications of the classification of patients at potential risk and of the incidence stratification of bacteremic dental procedures. There were no changes concerning suggested antibiotics or antibiotic regimens. The 2003 statement concludes that antibiotic prophylaxis is not indicated for dental patients who have pins, plates, or screws, nor is it recommended for most patients who have undergone total joint replacements. Premedication is recommended in a small number of patients who may be at increased risk for hematogenous total joint infection.

▶ Postoperative control of infection in patients with total joint replacement is easily controlled, for the most part, by the administration of antibiotics in the immediate postoperative period. Currently, there appears to be an overuse of antibiotic prophylaxis for patients who have had total joint replacements. In general, antibiotic prophylaxis is not indicated for dental patients with pins, plates, or screws or for patients with total joint replacement. There are several specific exceptions to this general rule: (1) patients within the first 2 years after total joint replacement; (2) immunocompromised patients; and (3) patients with comorbidities (eg, previous prosthetic joint infections, hemophilia, type 1 diabetes mellitus, and malignancy).

Antibiotic administration simply "to be on the safe side" is inappropriate justification for prophylaxis, as the risk/benefit and cost/effectiveness ratios are not in the patient's best interest. When a patient demands antibiotic prophylaxis or the patient's physician demands that the dentist provide antibiotic prophylaxis when medically unnecessary, the dentist is still ultimately responsible for the outcome.

D. P. Lynch, DDS, PhD

Adult Hemopoietic Stem Cell Transplantation
Westbrook SD, Paunovich ED, Freytes CO (Univ of Texas, San Antonio)
J Am Dent Assoc 134:1224-1231, 2003   9–7

Introduction.—Refinements in transplantation techniques and supportive care have enhanced posttransplantation survival rates. Hemopoietic stem cell transplantation (HSCT) is an important component in modern cancer treatment. Dental care has an important role in both pretransplantation and posttransplantation care in these patients. Oral complications and required supportive dental care in patients with HSCT were reviewed.

Supportive Care.—Transplantation candidates need to undergo dental screenings and be adequately treated before transplantation. Their dental care should be carefully managed during the transplantation process, with dental support being administered as soon as recovery permits. Dentists

---

BOX 2.—Common Prophylactic Medications for Patients
Who Undergo Hemopoietic Stem Cell Transplantation

ANTIVIRAL MEDICATIONS

For Herpes Simplex Virus
- Acyclovir
- Valacyclovir

For Cytomegalovirus
- Foscarnet
- Ganciclovir

ANTIMICROBIAL MEDICATIONS

For *Pneumocystis carinii* Pneumonia
- Trimethoprim/sulfamethoxazole
- Dapsone
- Pentamidine

For Gram-Positive Bacteria
- Ciprofloxacin
- Levofloxacin
- Gatifloxacin
- Penicillin

ANTIFUNGAL MEDICATIONS

- Fluconazole
- Itraconazole
- Amphotericin B

(Courtesy of Westbrook SD, Paunovich ED, Freytes CO: Adult hemopoietic stem cell transplantation. *J Am Dent Assoc* 134:1224-1231, 2003. Copyright 2003, American Dental Association. Reprinted by permission of ADA Publishing, a division of ADA Business Enterprises, Inc.)

---

need to consult with the patient's oncologist or primary physician to determine the appropriate timing and intensity of dental support.

Complications.—Some of the side effects of the patient's treatment regimen may be severe, and the dentist may encounter these in patient care. The most common and obvious oral complication in patients undergoing HSCT is mucositis caused by radiotherapy or chemotherapeutic agents. Patients with ulcerative mucositis are up to 3 times more likely to develop α-hemolytic streptococcal bacteremias than those without ulcerative mucositis. Standard transplantation protocols allow for the prophylactic use of antiviral, antifungal, and antimicrobial agents, since HSCT patients are at increased risk for life-threatening infections (Box 2). Oral hygiene regimens need to be modified in patients with neutropenia to avoid trauma to oral tissues. About 30% to 50% of patients may experience adverse immunologic responses that could lead to the development of acute graft-versus-host disease (GVHD). Oral manifestations of GVHD include xerostomia, mucosal lichenoid and papular lesions, erythema, atrophy, and ulcerations; these patients have an increased incidence of oral manifestations of squamous cell carcinoma, particularly in males. Transplant recipients need to be monitored for acute myelogenous leukemia and other solid tumors. Salivary gland dysfunction (increasingly mucinous saliva and marked xerostomia) may result from direct toxicity of conditioning agents and anticholinergic medications. Mucosal color changes may occur, including increased whiteness or erythema, atrophy, and vascularity and ulceration.

Conclusion.—Because of improved transplantation survival rates, more patients may seek supportive outpatient dental care after transplantation, which necessitates special management considerations. Dental professionals need to be informed concerning modern HSCT.

▶ HSCT, which includes both bone marrow transplantation and peripheral stem cell transplantation, has become a routine treatment modality for a number of malignancies. Tumoricidal doses of both chemotherapeutic agents and radiotherapy often result in substantial myelosuppression that can be as serious and severe as the original malignancy for which the patient is being treated. Fortunately, HSCT is a predictable way to reconstitute bone marrow after toxic tumoricidal chemotherapy or radiotherapy.

Patients who are scheduled to undergo HSCT must receive appropriate medical therapy before their transplant, as well as specialized dental management after transplantation. In addition to the side effects associated with preparation for engraftment (eg, pancytopenia, thrombocytopenic hemorrhage, fluid and electrolyte imbalance) secondary oral complications of mucositis, hemorrhage, GVHD, and salivary gland dysfunction can all result in significant morbidity. Familiarity with the complications associated with adult HSCT and the therapies available to deal with them are important additions to the clinician's armamentarium.

D. P. Lynch, DDS, PhD

Oral Candidiasis in Hematopoietic Cell Transplantation Patients: An Outcome-Based Analysis
Epstein JB, Hancock PJ, Nantel S (Univ of Illinois, Chicago; Univ of Washington, Seattle; Univ of British Columbia, Vancouver, Canada, et al)
Oral Surg Oral Med Oral Pathol Oral Radiol Endod 96:154-163, 2003   9–8

Introduction.—Even in the presence of aggressive antifungal prophylaxis, the risk of systemic fungal infection is increased in recipients of hematopoietic cell transplants (HCT). This is of concern since *Candida* infection can cause morbidity and mortality in these patients. The relationship between oral colonization by *Candida* species and systemic infection, mortality, and the impact of antifungal treatment was examined in a population of HCT recipients.

Methods.—A total of 115 consecutive patients undergoing HCT were assessed. Oral examinations and cultures for *Candida* were performed before transplantation and on a weekly basis until discharge. During oral examinations, the level of mucositis was scored by using the National Cancer Institute grade. Systemic antifungal prophylaxis was administered to all patients, and chlorhexidine oral rinses were routinely provided (Tables 5 and 6).

Results.—Colonization by *Candida* occurred in 31% of the cohort, 56% of whom had evidence of oral candidiasis. Significantly reduced *Candida*

TABLE 5.—Systemic Antimicrobial Agents Prescribed During Admission
for Transplantation

Drug	Total Doses (mg) All Patients ($N = 115$)				Total Doses (mg) *Candida*-Positive Patients ($n = 36$)		
	No. (%)	Range	Mean	Median	Range	Mean	Median
Amphotericin	113 (98%)	40-8400	647	400	135-8400	1086	655
Fluconazole	44 (38%)	50-7700	2669	2000	800-7700	3025	2400
Vancomycin	105 (91%)	1000-81,750	22,866	20,875	2000-64,000	25,293	22,000
Tobramycin	96 (83%)	100-18,250	3239	2660	420-18,250	3700	2790
Cephalosporin	93 (81%)	3750-38,300	74,824	60,000	12,000-38,300	94,195	8100
Acyclovir	106 (92%)	600-86,200	23,459	19,800	1000-86,200	28,245	21,600

(Reprinted by permission of the publisher from Epstein JB, Hancock PJ, Nantel S: Oral candidiasis in hematopoietic cell transplantation patients: An outcome-based analysis. *Oral Surg Oral Med Oral Pathol Oral Radiol Endod* 96:154-163, 2003. Copyright 2003 by Elsevier.)

colonization was observed in patients who used chlorhexidine alone, compared with those who used chlorhexidine and nystatin together ($P < .046$). Twenty-five patients died during the immediate posttransplant period. Of these, 17 were *Candida* positive. The length of hospital stay was 15 to 153 days; increased stay was linked with *Candida* colonization ($P = .04$). Ulcerative mucositis occurred in 74% of patients. The most severe mucositis occurred in patients undergoing chemotherapy and radiation therapy. No significant difference was observed between *Candida colonization and the presence or severity of mucositis.*

Conclusion.—Oropharyngeal colonization by *Candida* species occurred frequently in HCT recipients, despite systemic and topical antifungal prophylaxis. Candidiasis was often present in patients who did not survive the early transplant period. Among the 25 patients who died early after HCT, 92% had ulcerative mucositis versus 70% of survivors. There was a significant association between allogenic and autologous HCT, length of stay, and

TABLE 6.—Topical Antifungal Agents Prescribed During Admission for Transplantation

Medication	Positive *Candida* Number (Row %) Column %	Negative *Candida* Number (Row %) Column %	Total Cases Number (Row %) Column %	
Chlorhexidine	20 (23%) 56%	65 (77%) 82%	85 (100%) 74%	
Nystatin suspension	2 (100%) 6%	0 (0%) 0%	2 (100%) 2%	
Chlorhexidine and nystatin	12 (46%) 33%	14 (54%) 18%	26 (100%) 23%	$P = .046$
No topical agents	2 (100%) 6%	0 (0%) 0%	2 (100%) 2%	
			Total	$P = .002$

Note: Chlorhexidine versus nystatin, $P = .062$.
Nystatin versus chlorhexidine + nystatin, $P + .482$.
Chlorhexidine versus chlorhexidine + nystatin, $P = .046$.
Overall, $P = .002$.
(Reprinted by permission of the publisher from Epstein JB, Hancock PJ, Nantel S: Oral candidiasis in hematopoietic cell transplantation patients: An outcome-based analysis. *Oral Surg Oral Med Oral Pathol Oral Radiol Endod* 96:154-163, 2003. Copyright 2003 by Elsevier.)

colonization of *Candida*. In patients undergoing systemic antifungal prophylaxis, chlorhexidine rinse was significantly more effective in decreasing colonization by *Candida* than chlorhexidine and nystatin together.

▶ The previous review (Abstract 9–7) addressed the issue of adult hemopoietic stem cell transplantation and the side effects and oral complications associated with the procedure. This article addresses a particularly common problem in hemopoietic cell transplantation recipients and other immunosuppressed patients—that is, oral candidiasis. The article illustrates the fact that up to one half of patients who receive bone marrow transplants eventually develop systemic candidiasis, with a mortality rate approaching one third of infected patients.

Patients in this study were treated prospectively with chlorhexidine oral rinse, systemic antifungal medication, and in some cases, topical antifungal medication. In spite of aggressive antifungal therapy, one third of patients who developed systemic candidiasis died, in part, due to this infection. Hopefully, as we become more proficient in dealing with opportunistic infections in immunosuppressed patients, this level of mortality will decrease substantially.

D. P. Lynch, DDS, PhD

Fungal Load and Candidiasis in Sjögren's Syndrome
Radfar L, Shea Y, Fischer SH, et al (NIH, Bethesda, Md)
Oral Surg Oral Med Oral Pathol Oral Radiol Endod 96:283-287, 2003   9–9

Background.—The reduced salivary flow characteristic of the autoimmune disorder Sjögren's syndrome (SS) leads to oral and dental complications, including infection with *Candida albicans*. Patients with SS have high rates of oral *Candida* carriage. The association between salivary flow rate and oral *Candida* load was examined in a group of patients with SS.

Methods.—The study included 103 patients with SS, as defined by European criteria. There were 96 women and 7 men with a mean age of 55 years; SS was primary in 91 cases and secondary in 12 (Table 1). Oral rinse cultures were performed to assess the oral *Candida* load. Other evaluations included Gram's staining and wet-mount testing.

Results.—Seventy-seven percent of patients had positive oral rinse culture findings for *Candida*, but most positive culture findings yielded only scant growth. *C albicans* predominated, but other fungi were cultured as well. Colony counts of the oral rinse cultures were significantly and inversely correlated with the patients' total stimulated salivary flow rates but were unrelated to unstimulated salivary flow. The colony counts were also positively correlated with levels of anti-SSA and anti-SSB antibodies, the IgG level, and the focus score. Gram's staining resulted in positive findings in 38% of patients, and wet-mount testing resulted in positive findings in 49%.

Conclusions.—This study finds a 77% rate of oral *Candida* carriage among patients with SS, which is similar to the values reported in previous

TABLE 1.—Characteristics of the Study Population*

Variables	Values
Age	Mean, 55 y (range, 51-57y)
Women (no., %)	96 (94)
Dry-mouth symptoms (no., %)	102 (99)
Difficulty swallowing (no., %)	82 (80)
Denture (no., %)	10 (8)
Keratoconjunctivitis sicca (no., %)	100 (97)
Dry-eye symptoms (no., %)	99 (96)
Unstimulated parotid saliva flow rate (mL/min)	0.008 (0.002-0.013)
Stimulated parotid saliva flow rate (mL/min)	0.526 (0.416-0.637)
Unstimulated submandibular saliva flow rate (mL/min)	0.057 (0.017-0.096)
Stimulated submandibular saliva flow rate (mL/min)	0.260 (0.192-0.327)
Focus score	7 (6-8)
Anti-SSA + (no., %)	60 (59)
Anti-SSB + (no., %)	33 (32)
Rheumatoid factor (IU/mL)	141 (85-198)
Erythrocyte sedimentation rate (mm/h)	41 (35-48)
IgG (mg/dL)	1539 (1411-1668)
Antinuclear antibody (no., %)	79 (77)

*All values are given as means (95% CI), except where number (%) is specified.
Abbreviation: SS, Sjögren's syndrome.
(Reprinted by permission of the publisher from Radfar L, Shea Y, Fischer SH, et al: Fungal load and candidiasis in Sjögren's syndrome. *Oral Surg Oral Med Oral Pathol Oral Radiol Endod* 96:283-287, 2003. Copyright 2003 by Elsevier.)

studies. The candidal load is inversely related to stimulated total salivary flow but unrelated to unstimulated flow.

▶ As described in the previous article (Abstract 9–8), oral candidiasis is a common sequela of immunosuppression. This article illustrates oral candidiasis resulting from another common occurrence, xerostomia, in this case associated with SS. Xerostomia from SS is much less common than xerostomia found as a side effect of drug therapy, but the relationship with an increased risk of oral candidiasis is essentially identical.

Many otherwise healthy individuals carry *Candida* species intraorally with no ill effects. However, in xerostomic individuals, the rate of *Candida* carriage increases substantially. In this particular study, 77% of patients with SS had positive *Candida* cultures. In most cases, the predominant species was *C albicans*. This is despite the fact that the patients had excellent oral hygiene and were under the regular, routine care of dentists. Interestingly, an association was noted between the carriage of *Candida* and stimulated salivary flow. This most likely relates to lower levels of antimicrobial factors normally found in saliva.

D. P. Lynch, DDS, PhD

Differential Injury Responses in Oral Mucosal and Cutaneous Wounds

Szpaderska AM, Zuckerman JD, DiPietro LA (Loyola Univ, Maywood, Ill)
J Dent Res 82:621-626, 2003   9–10

Introduction.—Wounds of the oral mucosa and the skin heal through similar stages, yet oral mucosal wounds heal more rapidly and with less scarring. Many studies have examined the scarless wound repair process of fetal skin but few have compared wound repair at oral mucosal versus cutaneous sites. The inflammatory phase of wound repair in oral mucosal wounds was compared with that in dermal wounds in an animal excisional wound model.

Methods.—One-millimeter punch-biopsy wounds were made in the skin and oral mucosa of Balb/c mice. The wounds and surrounding tissues were removed after various healing intervals. Differences in the inflammatory phase were compared, including the inflammatory cell infiltrate and cytokine production.

Findings.—Compared with skin wounds, oral mucosal wounds had significantly reduced neutrophil, macrophage, and T-cell infiltration. Levels of inflammatory cytokines, including interleukin-6 and a mouse homologue of interleukin-8, were also lower in the oral mucosal wounds. In addition, the mucosal wounds had a lower level of transforming growth factor-β1, a fibrosis-promoting cytokine. Levels of the anti-inflammatory cytokine interleukin-10 and certain modulators of transforming growth factor-β1 were also reduced.

Conclusions.—Findings in this mouse model suggest that oral mucosal wound healing occurs with a significantly reduced inflammatory phase compared with that of dermal wounds. More research will be needed to determine the mechanism by which inflammation is reduced in oral wounds and how this contributes to rapid, scarless wound repair.

▶ As a surgically based health care profession, dentistry involves both intentional and unintentional damage to oral mucosa. Given the amount of trauma sustained by oral mucosa, both idiopathic and iatrogenic, and the ecology of the oral environment in which such injury takes place, it is a constant source of amazement that oral mucosa heals as well and as rapidly as it does. This article evaluates, at the cellular and molecular level, why oral mucosal wounds heal with greater rapidity and less scar formation than analogous cutaneous injuries.

Utilizing a mouse model, the authors made experimental cutaneous and oral mucosal wounds. After wounding of the animals, a number of molecular compounds associated with injury and inflammation were measured. Interestingly, the absolute numbers of inflammatory cells were lower in oral wounds than in skin wounds. In addition, several molecular compounds present in inflammation were found in higher concentrations in skin wounds than in oral mucosal wounds. This particular situation might be fortuitous, but it does allow us to perform some relatively aggressive surgical procedures with the expectation of rapid healing and minimal scar formation.

D. P. Lynch, DDS, PhD

Formation of Mucogingival Defects Associated With Intraoral and Perioral Piercing: Case Reports

Brooks JK, Hooper KA, Reynolds MA (Univ of Maryland, Baltimore)
J Am Dent Assoc 134:837-843, 2003   9–11

Objective.—As part of the fashionable body-piercing trend, piercing of the tongue, lip, and other intraoral and oral sites has become popular. Dentists and other health care professionals have reported various adverse events associated with oral piercings. Periodontal adverse effects of intraoral or perioral piercings are reported in 5 young women.

Patients.—The patients ranged in age from 19 to 25 years and had piercings of the tongue or lip in place for several months to a few years. All were seen for routine or emergency dental care. Examination showed gingival recession and mucogingival defects associated with their piercings (Fig 1). In 3 of the 5 cases, these changes were associated with probing depths of 5 to 8 mm. The most severe periodontal pocketing was associated with minimal gingival recession.

Discussion.—This report adds to the literature documenting the potential for mucogingival injury caused by intraoral and perioral piercings. These sites sometimes show severe attachment loss in the presence of minimal gingival recession. Patients with oral piercings should receive regular periodon-

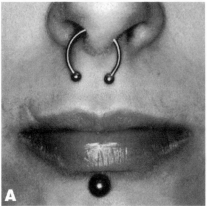 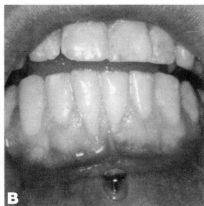

FIGURE 1.—Case 1. **A**, Nose and lip jewelry. **B**, View of gingival recession along the facial aspects of teeth nos. 24 and 25 induced by the flattened stud attachment on the lip. (Courtesy of Brooks JK, Hooper KA, Reynolds MA: Formation of mucogingival defects associated with intraoral and perioral piercing. *J Am Dent Assoc* 134:937-843, 2003. Copyright 2003 American Dental Association. Reprinted by permission of ADA Publishing, a division of ADA Business Enterprises, Inc.)

tal evaluations, along with education regarding the potentially harmful effects of intraoral jewelry to the teeth and oral tissues.

▶ Over the past several years, a marked increase in intraoral and perioral piercings has occurred. This body adornment is usually performed by untrained lay individuals with minimal knowledge of anatomy and sterile techniques. Recipients of such piercings do so for a variety of reasons, including personal perception of enhanced attractiveness, rebellion against authority, and enhanced sexual pleasure.

As with most trendy activities, there is a definite downside to participating. In the case of intraoral and perioral piercings, there are well-described incidents of damage to both teeth and gingiva. This article presents 5 cases of such damage and provides compelling evidence regarding the potential for significant dental and periodontal injury.

D. P. Lynch, DDS, PhD

Association Between Level of Education and Oral Health Status in 35-, 50-, 65- and 75-Year-Olds
Paulander J, Axelsson P, Lindhe J (Göteborg Univ, Sweden)
J Clin Periodontol 30:697-704, 2003   9–12

Purpose.—Epidemiologic studies have linked lower education to poor oral hygiene, missing teeth, and periodontal disease. However, this relationship may be confounded by other sociodemographic variables. The association among educational level and dental disease, treatment needs, and oral hygiene was evaluated in a previously studied sample of adults ranging from middle age to old age.

Methods.—The analysis included 1093 participants from a stratified, randomized sample of Swedish adults: 155 participants aged 35 years, 510 aged 50 years, 310 aged 65 years, and 310 aged 75 years. Patients who attended no more than elementary school were classified as having low education (LE); all others were classified as having higher education (HE). The educational status was compared with indicators of oral health status, including number of teeth, periodontal attachment level, caries, and occlusal functioning. The contribution of self-reported oral hygiene and dietary factors was assessed as well.

Results.—For all but the youngest age group, the number of remaining teeth was lower in the LE group than in the HE group: 21.1 versus 24.5 for 50-year-olds, 15.7 versus 18.9 for 65-year-olds, and 13.3 versus 16.6 for 75-year-olds. Periodontal attachment loss was also greater in the LE group, but no significant difference was found among the 65-year-old participants. Except among the 75-year-olds, the number of healthy gingival units was lower in the LE groups. Across age groups, LE status was associated with a lower number of intact tooth surfaces and with poorer occlusal functioning. Oral hygiene and dietary factors were similar between the 2 education groups.

Conclusions.—Education is significantly related to the number of missing teeth and other indicators of oral health status in adults of varying ages. This is despite the apparent lack of relationship between educational status and oral hygiene practice. Educational level may be an important factor to include in risk assessment and preventive planning.

▶ In oral medicine and pathology, it's easy to forget that dental caries and periodontal disease are the 2 most common infectious diseases that are dealt with in dentistry. As patients age, the prevalence of dental caries and periodontal disease also increases. This article assesses the relationship of the level of education to oral health status in adult and geriatric individuals.

Most individuals would assume that there would be a direct correlation between the level of education and the maintenance of increased oral health, especially in adulthood; however, a host of other factors influence the eventual outcome. This article reaffirms the findings of earlier articles that less educated individuals are more likely to have edentulism. Periodontal disease seems to be more strongly influenced by age than level of education. Nevertheless, a higher educational level correlated more closely with a decreased need for periodontal treatment. Both DMFS scores and occlusal function were found to be adversely affected by the educational level; however, oral hygiene and dietary habits were not significantly influenced.

D. P. Lynch, DDS, PhD

Tooth Loss and Dietary Intake
Hung H-C, Willett W, Ascherio A, et al (Harvard School of Dental Medicine, Boston; Harvard School of Public Health, Boston)
J Am Dent Assoc 134:1185-1192, 2003   9–13

Background.—Tooth loss has been linked to impaired nutritional status, likely because reduced chewing ability affects food selection. However, because most studies of this issue have been cross-sectional in nature, the exact sequence of events is unclear. Long-term follow-up of a sample of male health professionals was used to clarify the relationship between tooth loss and dietary changes, the focus of which was on fruits, vegetables, and nutrients important to general health.

Methods.—The analysis included 31,813 men from the Health Professionals' Follow-up Study, a prospective cohort study of dentists and other health professionals. At enrollment in 1986 and at follow-up assessments, participants completed a food frequency questionnaire to assess dietary factors. Self-reported tooth loss was evaluated every 2 years. All men included in the final analysis had at least 11 teeth at baseline; they were followed up through 1994.

Results.—About 22% of men lost teeth during follow-up, including 3% who lost 5 or more teeth. Tooth loss occurred in nearly half of the participants with 11 to 16 teeth at baseline versus 20 of those with 25 to 32 teeth at baseline. In general, the men in the cohort showed a trend toward a healthier diet during the period studied. Men without tooth loss had a greater improvement in diet during follow-up, after adjustment for change in total energy intake and for age, dietary intake, and number of teeth at baseline. Dietary changes were particularly apparent for men who lost 5 or more teeth. Compared with men with no tooth loss, those losing 5 or more teeth had lesser reductions in dietary cholesterol and vitamin B12 consumption, a greater reduction in consumption of polyunsaturated fats, and smaller increases in consumption of fiber and whole fruit. Men with tooth loss were more likely to stop eating certain fruits and vegetables, including apples, pears, and raw carrots. For most dietary factors, the outcomes of men who lost 1 to 4 teeth were no different from those of men without tooth loss.

Conclusions.—Men with decrements in dental status, particularly those losing 5 or more teeth during 8 years' follow-up, show significant reductions in dietary intake of nutrients important for health. These dietary changes may help to account for the increased risk of chronic disease observed in individuals with reduced dental status. The effects of tooth loss in the general population are likely even greater than that in the study cohort of health professionals.

▶ The role of diet in health promotion and disease prevention has been known for decades, including the association of nutritional intake with tooth loss. Most studies of this nature are cross-sectional and do not address the time frame in which tooth loss and altered dietary intake take place.

This article illustrates, with strong statistical significance, that patients who have lost at least 5 teeth have a significantly poorer diet in terms of intake of dietary fiber and whole fruits. Unfortunately, those individuals who lost some teeth were more likely to loose additional teeth. The study does not evaluate whether additional tooth loss is due to continued poor oral hygiene or specific nutritional factors, but the fact remains that once tooth loss begins, it is a "slippery slope" that can have some substantial negative outcomes.

D. P. Lynch, DDS, PhD

Maxillary Odontogenic Keratocyst: A Common and Serious Clinical Misdiagnosis
Ali M, Baughman RA (Univ of Florida, Gainesville; AmeriPath/Central Florida, Hawthorne)
J Am Dent Assoc 134:877-883, 2003   9–14

Introduction.—An odontogenic keratocyst (OKC) is a common, noninflammatory odontogenic cyst arising from dental lamina cell rests. The mandible, especially the posterior mandible, is the most common site of presentation. Questions remain about the presentation of maxillary OKCs. Pathology files were reviewed to determine the most frequent location of OKCs in the maxilla.

Methods and Findings.—An 8-year review of pathology files identified 398 OKCs from 393 patients. About two thirds of OKCs occurred in the mandible, and about one third overall were in the mandibular third molar and ramus area.

Just under one third of OKCs were found in the maxilla. The most common location of maxillary OKCs was the canine area and accounted for about 14% of all lesions. Other maxillary sites included the third molar and tuberosity region (7.5%), the anterior area (7.0%), the first and second molar area (3%), and the premolar area (2%). Of all OKCs in the maxillary canine region, the clinical diagnosis was correct in just 31.5%. The most common incorrect diagnoses were lateral periodontal cyst and periapical cyst/granuloma.

Conclusions.—The maxillary canine region is a common location of OKCs, second only to the mandibular third molar/ramus area. Maxillary canine OKCs are commonly misdiagnosed: the usual clinical impression is of an apical inflammatory lesion or lateral periodontal cyst. Histologic examination of surgically removed tissue may be needed for a definitive diagnosis, especially for lesions that do not respond to conservative endodontic treatment.

▶ OKCs are relatively common jaw cysts, exceeded in number only by periapical and dentigerous cysts. This article presents a review of odontogenic cysts in general and OKCs in particular. Because OKCs are indistinguishable from other odontogenic cysts and neoplasms, it is critical that clinicians be aware of where OKCs are most likely to occur and how they are most likely to present clinically and radiographically. The significance lies primarily in knowing when to be aggressive when enucleating potential OKCs; this article illustrates, once again, the need for submission of all surgically removed tissue for clinical and microscopic evaluation.

D. P. Lynch, DDS, PhD

General Medicine and Surgery for Dental Practitioners: Part 4. Neurological Disorders

Greenwood M, Meechan JG (The Dental School, Newcastle upon Tyne, England)
Br Dent J 195:19-25, 2003   9–15

Purpose.—A wide range of neurologic problems may be seen in dental patients. These conditions can have important effects on dental treatments, as well as on the provision of anesthesia and analgesia. Neurologic conditions affecting dental practice are reviewed.

Neurologic Conditions in Dental Practice.—A number of points from the patient history are important in highlighting dental patients with important neurologic disorders, including syncope or "blackouts" resulting from a wide range of problems, epilepsy and various types of seizures, strokes or transient ischemic attacks, and multiple sclerosis. Facial pain is a commonly encountered problem, especially in older adults. Neurologic causes include trigeminal neuralgia, postherpetic neuralgia, and atypical facial pain. Other important conditions include the movement disorder Parkinson's disease, various motor neuron diseases, CNS tumors, and myasthenia gravis. If facial palsy is idiopathic, it may be described as Bell's palsy. A wide range of other causes of facial weakness are possible as well, including infections, trauma, tumors, and metabolic conditions. Various types of cranial nerve dysfunction, with a wide range of causes, may also be observed. A systematic approach to assessing the sense of smell, eyes, face, mouth, neck, and ears is needed for evaluation of the cranial nerves (Table 4).

Management Considerations.—Many neurologic conditions are best managed with modifications to dental care. For patients with epilepsy, the epileptogenic anesthetics methohexitone and enflurane should be avoided, whereas IV sedation may help to reduce the chance of seizures. For patients with strokes, loss of the gag reflex or other neurologic changes may have an important impact on the anesthetic approach. Patients with multiple sclerosis may have limitations in their ability to comply with treatment. Those with Parkinson's disease may have trouble with excessive salivation; antimuscarinic agents may be useful in this situation. For patients with myasthenia gravis, treatment is best performed with the use of local anesthesia and should be performed early in the day. Treatments for neurologic diseases may also affect patients' dental status. For example, phenytoin and other an-

TABLE 4.—Cranial Nerve Dysfunction and Signs Arising From It

Cranial Nerve		Possible Problem	Sign
I	Olfactory	Trauma Tumour	Decreased ability to smell
II	Optic	Trauma, Tumour MS, Stroke	Blindness, visual field defect
III	Oculomotor	Diabetes, increased intracranial pressure	Dilated pupil Ptosis
IV	Trochlear	Trauma	Diplopia
V	Trigeminal	Sensory—idiopathic, trauma, IDN/Lingual nerve damage	None, sensory deficit on testing
		Motor—Bulbar palsy	Signs in IX, X, XI, XII
		Acoustic Neuroma	May be decreased facial sensation. Affects VIII also
VI	Abducens	MS, some strokes	Inability of eye to look laterally Eye deviated towards nose
VII	Facial	LMN—Lower motor neurone Bell's Palsy, Skull fracture Parotid tumour	Total Facial weakness
		UMN—Upper motor neurone Stroke, Tumour	Forehead sparing weakness
VIII	Vestibulo-cochlear	Excess noise; Paget's acoustic neuroma	Deafness
IX	Glosso-pharyngeal	Trauma, Tumour	Impaired gag reflex
X	Vagus	Trauma, brainstem lesions	Impaired gag reflex Soft palate moves to 'good' side on saying 'aha'.
XI	Accessory	Polio, stroke	Weakness turning head away from affected side (sternocleidomastoid). Weakness shrugging shoulders (trapezius)
XII	Hypoglossal	Trauma Brainstem lesions	Tongue deviated to affected side on protrusion

(Courtesy of Greenwood M, Meechan JG: General medicine and surgery for dental practitioners: Part 4. Neurological disorders. *Br Dent J* 195:19-25, 2003.)

ticonvulsant drugs may lead to gingival overgrowth and taste disturbances; antimuscarinic agents may cause a patient to have a dry mouth.

Discussion.—A wide range of neurologic diseases may be seen in dental practice. The dentist should be aware of the major signs of these diseases and appropriate modifications for dental care.

▶ This article is 1 of a series of 10 manuscripts published in the *British Dental Journal* that review general medicine and surgery for dental practitioners. This particular article was selected because of the number of neurologic conditions that may be encountered in the practice of dentistry. In some cases, the neurologic symptoms are anatomically localized (eg, trigeminal neuralgia and atypical facial pain). In other cases, extraoral manifestations (eg, Sturge-Weber syndrome) and intraoral manifestations (eg, uvular deviation) represent widespread neurologic involvement.

Dentists are not trained neurologists, but they should be able to detect fairly typical neurologic signs and symptoms and make appropriate referrals to qualified medical specialists.

D. P. Lynch, DDS, PhD

10 Pediatric and Preventive Dentistry

Section A

INTRODUCTION

The content of this chapter includes abstracts that represent a diverse cross-section of the literature related to the field of pediatric dentistry. The chapter was developed with an emphasis on clinical relevance pertaining to subjects such as early childhood caries etiology, treatment methods (clinically and in the hospital setting), factors influencing utilization of dental services in low-income children, the role of culture on treatment delivery, effects of acidulated phosphate fluoride (APF) foam on resin materials, and the effect of laser versus light-cure polymerization at the enamel-resin interface. Microleakage was also investigated in relation to the use of acid primer versus conventional acid etching. The eutectic agent EMLA (eutectic mixture of local anesthetics) may prove to be a promising pain obtundant.

It was interesting reading of the attempt to find an association in periodontal-related changes among adolescents with asthma. The effects of therapy on dentofacial development in individuals treated with rhabdomyosarcoma were also informative. The information contained in the abstracts cover diagnosis, clinical technical issues, and clinical studies.

These articles will hopefully raise questions in the minds of readers and stimulate further exploration of the literature, and, at the same time, lead to improved oral health for our children.

Seth B. Canion, DDS, MS

Access/Disparities

The Impact of Dental Benefits on the Utilization of Dental Services by Low-Income Children in Western Pennsylvania
Lave JR, Keane CR, Lin CJ, et al (Univ of Pittsburgh, Pa)
Pediatr Dent 24:234-240, 2002   10–1

Introduction.—Most attention concerning the uninsured has focused on uninsurance in general versus dental coverage specifically. The Pennsylvania Children's Health Insurance Program and The Caring Program are 2 programs that cover children up to age 19 years in families with incomes below 235% of the Federal poverty level. The impact of this dental coverage on the use of dental services in Western Pennsylvania was examined by a study using a before-and-after design and including a control group.

Methods.—Families of newly enrolled children were contacted at the time of enrollment for telephone interviews and at 6 and 12 months after enrollment. Both structured and open-ended questions were used concerning the use of health care services, unmet need/delayed care, and causes and consequences of unmet need/delayed care. A second group of families were interviewed 12 months after the study group was initially interviewed to provide a comparison sample. The study included 750 children who were continuously enrolled for 12 months and 460 comparison children.

Results.—After enrollment, the proportion of children with a regular source of dental care rose 42% and the proportion of children who had a preventive dental visit rose 50%. The proportion of children with unmet need/delayed care for dental service dropped from 43% to 10%. The program had a greater impact on the use of dental services than on the use of medical services.

Conclusion.—The extension of dental benefits to low-income children in Western Pennsylvania increased their access to dental care and to preventive dental services.

▶ Oral health is unquestionably a part of total health and it is essential to the well-being of all Americans. Much attention has been given to reasons for disparities in oral health care seen in minorities and uninsured children. There may be many other reasons that negatively impact on oral health care availability for underserved children, but lack of dental benefits remains a compelling factor limiting access to care. This study presents the positive impact of extending dental benefits to State Children's Health Insurance Program–eligible children in Western Pennsylvania. When dental benefits are made available combined with an equitable level of provider payments, good things can occur in a population that has been deprived of oral health care benefits.

S. B. Canion, DDS, MS

Assess ABCD to Ascertain the Level of Cultural Influence in Pediatric Dental Families
Nelson LP (Harvard School of Dental Medicine, Boston)
Pediatr Dent 25:26-28, 2003   10–2

Introduction.—Attitudes concerning pediatric dentistry may be influenced by cultural beliefs. The potential consequences of ignoring cultural attitudes include anger, mistrust, and even removal of the child from the health care system if the pediatric dentist insists on treatment modalities against the wishes of the family. Strategies the pediatric dentist can use to address cultural issues in pediatric dental families were discussed.

Strategies.—To avoid the dual pitfalls of cultural stereotyping and ignoring the potential influence of culture, the pediatric dentist can use ABCD (attitudes, beliefs, communication/language barriers, and decision-making styles) to deal with issues of cultural influence. It is important for the clinician to become educated concerning the attitudes common to the ethnic groups being treated. The use of open-ended questions can be employed to gain understanding about parents' expectations and beliefs.

Trust must be gained in ethnocultural relationships before beliefs can be addressed. It is beneficial for the dental clinician to be explicit so that the clinician and the child's family will work together to achieve the best possible care for the child. Frequently ask parents to explain their understanding of what they are being told to determine whether communication has occurred. It is important to remember that an interpreter wields considerable power. Placing a child in the position of interpreter for parents inverts the role most cultures ascribe in the family hierarchy by putting the child in a temporary superior position. This can be frustrating to the child, the parents, and the clinician. It is better to hire bilingual and bicultural staff to prevent bidirectional misunderstandings in communication.

The familial mode of decision making is the norm in many cultures, and ignoring this can create disagreement and conflict within the family and between family and dental staff. Asking "Is there anyone else that I should talk to about your child's care?" may prevent many problems. It is important to realize that the importance of "time" in the American culture may be seen in other cultures as more concern with getting things accomplished than with developing deep interpersonal relationships and quality of work. Tardiness may be cultural. Saying "yes" in some cultures may be a universal answer, even when the answer is really "no."

Conclusion.—Failure to take culture seriously means that the dentist's own values are elevated above those of others and the dentist fails to understand the value systems of persons from different backgrounds. It is important for the dentist to recognize manifestations of prejudice in himself/herself and in the dental staff.

▶ As the American population demographics gradually change, it is important that the health care provider asks questions and respectfully acknowledges the differences of his or her changing population base. This will enhance the trust between practitioner and family. Acculturation may not be necessary, but recognition and appreciation of differences is essential.

S. B. Canion, DDS, MS

Multicultural Influences on Child-Rearing Practices: Implications for Today's Pediatric Dentist

Ng MW (Children's Natl Med Ctr, Washington, DC)
Pediatr Dent 25:19-22, 2003   10–3

Introduction.—Parenting practices have, in general, been undergoing changes that likely affect how a dentist practices, yet there are few published data concerning child-rearing practices and even less on the role of cultural influence on child-rearing practices. The implications of multicultural influences on child-rearing practices in today's pediatric dentistry were discussed.

The Impact of Beliefs/Practices on Dental Care.—Most of the currently accepted views of child-rearing practices in the United States are based on European American traditions. The 2-parent nuclear family continues to be considered the ideal family unit, yet 1 of 4 children in the United States today lives in a single-parent home. One half of African American children live in female-headed households and 9 of 10 babies born in African American households live in 3 generational households. In these families, child-care responsibilities are likely to be dispersed in an authoritative-parenting style.

African American and white mothers who are poor tend to value obedience and are likely to hit and scold their children. The grandmother is likely to have a dominant role in infant-feeding decisions. Prolonged bottle feeding is usual in the Native American culture. Many Native American parents believe that early childhood caries is a normal childhood disease that affects all children.

Latinos are expected to surpass African Americans as the largest minority group in the United States by 2005. Pacifying young children with the nursing bottle is a commonly accepted practice among Latino immigrants who work long hours and have little sleep. Juice is frequently offered to children because of high acceptance; chocolate syrup in milk is commonly used to increase the child's acceptance.

Vietnamese immigrants are likely to live in large family units in which parents may pacify their children at nighttime with a nursing bottle containing formula. Prolonged bottle feeding may be considered the best source of nutrition for young children. The oral hygiene recommendations of health care providers may not be considered seriously due to a philosophy that there is little an individual can do to change fate.

Conclusion.—Educating parents from varying cultural backgrounds necessitates an understanding of the life circumstances that are unique to particular cultural groups. Many persons belonging to minority groups or of low economic status do not have the knowledge regarding how to prevent oral diseases. Cultural values and beliefs are important factors that impact care-seeking behaviors. Clinicians need to understand the multicultural factors affecting the United States today to improve the oral health care of all children.

▶ This article presents diverse cultural beliefs and child-rearing behaviors that may influence the delivery of health care to children within these families. The better we understand cultural diversity and its role in health care perception and willingness to change, the better we can address the challenges of underserved populations.

S. B. Canion, DDS, MS

Early Childhood Caries

Causes, Treatment and Prevention of Early Childhood Caries: A Microbiologic Perspective
Berkowitz RJ (Univ of Rochester, NY)
J Can Dent Assoc 69:304-307, 2003   10–4

Introduction.—Early childhood caries (ECC) is a public health problem that affects babies and preschool children throughout the world. In North America, the high-risk populations include Hispanic and Native American children, along with children enrolled in Head Start, a federally funded program for preschool children who are living in poverty. The incidence of ECC in these children ranges between 11% to 72%. The causes, treatment, and prevention of ECC were discussed.

Causes.—The most likely causative agent of ECC is *Streptococcus mutans*. Its early acquisition is a key element in the natural history of the disease. Acquisition may occur through vertical or horizontal transmission. The primary colonization of *S mutans* coupled with caries-promoting feeding behaviors produces accumulation of these organisms to levels surpassing 30% of the total cultivable plaque flora, which in turn produces rapid demineralization of tooth structure.

Treatment.—Treatment of ECC is usually costly because general anesthesia is needed for infants and preschool children. Treatment usually involves restoration or surgical removal of carious teeth and recommendations concerning feeding habits. This approach is associated with unacceptable clinical outcomes, with reports of relapse rates of about 40% within the first year after dental surgery.

Prevention.—Primary prevention of ECC typically involves counseling children concerning caries-promoting feeding behaviors. This approach has also been minimally successful. Newer strategies using topical antimicrobial therapy seem promising.

Conclusion.—The success of current approaches to the treatment and prevention of ECC have been disappointing. A promising approach is the development of strategies that target the infectious component of ECC by preventing or delaying the primary acquisition of *S mutans* at an early age through the suppression of maternal reservoirs of the organism.

▶ The author recognizes that this alternative strategy is in the preliminary stages and that larger and more in-depth clinical trials are necessary to evaluate the true efficacy of this approach. Issues of reimbursement for frequent visits for bimonthly application of antimicrobial agents and patient and parent compliance must also be addressed concerning the actual efficacy of the approach after the antimicrobial agent is withdrawn. This may prove to be an adjunctive therapy for high-risk patients being treated in ambulatory centers or hospitals.

S. B. Canion, DDS, MS

Preschool Caries as an Indicator of Future Caries: A Longitudinal Study
Peretz B, Ram D, Azo E, et al (Hebrew Univ, Jerusalem; Tel-Aviv, Israel)
Pediatr Dent 25:114-118, 2003   10–5

Introduction.—Early childhood caries (ECC) is a distinctive form of rampant caries that develops in the primary dentition soon after eruption of the first teeth. There is some evidence in the dental literature that children who experience ECC continue to be at increased risk for new lesions in both the primary and permanent dentitions as they get older. The increment of carious surfaces per year in children who had ECC was compared with that of children who had posterior caries only and caries-free children after 7 to 10 years.

Methods.—Data from 150 files of children who underwent an initial examination between the ages of 3 and 5 years (T1) and were treated in 2 private pediatric dental clinics were obtained. These children were treated, if necessary, and were seen for follow-up visits at least 7 years after the initial visit (T2). Clinical and radiographic examinations (2 bite-wing radiographs) were reviewed from T1 and T2. There were 3 groups of 50 children each: caries-free children (CF), children with ECC, and children with posterior caries only (PC).

Results.—Children with ECC had a mean of 1.15 new affected surfaces per year; CF children had a mean increment per year of 0.41, and children with PC had a mean increment per year of 0.74. Statistically significant differences were observed between the ECC and CF groups and between the ECC and PC groups. The high increment in the ECC group was impacted by the high number of affected surfaces in the primary teeth.

Conclusion.—Children with ECC may be at increased risk for future carious lesions, compared with CF children. Those with PC have less carious lesions by age 12 years. They resemble ECC children when they are in their mid teens.

▶ This large study over a longer research period of time confirms that ECC is a high-risk indicator for future caries development. Aggressive intervention may be the only viable answer to treating this condition.

S. B. Canion, DDS, MS

Prevalence of Dental Caries and Enamel Defects in Connecticut Head Start Children
Montero MJ, Douglass JM, Mathieu GM (Univ of Illinois, Chicago; Univ of Connecticut, Farmington)
Pediatr Dent 25:235-239, 2003   10–6

Background.—The incidence of caries is higher among children of low-income families, and this has been attributed to a variety of factors, including lack of access to dental care, poor nutrition, and more fatalistic health beliefs among some populations. However, a more tangible cause of the higher incidence of caries among low-income children may be a higher incidence of dental defects, which has been suggested as predisposing teeth to an increased risk of caries and has been associated with increased levels of dental caries. The prevalence of dental caries and enamel defects was investigated in a sample of predominantly African American and Hispanic children in an inner city Head Start program in Connecticut.

Methods.—A total of 517 children aged 2.7 to 4.9 years and enrolled in the federally funded Head Start preschool program in Hartford, Connecticut, were examined for the presence of dental caries and enamel defects. Caries experience was described by means of the dmfs/t indexes, and dental defects were described by using a modified developmental defects of enamel index.

Results.—The mean dmfs in this population was 3.0; caries was present in 38% of the children. The prevalence of enamel defects was 49%. No significant differences in dmfs scores or in the prevalence of defects were observed on analysis by race and ethnicity. Most of the defects were located on anterior teeth, and the type of defect varied with the location. Hypoplasia accounted for 50% of the lesions on the buccal surface of canines, while linear opacities accounted for 50% of the lesions on maxillary anterior teeth. A positive association was observed between enamel defects and caries.

Conclusions.—There was a high prevalence of caries and defects in a population of Head Start children in Connecticut, with most of these defects located on anterior teeth. An association was identified between enamel defects and an increased incidence of caries.

▶ This study confirms previous findings that a small percent of the population (10%) manifests a significant amount of disease (70%). However, there was no difference between the prevalence of caries in African American or Hispanic children. The study also suggests an association between enamel defects and caries, with children with enamel defects having more than twice the level of caries compared with those without enamel defects.

S. B. Canion, DDS, MS

Progression of Proximal Caries in the Mixed Dentition: A 4-Year Prospective Study

Vanderas AP, Manetas C, Koulatzidou M, et al (Univ of Athens, Greece; Athens, Greece)

Pediatr Dent 25:229-234, 2003   10–7

Background.—The progression of caries through the enamel of posterior proximal surfaces of permanent teeth has been reported to be a slow process. There is also evidence that the criteria for restoration of dentin proximal caries are changing, and a new strategy for monitoring lesion progression has been suggested. The results of previous studies showed that an average of 4 years was needed for a lesion to progress through the enamel of permanent teeth, with slower progression for older persons, particularly those with long-term exposure to fluorides. To determine when to apply a restorative treatment on proximal caries, it is necessary to develop more longitudinal knowledge concerning the progression of caries through the enamel and into the dentin of permanent teeth. The survival rate and median survival of different stages of proximal caries were investigated in children aged 6 to 8 up to 10 to 12 years.

Methods.—Proximal caries and caries progression were diagnosed from bite-wing photographs obtained at 1-year intervals for 4 years from 196 children age 6 to 8 years at baseline. The examinations included the mesial surface of the first permanent molars, the mesial and distal surfaces of the first and second primary molars, and the distal surface of the primary canine. In addition, records were made of sound surfaces; caries lesions in the external and internal half of the enamel and external, middle, and internal third of the dentin; and filled, extracted, and exfoliated teeth. Life table analysis was used to estimate the annual and cumulative survival rates and the median survival time of each stage of proximal lesions.

Results.—The cumulative survival rate for the sound mesial surfaces of the first permanent molars was 76%, and the median survival time was over 48 months. The corresponding values for the external half of the enamel lesions were 41% and 45 months. The cumulative survival rate for the sound mesial and distal surfaces of the primary teeth was 92%, and the median survival time was more than 48 months. For the external and internal half of the enamel lesions, the corresponding values were 40% and 31 months and 29% and 22 months, respectively. The value of the cumulative survival rate for the external third of dentin lesions was 42%, with a median survival time of 34 months. The value for the middle third of the dentin was 38%, with a median survival time of 17 months.

Conclusion.—There is a low risk of carious lesions developing in the sound proximal surfaces of both primary teeth and first permanent molars during the mixed dentition period. The progression of the external half of enamel lesions in the first permanent molars is low for the first 3 years and then accelerates. As the duration of exposure to cariogenic factors increases, the progression of the proximal caries is faster for all stages of the lesion in primary teeth.

▶ This study measured the progression of carious lesions in the surfaces of primary molars and first permanent molars. The decision on when to employ demineralization techniques versus restorative measures remains a clinical decision. This study suggests that in the permanent dentition, the progression of decay is low but after the first 3 years, the rate becomes faster and in primary dentition, the greater the exposure time the greater the rate of progression. Thus, the clinician may want to be more aggressive in using treatment modalities.

S. B. Canion, DDS, MS

Interdental Spacing and Caries in the Primary Dentition
Warren JJ, Slayton RL, Yonezu T, et al (Univ of Iowa, Iowa City; Oregon Health and Science Univ, Portland; Tokyo Dental College, Chiba City, Japan)
Pediatr Dent 25:109-113, 2003   10–8

Introduction.—In pediatric dentistry, it is widely believed that the absence of interdental spaces in the proximal dentition increases the risk for interproximal dental caries. The association between interdental spacing patterns and caries experience in the primary dentition was examined in a large sample of US children.

Methods.—Caries examinations were performed in 356 children aged 4 to 6 years. Alginate impressions were obtained and poured in yellow stone at the time of evaluation. Each interdental area from the stone casts was categorized as either: space greater than 1 mm; space less than 1 mm; no space, teeth in contact; or no space, teeth overlapped. These categories were collapsed into presence or absence of space for each interdental site, then counted for each participant. Analyses assessed the associations between interdental spacing and caries experience with separate analyses for anterior spacing, posterior spacing, and total spacing.

Results.—Participants with more total interdental spaces had less decay experience and less untreated decay, compared with children with fewer interdental spaces. Those with more molar spacing had less molar decay experience. Both associations were weak. Correlation analyses showed significant associations between the number of decayed surfaces and the total number of interdental spaces ($r = -1.1$; $P = .04$) and the number of molar sites with interdental spaces ($r = -0.13$; $P = .02$). Multivariate analyses demonstrated that the total number of interproximal spaces were weakly linked with interproximal caries experience; fluoride exposure was a much stronger predictor.

Conclusion.—The absence of interdental spaces is weakly linked with an increased risk of dental decay in the primary dentition.

▶ This study confirms the association between less interdental spacing and greater caries experience. The weakness of the relationship observed in this cohort may relate to the low caries prevalence. For children lacking interproximal spacing, this study supports the rationale for bite-wing radiographs.

S. B. Canion, DDS, MS

Effects of Oral Health Education and Tooth-Brushing on Mutans Streptococci Infection in Young Children
Seow WK, Cheng E, Wan V (Univ of Queensland, Brisbane, Australia)
Pediatr Dent 25:223-228, 2003   10–9

Background.—Dental caries is an infectious disease caused by mutans streptococci bacteria; thus, the presence of this bacteria in the mouth of a child is an important risk factor for caries. There are 2 main cariogenic species of mutans streptococci—*Streptococcus mutans* and *Streptococcus sobrinus*. It has been well established that mutans streptococci is usually transmitted from the mother and that reduction of her bacterial counts may delay this transmission. Earlier introduction of tooth brushing has also been correlated with less caries in young children. The effects of maternal dental health education and early introduction of tooth brushing on the levels of mutans streptococci in children were investigated.

Methods.—One hundred seven children (mean age, 20.5 months) were randomly selected from a child health clinic for participation in this study. Medical, dental, and dietary information was obtained by questionnaire. The children's mouths were clinically examined, and plaque samples were obtained by swabbing the teeth and mucosa. A commercial microbiological kit was used to determine the presence of mutans streptococci. The mothers of these children were instructed in tooth brushing with the soft-scrub method. A second evaluation of the mutans streptococci levels was performed at the same clinic after 4 weeks.

Results.—In the first visit, 69 of 107 children (64%) showed positive infection with mutans streptococci. Of the original 107 children examined, 90 (84%) returned for the follow-up visit. At that examination, only 44 (49%) of the 90 children tested positive for mutans streptococci. This difference was statistically significant. The children who did not show infection with mutans streptococci in the first visit were those who reported greater frequency of tooth brushing and less snacking. Twenty-six children (29%) converted from positive to negative results for mutans streptococci infection between the first and second visits; the conversion was attributed mainly to increased tooth brushing.

Conclusion.—Infection with mutans streptococci in young children is associated with increased frequency of snacking and inadequate tooth brushing. In this study, a single dental health education session and instructing young mothers in tooth brushing provided a reduction of approximately 25% in mutans streptococci infection in young children of relatively high socioeconomic status.

▶ Some have downplayed the effectiveness of patient education and the teaching of tooth brushing as perfunctory behavior, but this study, at least for the short term, demonstrates that education of mothers to start tooth brushing for their children can be successfully achieved through a single health education session and result in mutans streptococci reduction.

S. B. Canion, DDS, MS

Caries Management Under Sedation and General Anesthesia

Mortality Risks Associated With Pediatric Dental Care Using General Anesthesia in a Hospital Setting

Lee JY, Roberts MW (Univ of North Carolina, Chapel Hill)

J Clin Pediatr Dent 27:381-384, 2003   10–10

Introduction.—General anesthesia (GA) may be needed to perform invasive dental procedures in children who are developmentally or medically compromised, or those who are acutely anxious in the dental environment. It may also be appropriate for preschool-aged children with extensive dental needs who have not developed the language skills or attention span necessary for coping with conventional dental care. GA is associated with risks that must be considered when planning dental care in the aforementioned patients. The risk of mortality linked with GA in children in a hospital setting was examined.

Methods.—An 8-item, 1-page survey was mailed to all 928 southeast region hospital members of the American Hospital Association. Questions in the survey addressed the type of institution, availability of dental services, number of pediatric dental cases completed between 1987 and 1997, the American Association of Anesthesiology classification of cases, and the number of dental GA cases that resulted in death. The survey was restricted to children between 1 and 6 years of age.

Results.—The response rate was 41% (376 of 928 member institutions). Of these, 10% reported any pediatric cases in which GA was used between 1987 and 1997. There were 22,615 dental cases using GA for children aged 1 to 6 years during the evaluation period. No deaths were associated with use of GA among respondents.

Conclusion.—There were no deaths linked with the use of GA among responding hospitals between 1987 and 1997 in children aged 1 to 6 years undergoing dental procedures. It appears that use of GA in a hospital setting is a safe alternative in these patients.

▶ Although there can be no guarantees when taking a patient under GA for dental treatment, this study will assist the practitioner in answering the questions regarding mortality risks. However, this study does not remove the ever pervasive element of risk and it specifically does not address the question of morbidity.

S. B. Canion, DDS, MS

Outcomes of Dental Procedures Performed on Children Under General Anesthesia

Al-Eheideb AA, Herman NG (Dental Ctr, King Abdulaziz Med City, Natl Guard, Riyadh, Saudi Arabia; New York Univ)
J Clin Pediatr Dent 27:181-184, 2003   10–11

Introduction.—The ability to treat children with comprehensive dental care in the hospital environment with general anesthesia (GA) is a useful option for pediatric dentists. The durability of the restorative materials must be considered to avoid a second procedure under GA. The integrity and longevity of restorative and pulpal procedures performed on primary teeth under GA were examined in children undergoing comprehensive dental treatment.

Methods.—Fifty-four of 92 children who underwent dental procedures under GA between 1993 and 1995 responded to a request for recall examination. Medical and dental histories were reviewed. Background data were gathered from dental records. Patients underwent an oral examination to rate the quality of the restorative pulpal treatments.

Results.—The range of the postoperative examination period was 6 to 27 months. The primary reasons for treatment under GA were behavior problems and inability to cooperate. Restoration of posterior teeth with stainless steel crowns were more successful (95.5%) than were amalgam or composite restorations (50%). In the anterior teeth, strip crowns had a success rate comparable to that of class III, IV, and V composite resin materials. Pulpotomies had an extremely high success rate (97.1%). Sealants were retained in 68.3% of procedures.

Conclusion.—Stainless steel crowns were more likely to be successful and last longer, compared with multisurface amalgam or composite restorations in children treated under GA. The failure rate of both strip crowns and composite restorations was 30% in the anterior teeth. Definitive treatment is more likely to assure a positive outcome for children treated under GA since it is linked with less frequent complications from failed restorations.

▶ This study confirms the findings of others regarding effective treatment of high-risk patients treated under GA. Conservative dentistry applied to high-risk compromised patients will inevitably end in a poor treatment outcome and necessitate frequent repair of restorations or outright failure of the restoration.

S. B. Canion, DDS, MS

Evidence-Based Restorative Dental Care for High-Risk Children

Mueller WA (Aurora, Colo)
J Dent Child 70:61-64, 2003   10–12

Introduction.—Most general practitioners base their decision concerning intracoronal versus metal crown restorations upon the extent of carious destruction of an individual tooth. There is a need for greater accountability and justification of treatment plans to government and insurance carriers, making it important that treatment plans be based on evidence rather than opinion. The evidence available to clinicians regarding restorative dental care for high-risk children was reviewed to ascertain which approach should be used in planning treatment for these patients.

Methods.—A literature review was performed to determine the areas of population risk, individual risk, treatment outcomes, and decision making. Information from these areas was integrated to construct a plan of action for practitioners.

Results.—Caries is a transmissible infectious disease acquired by children during a specific time frame and is site-specific and symmetrical in a predictable pattern. This makes it possible for clinicians to anticipate subsequent occurrences. High-risk groups include immigrant and low-income children. Children with caries or extensive visible plaque on primary anterior teeth on initial examination are highly likely to have caries lesions develop at specific sites and in specific patterns associated with stages of dental development.

Efforts at prevention directed to these high-risk children are unproven. Evidence suggests that in these high-risk groups, restorations that just restore the damage already done with a multisurface amalgam or composite restoration are likely doomed to failure. Preformed metal crowns have greater longevity and reduced treatment need in primary molars that require multisurface restorations. Caries recurrence is highly predictable.

Conclusion.—Evidence available to clinicians regarding restorative dental care for high-risk children needs to be reviewed by the clinical practitioner and included in the decision-making process when creating treatment plans for high-risk groups.

▶ Treatment for high-risk populations should be definitive, durable, comfortable, and functional, and ideally the restoration should last the life of the primary tooth through exfoliation.

S. B. Canion, DDS, MS

Adverse Events and Outcomes of Conscious Sedation for Pediatric Patients: Study of an Oral Sedation Regimen
Leelataweedwud P, Vann WF Jr (Mahidol Univ, Bangkok, Thailand; Univ of North Carolina, Chapel Hill)
J Am Dent Assoc 132:1531-1539, 2001   10–13

Background.—Conscious sedation has for many years been a popular approach to the management of young uncooperative children in need of invasive dental and medical procedures. Conscious sedation is thought to be widely used by general dental practitioners, but the frequency of its use is not well documented in this population. However, the frequency of use of conscious sedation among pediatric dentists is well documented in the literature. The use of conscious sedation is associated with a risk of potential adverse side effects, including nausea and vomiting (as can occur with sedation agents such as chloral hydrate, meperidine, and nitrous oxide) and respiratory compromise. This study reported on the adverse events and sedation outcomes for an oral sedation regimen comprising chloral hydrate, meperidine, and hydroxyzine with 100% oxygen supplementation.

Methods.—Records for 111 healthy children (aged 24-48 months) were reviewed in this 5-year retrospective study. The records were analyzed for age, sex, weight, methods of drug delivery, waiting time after drug administration, treatment rendered, treatment time, adverse events, sedation outcomes, and the number of visits needed to complete treatment.

Results.—Adverse events occurred in 3% of all sedations and were minor in nature. They consisted of vomiting, desaturation, prolonged sedation, and an apneic event. Satisfactory behavior outcomes were noted in 72% of sedations, while 23% had unsatisfactory behavior outcomes, and 5% of procedures were discontinued as a result of the disruptive behavior of the patient. Better sedation outcomes were obtained with patient compliance with oral medications and a longer waiting time after medication intake.

Conclusion.—Only a few minor adverse events occurred with a sedation regimen of chloral hydrate, meperidine, and hydroxyzine with 100% oxygen supplementation. The use of this regimen provided reasonable outcomes with minimal adverse events. Patient compliance with oral medications and a longer waiting time appeared to be important factors contributing to the success of this regimen.

▶ This conscious sedation regimen is not a panacea, but utilization in a strict protocol has a reasonable outcome with minimal events.

S. B. Canion, DDS, MS

Pain Management

The Relationship of Application Time to EMLA Efficacy
Barcohana N, Duperon DF, Yashar M (Beverly Hills, Calif; Univ of California, Los Angeles)
J Dent Child 70:51-54, 2003   10–14

Background.—New advances in dental technology have facilitated dental operative procedures on patients without the use of local anesthesia. However, the use of rubber dam clamps or matrix bands with these patients is often uncomfortable, and these procedures may require the use of a topical anesthetic that is effective at a practical application time. A previous study found that 5% eutectic mixture of local anesthetics (EMLA) cream significantly increased the pain threshold, followed by 1% dyclonine and 20% benzocaine. The efficacy of 5% EMLA cream at application times of 3, 5, and 10 minutes was compared to determine the most effective duration of topical anesthetic application on normal mucosa.

Methods.—Twenty volunteers (11 men, 9 women; ages 22-37 years) were recruited for this study. EMLA cream (20 mL) or placebo was placed on the maxillary anterior region with the use of Beckman paper wicks formed into disks. The gingiva was wiped dry to obtain the most effective absorption result. The disks were left on the gingiva for 3, 5, and 10 minutes and left off for another 3 minutes. A special instrument was used to apply progressive pressure on the gingiva to obtain a threshold level of discomfort in grams before and after topical application of EMLA or placebo.

Results.—There was a significant reduction in the pain threshold level with 5% EMLA cream compared with placebo at all application times, with no significant differences among the different application times.

Conclusion.—The use of 5% EMLA could be particularly beneficial to pediatric patients and to young adults with a fear of needles. Future research should be directed toward the development of an EMLA patch with the proper pediatric dosages to prevent possible overdose and side effects in children.

▶ EMLA cream has the ability to produce anesthesia through intact skin. It has been used primarily to produce anesthesia of the skin before the insertion of an IV cannula for sedation or general anesthesia. This study suggests that 5% EMLA could be beneficial to pediatric patients and young adults who are needle phobic. It also suggests development of an EMLA patch with the proper pediatric dosage to avoid possible overdosage and side effects. This agent does have promise, but I agree with the authors that future research is necessary. The best application time was not answered in this study.

S. B. Canion, DDS, MS

The Assessment of Pain Sensation During Local Anesthesia Using a Computerized Local Anesthesia (Wand) and a Conventional Syringe
Ram D, Peretz B (Hebrew Univ, Jerusalem)
J Dent Child 70:130-133, 2003   10–15

Background.—Anxiety is a significant issue in the delivery of dental treatment to children, and the most anxiety-provoking procedure for both children and adults is injection. However, the administration of injected local anesthesia in children can also be a source of significant anxiety for the dentist. It is thought that the fear of injection begins early in life, as anticipatory fear of sharp objects has been observed in children at about 1 year of age. Studies that have attempted to define the influence of duration of injection on pain have produced conflicting results, but it is thought that slower injections are less painful. In addition, it is generally recommended that a topical anesthetic agent be administered for at least 1 minute before administration of local anesthesia to minimize the sensation of pain from the injection; however, this procedure has not completely eliminated the pain associated with the use of local anesthesia.

A computerized local anesthetic delivery system has been developed and may be a solution to the problem of reduction of pain associated with local anesthesia. The reactions of children who received local anesthesia with a conventional syringe injection were compared with reactions to anesthesia received with a computerized device (Wand).

Methods.—The study group was composed of 102 children aged 3 to 10 years, divided into groups of 55 children aged 3 to 5 years and 47 children aged 6 to 10 years. All of the children needed at least 2 clinical sessions of operative procedures preceded by injection of local anesthesia, 1 injection on either side of the same jaw. The local anesthesia was delivered in a random crossover design using either the Wand or the traditional syringe.

Results.—Most of the children in both groups had a good reaction to both techniques, with no significant differences between boys and girls. The children's reactions to injection in the mandible or maxilla were similar for the traditional syringe and Wand techniques in regard to crying; facial expressions; and hand, leg, or torso movements. No statistically significant difference was found between the 2 techniques whether the maxillary infiltration was delivered to 1 or to multiple teeth. In addition, there was no significant difference whether the Wand was delivered during the first or second visit.

Conclusion.—It appears that there is no difference in the pain behavior of children during administration of local anesthesia with a conventional injection versus a computerized injection.

▶ The computerized local anesthesia (Wand) system holds promise for minimizing injection anxiety in adults, but it has not been proven to be significantly less painful relative to conventional injection by syringe in children.

S. B. Canion, DDS, MS

Restorative Materials and Techniques

The Effect of Acid Primer or Conventional Acid Etching on Microleakage in a Photoactivated Sealant

Perry AO, Rueggeberg FA (Med College of Georgia, Augusta)
Pediatr Dent 25:127-131, 2003   10–16

Background.—Dental sealants are an effective means of preventing pit and fissure caries. These sealants are either self-activated or light-activated, filled or unfilled resin systems bonded to etched enamel. However, the conventional methods of sealant placement involve numerous time-consuming steps. The self-etching primer, a new type of acid-priming material, has recently been introduced to the market. These self-etching primers make use of a combination of acidic resins that simultaneously demineralize both enamel and dentin and then are polymerized directly to the tooth. With this technique, no rinsing or drying is required, and the time to maintaining a dry field is lowered in comparison with conventional methods. The differences in microleakage in extracted human teeth when sealants were placed with the use of a conventional acid etching versus use of an acidic primer resin were examined.

Methods.—This study utilized 3 experimental groupings: conventional acid etching with placement of light-cured sealant (group 1); application of an acidic primer resin (Prompt L-Pop, ESPE, Seefeld, Germany) and light curing, followed by sealant placement (group 2); and photocuring of acidic primer and sealant after placement (group 3). Teeth in all 3 groups were thermocycled, stained, sectioned, and examined for marginal microleakage. *Results.*—In group 1, 94% of the enamel-sealant interfaces were free of microleakage. In groups 2 and 3, only 28% showed no leakage, with most leakage occurring at both margin and base areas. Nonparametric data analysis showed that acid etching demonstrated significantly lower microleakage compared with either treatment using the acidic primer resin and that leakage scores in the acidic primer groups were identical.

Conclusion.—The use of the acid resin primer in place of conventional acid etching resulted in a greater incidence of microleakage and thus is not recommended over traditional etching procedures.

▶ There are less steps involved in placing sealants when using the acidic primer, which would save both patient and clinician chairside time. However, this specific acidic primer resin did not compare to the conventional acid etch and sealant placement technique in preventing microleakage at the enamel-sealant interface.

S. B. Canion, DDS, MS

Restoration-Enamel Interface With Argon Laser and Visible Light Polymerization of Compomer and Composite Resin Restorations: A Polarized Light and Scanning Electron Microscopic In Vitro Study

Hicks J, Ellis R, Flaitz C, et al (Univ of Texas, Houston; Pueblo, Colo; Creighton Univ, Omaha, Neb; et al)
J Clin Pediatr Dent 27:353-358, 2003   10–17

Introduction.—The interface between enamel and a restorative material is important in preventing secondary caries formation. The ability to eradicate voids and microspaces along this interface is crucial in reducing the likelihood of secondary caries development. A synergistic effect between topical fluoride and argon laser (AL) irradiation has been identified, with dramatic decreases in enamel and root surface caries formation. The effect of AL and visible light (VL) polymerization of compomer and composite resin materials on the restoration-enamel interface was examined in this polarized light and scanning electron microscope (SEM) in vitro investigation.

Findings.—Surface topography by SEM demonstrated a smooth transition between the restorative materials and adjacent enamel surfaces, with no microspaces between the restorations and enamel surfaces. The enamel surfaces revealed relatively smooth surface coatings with AL curing versus exposure of etched prism endings with VL curing. The restoration-enamel interface by polarized light demonstrated an intimate association between the restorative materials and the cavosurface enamel. No differences were seen between AL and VL polymerization. With the restoration-enamel interface by SEM, compomers, and composite resins were adapted closely to the cavosurface enamel and tags of restorative material protruded into the adjacent cavosurface material.

Conclusion.—Both VL and AL polymerization of compomers and composite resin restorations in vitro provided closely adapted restorations with intimate restoration-enamel interfaces. These restoration-enamel interfaces may offer some resistance against secondary caries formation, which may be enhanced by the caries protective effect of AL irradiation.

▶ AL polymerization of compomers and composite resin restorations in vitro produced closely adapted restorations with intimate restoration-enamel interfaces, identical to those for VL polymerized compomers and composite resins. Although the adaptation of these materials was identical with the respective curing sources, the authors suggest that increased resistance against a cariogenic challenge may come from the surface coating overlying the enamel adjacent to the AL-cured restoration.

S. B. Canion, DDS, MS

Effect of APF Minute-Foam on the Surface Roughness, Hardness, and Micromorphology of High-Viscosity Glass Ionomers
García-Godoy F, García-Godoy A, García-Godoy F (Nova Southeastern Univ, Fort Lauderdale, Fla)
J Dent Child 70:19-23, 2003   10–18

Introduction.—Restorative materials—including porcelain, resin-based composites, sealants, and glass-ionomer cements (GICs)—are susceptible to alterations in surface morphology when treated with topical fluoride gels. Topical applications of acidulated phosphate fluoride (APF) gels may change the surface texture of resin-based restorative materials. The daily use of fluoride may affect the stability and structure of the GICs. The effect of Oral-B APF Minute-Foam on the surface roughness, hardness, and morphology of high-velocity GICs was examined.

Methods.—The GICs were Fuji IX GP and Ketac-Molar; the controls were Vitremer resin-modified GIC and Fuji II conventional GIC. The materials were mixed to a restorative consistency. The encapsulated GICs were mixed by a Rotomix for 10 seconds. For each GIC, 14 specimens (6 mm in diameter and 3 mm thick) were created, with a Teflon mold and a fresh mix used for each sample. The specimens set at room temperature for 15 minutes, then were stored in water at room temperature for 48 hours. Profilometry and microhardness measurements (Knoop) were determined on untreated specimens as baseline data.

Specimens were rinsed with water and gently air-dried; 1.23% APF Minute-Foam was applied for 1 minute with a brush, rinsed with water, and gently air-dried. Hardness and roughness were remeasured. In another set, similar measurements were taken and a 4-minute application of the APF foam was used. In yet another set, similar measurements were obtained as before after a simulated 2-year application of the APF foam. The APF effects on the surface micromorphology of the materials were evaluated.

Results.—Foam application time had no statistically significant effect on the surface roughness of Ketac-Molar or Vitremer. Fiji IX GP demonstrated that 1- and 4-minute applications had lower values compared with those after 2 years. Fuji II had similar roughness for the control at 1 and 4 minutes, yet higher values after 2 years. Fuji IX GP showed no significant difference in hardness after the different application times. Ketac-Molar had less hardness than the control at 1 and 4 minutes, yet hardness was higher after 2 years. Foam application time had no statistically significant influence on the surface hardness of Vitremer. For Fuji II, 1 minute produced harder values versus 4 minutes and 2 years; the control was harder than 2-year specimens.

Conclusion.—Surface morphology was not significantly affected by the use of Oral-B APF Minute-Foam. Treatment with the APF foam tested may be material dependent. Application for shorter times (1 vs 4 minutes) appears to be preferable to diminish any adverse effect.

▶ The application times (1 and 4 minutes) were chosen because these were the recommended application times for APF agents. With the increasing use of esthetic restorative materials in dentistry, the dental team must be careful with the application of topical APF agents in their efforts to prevent future disease. In the case of this particular APF foam, the shorter application times appear to be less deleterious.

S. B. Canion, DDS, MS

Pediatric Medical Concerns

The Prevalence of Periodontal-Related Changes in Adolescents With Asthma: Results of the Third Annual National Health and Nutrition Examination Survery

Shulman JD, Nunn ME, Taylor SE, et al (Baylor College of Dentistry, Dallas; Boston Univ)
Pediatr Dent 25:279-284, 2003   10–19

Introduction.—The prevalence of asthma has been increasing in the United States, particularly among children younger than age 14 years. There is concern regarding a link between asthma and periodontal disease that may involve either pathologic activation of the immune and inflammatory processes, anti-asthmatic medications, or the interaction between them. The relationship between asthma and periodontal disease in adolescents was assessed by means of oral examination and health interview data from the Third National Health and Nutrition Examination Survey (1988-1994).

Methods.—A total of 1596 adolescents aged 13 to 17 years were evaluated. Of these, 253 (16%) had asthma and 1358 (84%) acted as control subjects. All participants were examined for bleeding on probing, subgingival calculus, supragingival calculus, probing depth of 3 mm or greater, and loss of periodontal attachment of 2 mm or greater. Adjustments were made for parents' income, gender, race, exposure to potentially xerogenic drugs (antihistamines, corticosteroids, and inhalers), tobacco exposure, and dental examination within the past year.

Results.—None of the periodontal measures was linked with asthma severity or with use of any of the anti-asthmatic drugs. Several covariates had statistically significant odds ratios ($P < .05$).

Conclusion.—No evidence was identified to support an association between asthma and periodontal health in the adolescent population.

▶ The increasing prevalence of asthma in the population has given rise to multiple questions regarding the association of it and oral health problems. This study provides no evidence to support the association between asthma and periodontal health in the adolescent population.

S. B. Canion, DDS, MS

Effects of Therapy on Dentofacial Development in Long-term Survivors of Head and Neck Rhabdomyosarcoma: The Memorial Sloan-Kettering Cancer Center Experience
Estilo CL, Huryn JM, Kraus DH, et al (Mem Sloan-Kettering Cancer Ctr, New York)
J Pediatr Hematol Oncol 25:215-222, 2003   10–20

Introduction.—About 150 per 1 million children in the United States who are younger than 20 years will be diagnosed with cancer each year. Of these, 4.6 per million will be diagnosed with rhabdomyosarcoma, the most common malignant tumor of the soft tissues in infants and children. The potential impact of multimodal therapy on dental and facial development in long-term survivors of head and neck rhabdomyosarcoma was examined retrospectively.

Methods.—The medical records of all patients aged 20 years or less seen between December 1, 1984, and December 31, 1996, with a diagnosis of rhabdomyosarcoma and treated by protocol were examined. Data were gathered from the pediatric database, office records, and medical and dental records. Patients with head and neck rhabdomyoscarcoma who were alive and free of disease at a minimum of 5-year follow-up were included. Ten patients satisfied inclusion criteria. The median age of these 10 patients at diagnosis was 4.3 years (range, 10 months to 19.5 years). All patients were treated with chemotherapy, 2 underwent surgery, and all except 1 received external beam radiation therapy.

Results.—Clinical or radiographic dentofacial abnormalities were seen in 8 of the 10 (80%) patients and included enamel defects, bony hypoplasia/facial asymmetry, trismus, velopharyngeal incompetency, tooth/root agenesis, and disturbance in root development. Bony hypoplasia and disturbance in root formation were observed most frequently.

Conclusion.—Multimodal therapy for head and neck rhabdomyosarcoma can produce dentofacial abnormalities that impact on quality of life. The care of the long-term survivor necessitates a multidisciplinary approach, including early involvement of the dental team.

▶ The success in improving the survival rate of children with rhabdomyosarcoma presents a unique challenge for the oral health team. The critical role of prevention and dental education before, during, and after cancer therapy can decrease or even eliminate the need for invasive dental procedures in many pediatric oncology patients. Multidisciplinary early intervention is the key to enhancing the quality of life for long-term cancer survivors.

S. B. Canion, DDS, MS

Section B

INTRODUCTION

This year's selections reflect the shifting emphasis of dentistry to a medical model. Articles concerning treatment plans based on risk, how *Streptococcus mutans* is transmitted, and other major aspects of the infectious diseases we deal with every day are presented. This year's focus is primarily on dental caries. Since the advent of fluoride, the major affected teeth have changed from proximal surfaces of premolars to pit-and-fissure caries, primarily of molars. The diagnosis of pit-and-fissure decay remains a problem but is being addressed by new technology described here. These developments, along with an emphasis on clinical trial methodology as the basis for evidence-based dentistry, are also reflected here. Finally, the patient's role in self-care (compliance) and the profession's societal responsibility are described.

Stephen Wotman, DDS

A Pilot Study of Risk-Based Prevention in Private Practice
Bader JD, Shugars DA, Kennedy JE, et al (Univ of North Carolina at Chapel Hill; Univ of Connecticut, Farmington; Dental Delivery Systems Consultants, Lee's Summit, Mo; et al)
J Am Dent Assoc 134:1195-1202, 2003   10–21

Background.—Risk-based prevention strategies have been promoted as an effective management technique for dental caries and periodontal prevention, with dentists being encouraged to assess the level of caries risk for each patient and design interventions on the basis of risk level and reasons for the determination. A pilot study was undertaken in conjunction with a national insurance carrier to refine the study procedures needed to conduct a full-scale demonstration study of risk-based prevention in dental offices. Methods of communicating risk assessment from practitioner to insurance carrier and the practitioners' reasons for assigning risk levels and proposed preventive treatment plans were assessed.

Methods.—Clinicians in 15 dental offices volunteered to participate in a 6-month pilot study. Along with oral examinations of patients for the insurance carrier, patients with higher risk of developing dental caries and periodontitis were identified, including the risk indicators or reasons for elevated risk and the planned preventive treatment in response to risk. The information was documented and shared with the insurer using the claim form and stick-on notes. Data were available for 813 adult patients.

Results.—Thirty-four patients (4%) were identified as being at high risk for developing dental caries, with a range of 0% to 18% among the various offices. Twenty-nine percent of patients were identified as being at moderate risk, with a wide variation in the proportions reported by each office (7% to 88%). Two thirds of the patients were in the low-risk category, with a broad range of proportions among offices. The specific caries-preventive treatments planned for high- and moderate-risk patients included oral hygiene and/or dietary counseling, topical fluoride application, and more frequent prophylaxis and/or recall appointments, with the relative frequencies of these interventions similar regardless of risk category. Only small percentages of patients were scheduled to undergo patient-based preventive treatments such as the use of a prescription fluoride dentifrice or mouthrinse, prescription antimicrobial mouthrinse, over-the-counter fluoride rinse, or calcium phosphate dentifrice.

Fifty-eight patients (7%) were labeled as high risk for developing periodontitis, with a narrow range of proportions among the various offices. Moderate risk was assessed in 241 patients (30%). The indicators used most often for elevated periodontal risk were pocket depth and bleeding on probing; other risk indicators included smoking and increasing pocket depth. The predominant planned intervention for patients at high risk for periodontal disease was more frequent recall program; hygiene aids/enhanced instruction and the use of antimicrobial mouthrinse were planned less often.

Discussion.—The clinicians offered appropriate reasons for assigning patients to the high- and moderate-risk categories regarding the development of dental caries or periodontal disease. In addition, patients at elevated risk received more treatment than lower-risk patients. The preventive and maintenance interventions planned for patients at elevated risk were similarly appropriate. Additional consideration should be given to clarifying the criteria used to define moderate disease risk, as reflected by the wide variance noted among the volunteering offices.

▶ Studies carried out in the real world of dental practice provide substantial information about what is practical in the real world. This pilot study provides preliminary information on the ability of dentists to evaluate patients for risk and prescribe appropriate preventive measures, based on the risk status of the individual patient. Although this study provides evidence that a well-thought-out risk assessment program is feasible and probably will improve efficiency in the provision of oral health care, the next step would be to do a comparative study of oral health outcomes for the patients involved. The risk assessment approach is an important first step in the reorientation of the dentist's approach to the control of disease rather than the repair of the ravages of disease and the restoration of function.

S. Wotman, DDS

Acquisition and Transmission of Mutans Streptococci

Berkowitz RJ (Univ of Rochester, NY)
Calif Dent Assoc J 31:135-138, 2003   10–22

Background.—Dental caries is an infectious, transmissible disease. Streptococci and some *Lactobacillus* species are the infectious agents most strongly associated with dental caries. It was thought, on the basis of previous studies, that *Streptococcus mutans* could not colonize the predentate oral cavity because they have a feeble capacity to attach themselves to epithelial surfaces. It was shown in earlier studies that infants acquired *S mutans* from their mothers and that acquisition of the bacteria only occurred after the eruption of primary teeth. However, more recent clinical studies have demonstrated that *S mutans* is able to colonize the mouths of predentate infants. The latest findings in clinical research on acquisition of *S mutans* in the predentate infant are reviewed.

Overview.—Early colonization by *S mutans* is a major risk factor for future development of dental caries. The furrows of the tongue seem to be an important ecological niche. The major source of infection with *S mutans* in infants is the mother. However, horizontal transmission is also possible; studies among groups of nursery school children have found that many children harbored identical genotypes of *S mutans* strains, which indicates that horizontal transmission may be another vector for the acquisition of these organisms. Recent findings that reported the potential for *S mutans* to colonize the mouths of predentate infants imply that the timing of intervention strategies for the prevention or delay of transmission should consider that a nonshedding oral surface—the primary teeth—is likely not a requirement for oral colonization by these bacteria.

Conclusions.—It is clear that *S mutans* can colonize the predentate infant mouth and that horizontal and vertical transmission occur. Additional clinical studies are needed to facilitate the development of strategies for prevention and delay of infection by *S mutans* in infants, which will reduce the prevalence of dental caries.

▶ Understanding the dynamics of dental caries is necessary information if we wish to control this disease more effectively. The infectious character of the disease is being better defined with recent information concerning when and how *S mutans* is transmitted. Evidence quoted in this article suggests that organisms causing dental caries are transmitted to infants even before the eruption of teeth. Between the ages of 6 and 18 months, 70% of children had *S mutans* in tongue scrapings. Transmission from mother to child and between siblings has been demonstrated.

S. Wotman, DDS

Caries Vaccines for the Twenty-First Century
Smith DJ (Forsyth Inst, Boston)
J Dent Educ 67:1130-1139, 2003   10–23

Background.—Great progress has been made in understanding the etiology of dental caries. However, caries remains a significant disease in many parts of the world and in large segments of the American population, particularly the poor and the elderly. Developments in the ongoing struggle to conquer dental caries and the potential for development of a caries vaccine are reviewed.

Overview.—Molecular biological and cultural techniques have identified several bacteria involved in the process and extension of dental caries. However, *Streptococcus mutans* infection is, by far, the most important source of caries. The use of fluoride, sugarless products, and sealants and increased access to dental care have had a significant effect on the reduction of caries in the young and economically advantaged. However, economic, behavioral, or cultural barriers to their use have perpetuated the epidemic in many parts of the world and among some populations in the United States. At present, both passive and active immunization approaches for caries vaccination have shown success in animal models and in human clinical trials in adults. However, a number of challenges must be overcome in the development of an effective dental caries vaccine. One challenge involves the timing of vaccination, which ideally would occur in the second year of life to intercept initial colonizing events. However, studies have shown that children at 1 year of age are able to mount secretory responses to the proteins that have been suggested as vaccine components.

Conclusions.—The development of an effective dental caries vaccine would have a profound effect on the health of children, particularly for those who are at increased caries risk because of their economic or cultural position.

▶ Although the presence of fluoride and good dental care severely restricts the amount of dental caries seen by most dentists, populations not receiving regular dental care continue to have high caries rates. A recent experience in Cleveland in a program that provides sealants for 2nd and 6th graders in inner city schools found that more than 70% of these children have carious lesions.[1] Other findings suggest that the reduction in caries has reached a plateau. Smith's article suggests targeted populations for a vaccine—children during the window of infectivity are also good candidates for early dental care. It is well-known that it is extremely difficult to implant *S mutans* in the mouths of adults, so prevention of infection in children would be a major breakthrough.

S. Wotman, DDS

Reference

1. Bingham M, Lalumandier J, Nelson S, et al: Prevalence and severity of caries by school. *J Dent Educ* Feb 2004 (Abstract 29).

The Caries Balance: Contributing Factors and Early Detection

Featherstone JDB (Univ of California, San Francisco)

Calif Dent Assoc J 31:129-133, 2003   10–24

Background.—An overview of the process of dental caries, its management, and the role of early detection in the effective management of tooth decay is presented.

Overview.—Dental caries is a well-understood process. Much is known about demineralization, the role of fluoride in inhibiting or reversing dental caries, and the multiple roles of saliva and salivary components. It is also known that acidogenic bacteria, primarily *Streptococcus mutans* and the lactobacilli species, cause demineralization and, thus, caries and that fermentable carbohydrates in foods and beverages contribute to the caries process. The one area in which there is still much to learn involves the complex microbiological process that occurs in the dental plaque or biofilm on the surface of the tooth. Until recently, caries detection has involved visual, tactile, and radiographic methods. However, visual detection is difficult when the surface of the tooth is obscured and in occlusal surfaces, and lesions on occlusal surfaces can only be detected radiographically when they are advanced. The US Food and Drug Administration has recently approved a device (the DIAGNOdent) that shines a red laser into the tooth. The red light easily penetrates the tooth, and fluorescence occurs when the light interacts with a subsurface lesion that contains certain bacterial byproducts. More improvements and new techniques for early detection of caries will be available in the future, and the purpose of detection must be intervention, not justification of more drilling and filling. It is also anticipated that improved chairside bacterial testing and improved antibacterials will be available in the near future.

Conclusions.—The control of caries for individual patients is dependent on risk assessment, therapeutic analysis, and conservative management. The balance between the factors involved in the etiology of caries and those that protect the individual patient from caries progression is described, and the role of early detection in the clinical management of this disease is emphasized.

▶ Featherstone describes caries progression or reversal as the result of an important balance between pathologic and protective factors. It is the responsibility of the dentist to help tip this balance toward protection, thus controlling or eliminating progression of the disease. Risk assessment, therapeutic analysis, and conservative caries management are described as step-by-step techniques to accomplish disease control for individual patients. This process is assisted by recently developed methods for early caries detection.

S. Wotman, DDS

Occlusal Pit-and-Fissure Caries Diagnosis: A Problem No More: A Science-Based Diagnostic Approach Using a Laser-Based Fluorescence Device

Sanchez-Figueras A Jr (Glendale, Calif)

Compend Contin Educ Dent 24:3-11, 2003   10–25

Background.—There has been little change in the methodology of occlusal pit-and-fissure caries diagnosis in the past 100 years. Great strides have been made in caries prevention, but it remains a common health problem in the United States and throughout the world. The National Institutes of Health's Consensus Development Conference on Caries Prevention and Management in 2001 highlighted the need for more diagnostically specific caries management protocols and methods. The literature related to occlusal pit-and-fissure caries diagnosis is reviewed, and a relatively new diagnostic method that uses a laser fluorescence device is described.

Overview.—Many clinicians are surprised to discover the extent and severity of carious involvement of a specific tooth, particularly when radiologic and clinical examinations have indicated that little or no carious process should be present. However, the degree and extent of demineralization and compromised tooth structure are already significantly advanced by the time an explorer detects an occlusal catch. The result is the removal of significant amounts of tooth structure in the process of fashioning a functional restoration. Earlier detection of the carious occlusal lesion could have prevented the consequential structural weakening of the tooth. Laser fluorescence is a new technology in caries detection. Three cases are presented in this article to highlight the effectiveness of laser fluorescence, as part of a science-based diagnostic approach, in early detection of caries on occlusal surfaces.

Conclusions.—Occlusal pit-and-fissure caries is a ubiquitous disease that has not been affected much by fluoridation of the water supply. It is thought that fluoridation of the enamel has increased its resistance to demineralization such that an enamel "ceiling" may disguise carious lesions that cavitate much later in the course of the disease. The evidence presented here is supportive of the need for diagnostic tools and methods with greater sensitivity, such as laser fluorescence, to aid in the early detection of caries.

▶ Teeth are wonderful archeological artifacts. After the individual has died, they are often preserved for millennia. In life, they are subject to destruction, and the primary culprit is dental caries. Since the advent of fluoride as a primary preventive mechanism, the most prevalent remaining susceptible portion of the tooth are the occlusal pits and fissures. Early detection of occlusal caries is an essential element in any effective disease control program. By the time a lesion is detected with an explorer, it is often large enough to endanger substantial amounts of tooth structure or be very close to the pulp. Previous studies have even suggested that the intrusion of the explorer may itself be an untoward event in the progression of the disease. The recent development of a laser diagnostic device promises earlier detection of occlusal caries and offers the possibility of substantially greater tooth preservation through conservative management.

S. Wotman, DDS

Integration of a Laser Fluorescence Caries Detection Device in Dental Hygiene Practice
Guignon AN (Houston)
Compend Contin Educ Dent 24:13-17, 2003   10–26

Background.—It has been shown that most initial carious lesions are found on occlusal surfaces. The detection of occlusal caries continues to rely on methods that have remained the same for hundreds of years: visual and tactile inspection of a lesion suggestive of caries. Many studies have shown that radiographic evaluation of occlusal caries is much less effective than visual inspection in the detection of early lesions. Another factor complicating the management of dental caries is that the widespread use of fluoride has resulted in harder enamel surfaces, which effectively hide carious lesions until they are well advanced. In addition, there is evidence that an undetected carious lesion may continue to progress after a tooth is sealed, which leaves the tooth vulnerable to additional destruction. One promising technological development is laser fluorescence for early caries detection.

Overview.—The DIAGNOdent is a diode-laser caries detector that can be used to determine the soundness of the tooth structure on occlusal surfaces. This can aid clinicians in determining whether demineralization therapy, sealant application, or a more invasive restorative procedure is appropriate for an individual tooth. The integration of this technology into a dental hygiene practice is described. Hygienists have a genuine desire to contribute to the success of a dental practice and to the overall health of patients. The integration of laser caries detection can provide the hygienist with an opportunity to provide a more complete oral health evaluation and can provide the patient with reassurance that the final diagnosis is based on scientifically obtained, objective data. It has been estimated that 30% to 50% more occlusal caries will be detected at earlier stages with this technology. Laser fluorescence caries detection technology can also be used to monitor changes over time that may reflect remineralization and reversal of the caries process.

Conclusions.—The integration of laser fluorescence caries technology offers the opportunity for earlier detection of carious lesions on occlusal surfaces and provides the dental hygienist with an ideal tool for patient assessment.

▶ Dental hygienists have become ubiquitous in dental practices in most parts of the country. The dental hygienist assumes a large part of the preventive responsibility of the practice and manages the traditional recall visit, which is designed to detect any progression of disease. Guignon addresses how the use of the new laser diagnostic technology can be combined with appropriate therapeutic measures to control caries for individual patients through the diagnosis and therapeutic recommendations made as part of dental hygiene practice.

S. Wotman, DDS

Diagnosis of Approximal Caries: Bite-Wing Radiology Versus the Ultrasound Caries Detector. An In Vitro Study

Matalon S, Feuerstein O, Kaffe I (Tel Aviv Univ, Israel; Hebrew Univ, Jerusalem)
Oral Surg Oral Med Oral Pathol Oral Radiol Endod 95:626-631, 2003   10–27

Background.—Bite-wing radiographs are a widely accepted and an important adjunct in the diagnosis of approximal carious lesions. The validity, sensitivity, and specificity of bite-wing radiographs and high-frequency sound waves in providing a diagnosis of carious lesions on approximal surfaces were compared and measured.

Methods.—Thirty-six human premolars and molars were extracted and stored in phosphate-buffered saline solution. Each tooth was examined independently by 7 clinicians with the Ultrasound Caries Detector (UCD) (Novadent Ltd, Savyon, Israel), and bite-wing radiographs were also taken under standardized conditions.

Results.—The sensitivity (interpreting a lesion as being present) was 0.90 for all observers and the specificity (interpreting no lesion) was 0.92 for all observers compared to the UCD, which was 1.0 for both sensitivity and specificity.

Discussion.—The new UCD had better efficacy than bite-wing radiology in detecting approximal carious lesions and a similar level of accuracy to that of bite-wing radiographs.

▶ Although bite-wing x-rays have long been the sine qua non of diagnostic technique for interproximal caries, there are some important limitations to the use of this technique. There continues to be increasing public concern about the use of x-rays and the cumulative effect of x-ray diagnosis over a lifetime. X-ray equipment and shielded space are not often available in places where it is advantageous to screen populations or provide care for special patients. Public schools, preschools, nursing homes, and the homes of those confined due to illness, age, or infirmity are just a few of these locales. The development of an alternative US method for the detection of interproximal caries could be useful in a variety of settings. An in vitro study of a US system has been conducted, yielding promising results. Further in vivo studies should be of interest to private practitioners and public health dentists alike.

S. Wotman, DDS

Xylitol and Caries Prevention—Is It a Magic Bullet?
Maguire A, Rugg-Gunn AJ (Newcastle Univ, Newcastle upon Tyne, England)
Br Dent J 194:429-436, 2003   10–28

Background.—The value of xylitol in the prevention of caries has been the focus of several reports. Some reviewers are cautious and others are enthusiastic. Xylitol is one of the nonsugar sweetners now being used in the production of food products. The effectiveness of xylitol in the prevention of caries was reviewed.

Methods.—The review was of clinical trials that involved xylitol and other polyols; it was divided into 3 areas: total substitution of normal dietary sugars for xylitol, partial substitution, and supplementation of normal dietary sugars with xylitol and other polyols.

Results.—It has been shown that xylitol leads to the reduction of mutans streptococci in plaque. A number of xylitol-specific effects have been shown to include the following: a selective effect on mutans streptococci, resulting in the development of mutant xylitol-resistant strains; an increase in concentrations of ammonia and basic amino acids when plaque is exposed to xylitol; and conversion of xyliton to xylitol-5-phosphate that results in the development of intracellular vacuoles.

Discussion.—From the evidence of the clinical trials, xylitol in chewing gum is anticariogenic, it inhibits mother/child transmission of cariogenic oral flora leading to reduced caries development, and it has superior dental properties to other polypols.

► Xylitol has been shown to have specific effects on oral flora and especially on certain strains of strep mutans. Recently, efforts have been made to incorporate xylitol into candies as well as gum, eliminating the need for the sometimes objectional habit of gum chewing. Intriguing early studies have suggested that chewing xylitol gum by mothers may prevent transmission of strep mutans to their infants. Of course, that may require a lot of gum chewing by mothers.

S. Wotman, DDS

Manual Versus Powered Toothbrushes: The Cochrane Review
Niederman R (Boston Univ)
J Am Dent Assoc 134:1240-1244, 2003   10–29

Background.—The Cochrane Collaboration is an international, volunteer, nonprofit organization that focuses on the provision of peer-reviewed, systematic assessments of clinical data published in the scientific literature and maintenance of a database of controlled clinical trials. The Collaboration's findings from a systematic review of the effectiveness of powered versus manual toothbrushes for the reduction of gingivitis and plaque formation are presented.

Methods.—Data were obtained from the Cochrane Oral Health Group's Trial Register, the Cochrane Central Register of Controlled Trials, MEDLINE, and the Cumulative Index to Nursing and Allied Health Literature. Additional information was obtained from manufacturers. Trials were selected for analysis on the basis of several criteria, including comparison of powered versus manual toothbrushes, a randomized design, a study group drawn from the general population and without disabilities, availability of data regarding plaque and gingivitis, and length of study of at least 28 days. Only studies published in 2001 or earlier were selected. Data were extracted from the studies by 6 independent reviewers. Indexes for plaque and gingivitis were expressed as standardized values for data distillation, which was accomplished with the use of a meta-analysis. The main outcome measure was the mean difference between powered and manual toothbrushes.

Results.—From a total of 354 trials, only 29 were found to meet the inclusion criteria, none of which involved battery-powered toothbrushes. Approximately 2500 research subjects were involved in these studies. The findings indicated that only the rotating oscillating powered toothbrush consistently provided a modest but statistically significant clinical benefit over manual toothbrushing in terms of reduction of plaque and gingivitis.

Conclusions.—This analysis by an international team used international, rules-based standards to systematically review more than 3 decades of study of powered versus manual toothbrushes. Only 1 type of powered toothbrush, the rotating oscillating design, showed a statistically significant clinical benefit over manual toothbrushing. It should be noted that battery powered toothbrushes were excluded because no studies involving these brushes met the inclusion criteria of study duration of 28 days or longer.

▶ There has been a plethora of articles over the last several years comparing various mechanical toothbrushes to each other and to manual use. I have hesitated to include these articles because many of them seem to be concerned with the "best" product. As part of the movement to provide evidence for what dentists do on a daily basis, the Cochrane group has undertaken a major effort to provide a basis for evidence-based dentistry. This recent article in the *Journal of the American Dental Association* gathered data from 354 trials of mechanical toothbrushes. The group set rigid criteria for the validity and sensitivity of the studies reported. Only 29 of these studies met the criteria. The group conducted a meta-analysis of these studies and came to the conclusion that some powered toothbrushes achieve a significant but modest reduction in plaque and gingivitis compared with manual toothbrushes. The details of the analysis and the results for different types (brands) of toothbrushes are reported in the article.

S. Wotman, DDS

Comparative Clinical Trials and the Changing Marketplace for Oral Care: Innovation, Evidence and Implications
Gerlach RW, Biesbrock AR (Procter & Gamble Co, Mason, Ohio)
Am J Dent 15:3A-6A, 2002   10–30

Background.—Personal oral care has been significantly affected by 2 recent product introductions: a novel at-home tooth whitening system and a novel power toothbrush. Both of these Crest products have achieved widespread acceptance in the marketplace, as demonstrated by the fact that they garnered more than $200 million in sales just months after their entry into the market. These 2 products are reviewed, and the findings of comparative clinical trials conducted by the manufacturer are presented.

Overview.—The strip-based whitening system is a departure from conventional tray-based treatments. Bleaching is accomplished by means of a flexible polyethylene strip coated with an adhesive hydrogen peroxide bleaching gel. Each strip holds a uniform 150 or 200 mg of a 6.0% or 6.5% hydrogen peroxide whitening gel distributed across the surface of the strip. The strips are applied twice daily for 30 minutes for 14 to 21 days. The benefit of this approach is that it allows higher concentrations of peroxide at a lower dose than is possible with tray-based vital bleaching systems. Few complications have occurred, and previous clinical studies have indicated that less than 1% of strip users discontinue treatment early because of adverse effects related to the whitening strips. The powered toothbrush provides a combination of fixed and moving bristles to present a more traditional brush head size versus other powered brushes. The motorized circular portion of the brush provides additional cleaning beyond the manual head alone without modifying the brushing style. In addition to its low cost, this brush is reported to offer significant additional plaque removal in comparison with conventional brushes and may result in a 36% to 38% increase in toothbrushing time.

Conclusions.—The Crest Whitestrips and Spinbrush have achieved widespread acceptance in the marketplace and offer easy, low-cost options for personal oral care. The safety and efficacy of these products are supported by new clinical research.

▶ The movement toward evidence-based dentistry has stimulated the publication of more clinical trials. The National Institute of Dental Research has issued a request for proposals for a practice-based research network, which is seen as a potential laboratory for clinical trials in the real world of dental practice. The Gerlach and Biesbrock article is an example of the use of clinical trials by a manufacturer to test and market a new product. Dentists need to postpone conclusions based on these toothbrush studies and similar studies until they are repeated and analyzed by independent investigators.

S. Wotman, DDS

Oral Malodor

ADA Council on Scientific Affairs (Chicago)
J Am Dent Assoc 134:209-214, 2003   10–31

Background.—Oral malodor, or bad breath, is a common complaint with an uncertain prevalence in the adult population. However, it is believed that the prevalence of bad breath in the United States is high. Some authors have indicated that most adults have bad breath at some time, usually immediately on waking or after consumption of some foods. Others have stated that at least 50% of the sampled population have persistent oral malodor, and 25% of these individuals have chronic bad breath. The current knowledge regarding the causes, diagnosis and assessment, and treatment of oral malodor is reviewed.

Overview.—The etiology of oral malodor is complex and involves both intrinsic and extrinsic pathways. Intrinsic causes are oral and systemic in origin, whereas extrinsic causes include tobacco, alcohol, and certain foods such as garlic, onions, and some spices. Multiple sites within the oral cavity have been implicated in the formation of malodor, including the teeth, tongue, and periodontal pockets. However, it is clear that the most important source of oral malodor is microbial deposits on the tongue. Other sources of oral malodor include gram-negative anaerobic organisms, respiratory tract conditions, and carcinomas of the upper respiratory tract. A thorough medical, dental, and oral malodor history is necessary to determine whether the cause of a patient's bad breath is intraoral in origin. Eating, drinking, and oral hygiene procedures increase salivary flow and may temporarily decrease oral malodor, so patients should be instructed to refrain from these activities and from smoking for at least 2 hours before an appointment for evaluation of oral malodor. No ideal test exists for the objective measurement of oral malodor. Assessment techniques include the whole mouth or nose assessment, the spoon test, and the saliva odor test. In addition, a highly sensitive and specific gas chromatographic method, coupled with flame photometric detection, has been adapted for direct measurement of 3 volatile sulfur compounds that account for approximately 90% of the volatile sulfur compound content in the mouth. A relatively inexpensive, portable industrial sulfide monitor has been adapted to measure gases associated with oral malodor. The first step in the treatment of oral malodor is an assessment of all oral diseases and conditions that may be contributing factors. For patients who are disease-free, the treatment is based on the assumption that the oral malodor is a result of overgrowth of oral microorganisms. Improved oral hygiene procedures, particularly mechanical cleaning of the tongue, have been associated with reductions in oral malodor. Chemical control of malodor may be achieved with a number of oral active and antimicrobial metabolics.

Conclusions.—Further studies are needed to establish the actual prevalence of oral malodor, but it would appear that up to 25% of the population experiences chronic bad breath. It would also appear that about 90% of oral malodor is intraoral in origin. Improved oral hygiene, specifically tongue cleaning, has been shown to reduce oral malodor.

▶ With the current emphasis on cosmetic dentistry, it was inevitable that dentists would again be asked to look at the problem of oral malodor. This important article on malodor by the American Dental Association Council on Scientific Affairs discusses the complicated, currently understood origins of malodor. The Council suggests that the crypts and fissures on the posterior tongue may be as great or a greater factor in the harboring of these organisms, even though the teeth and gums are an important source of the anaerobic bacteria that seem to be the primary culprits. Many years ago, at Columbia University, a dental researcher was culturing oral anaerobic organisms in large quantities. While at lunch one day, a technician had a major spill of the culture medium containing these organisms. Because the laboratory was on the ninth floor of a large clinical research building, the administration of the dental school spent the afternoon hearing from the various ambulatory care clinics housed on the lower floors as the strong oral malodor smell invaded their spaces. Clearly, these organisms make their presence known. The Council also provides some suggestions for the treatment of this condition.

S. Wotman, DDS

How Can Oral Health Care Providers Determine if Patients Have Dry Mouth?
Navazesh M (Univ of Southern California, Los Angeles)
J Am Dent Assoc 134:613-620, 2003   10–32

Background.—Xerostomia and salivary gland hypofunctioning have been much studied in the past 2 decades. The significant role of saliva in protecting oral soft and hard tissues, in tooth remineralization, and in digestion and alimentation is known to oral health care providers. However, these important contributions are often underappreciated by other health care providers, health insurance carriers, and the general public. Salivary secretion may be altered by a variety of medical conditions and medications. Unfortunately, the diagnosis of hyposalivation is made only after damage has already occurred to the oral tissues. Among the serious consequences of a lack of or diminished saliva flow are restorative or endodontic treatment and potential treatment failure (as in recurrent dental caries), despite excellent dental care. Dental caries is the most common complication associated with salivary gland hypofunctioning. A series of clinical steps are described that, if followed properly, might aid in the early detection of salivary gland hypofunctioning and in the prevention of severe complications.

Overview.—Included in this 4-step program are identification of a patient's chief complaint and the symptoms that prompted the patient to seek treatment; a medical history, including a review of body systems; a clinical evaluation not only of the health and functioning of the salivary glands and oral soft and hard tissues but also of the patient's overall condition; and further diagnostic evaluations, if necessary.

Conclusions.—The recommendations provided in this article may improve the awareness of clinicians regarding objective methods for identification of patients with salivary gland hypofunctioning or those at risk of development of hypofunctioning. Early identification of asymptomatic, at-risk patients, as well as symptomatic patients, may reduce the incidence and prevalence of dental caries and fungal infections in this population.

▶ Dry mouth is another condition that is receiving more attention by the modern dentist. Problems of hydration, pharmacologic effects, obstruction of salivary ducts, and diseases such as Sjögren's syndrome are all possible contributing factors. Navazesh describes a systematic methodology for diagnosis that includes history taking, direct observation, and sialography that can be done by every dentist. Problems of dry mouth are often very uncomfortable and disturbing for patients, and a definitive diagnosis is a very important service. Prevention is the best treatment, but basic treatment options are also outlined in the accompanying box at the end of the article.

S. Wotman, DDS

Prevention: Part 3. Prevention of Tooth Wear
Holbrook WP, Árnadóttir IB, Kay EJ (Univ of Iceland, Reykjavik; Univ of Manchester, England)
Br Dent J 195:75-81, 2003   10–33

Background.—Archaeological evidence of the noncarious destruction of teeth exists in various parts of the world, and this process obviously predates the first appearance of dental caries. These other causes of tooth destruction have been largely ignored in affluent societies, which have emphasized the diagnosis, treatment, and prevention of dental caries. The diagnosis, treatment, and prevention of noncarious tooth destruction are reviewed.

Overview.—Reports of tooth erosion, particularly in young adults, adolescents, and children, have steadily increased in the past 10 to 15 years. This increase in tooth erosion has been attributed in large measure to the high (and steadily increasing) consumption of fruit juice and carbonated beverages. However, this link has been recognized mainly in Europe; little attention has been given to this problem in the literature originating in the United States. The diagnosis of tooth wear should include a careful recording of the location of wear and a grading of its severity. A history should be taken to aid in determining the likely etiologic factors. Good history taking is essential in determining the quantity of carbonated drinks and fruit juices consumed and other dietary factors that may contribute to tooth wear. Medication usage should also be checked, particularly frequent use of asthma inhalers containing steroids, as they may contribute to tooth erosion. Preventing tooth wear is not the same as preventing caries. Tooth wear may now be considered a community-wide problem, but population-based preventive strategies will likely be less effective than for dental caries. Fluoride seems to offer only a limited protective effect against tooth erosion. Drink modification has been found to be the most promising and realistic preventive measure. The addition of calcium lactate to Coca-Cola has been shown to reduce the erosive potential of carbonated beverages. However, manufacturers, rather than adopting this technique, have instead marketed drinks with added citric acid, which increases the erosive potential of carbonated beverages in vitro. Bonding agents have been shown to be effective in reducing sensitivity and in offering protection against further dissolution of erosive lesions.

Conclusions.—Tooth wear has significantly increased in recent years. Most of this tooth wear is the result of erosion, but other factors may be involved. Careful diagnosis and monitoring of progress are important in determining the etiologic factors involved in tooth wear. Population-based strategies for preventing tooth wear are largely ineffective; however, modification of erosive beverages, medicines, and foods may eventually be adopted by both manufacturers and consumers. Extensive restorative procedures may be avoided by careful monitoring of patients after diagnosis of tooth wear, elimination of causative factors, and the use of relatively simple dental treatments.

▶ This recent article in the *British Dental Journal* describes observations in the UK National Survey and in Europe of increased tooth wear in young adults, adolescents, and young children. This increased wear is ascribed to high consumption of soft drinks, both fruit juice and carbonated drinks, by these age groups. There have not been similar reports in the US literature, and the causal link has not been established based on data collected here. Several questions are raised by this article. Is this phenomenon of increased tooth wear in younger age groups seen in this country and other parts of the world? Does the case for the soft drink etiology hold up in other circumstances? What are the long-term oral health effects on these individuals as a result of these early wear patterns? Is there sufficient evidence to mount a major prevention program? Do you see cases of increased wear in young people's teeth in your practice?

S. Wotman, DDS

It's All About Compliance
Schlossberg M
AGD Impact February:9-15, 2003

10–34

Background.—Selecting a toothbrush today is not merely a question of selecting an inexpensive personal oral care device. The toothbrush has now become a trendy lifestyle accessory, thanks to the proliferation of toothbrushes in myriad designs. The oral care market in the United States is now a $3.4 billion industry. The evolution of this industry and the current trends in toothbrush design and marketing are reviewed.

Overview.—The growth in the oral care industry is being led by children's brushes that target specific age groups and encourage proper technique and by adult brushes that cater to specific brushing styles and esthetic sensibilities. The introduction of inexpensive battery-powered toothbrushes has resulted in significant gains in the powered brush market. Manufacturers have stressed that esthetics are secondary motivations to toothbrush redesign—the emphasis is on helping people to brush better. From 1963 to 1998, more than 3000 toothbrush designs were patented in the United States. Among the more radical designs is the Radius toothbrush, which retails for about $9. In the power brush market, the creation of battery-powered units has dropped prices from up to $130 a few years ago to less than $10 today. Other personal oral care products, such as whiteners and tongue scrapers, have also become popular with consumers.

Conclusions.—The explosive growth of the toothbrush market is reviewed and features the evolution of tooth care and interesting facts about the toothbrush. It is expected that manual toothbrushes will continue to have strong sales, despite the increasing popularity of battery-powered toothbrushes. As this article demonstrates, esthetics have now become an important factor in the design of personal oral care products, and toothbrushes are achieving the status of a lifestyle accessory. However, ultimately, the consumer's quest for a better-cleaning toothbrush that provides a better fit for the mouth and hand will continue to provide the impetus for innovation in toothbrush design.

Selling Patients on Brushing: Consumer Education, Gift Ideas, Partnerships Go a Long Way
AGD Impact February:14, 2003   10–35

Background.—Americans are more interested than ever in improving their oral health. Whether the motivation is concern for general oral health or mainly esthetic, this increased interest in oral health has transformed the dental product industry into a multibillion dollar industry in a market that is rewarding manufacturers with soaring profits. However, the most innovative, inexpensive, or trendy toothbrush is only effective if the consumer actually uses it. Today, the likelihood of finding the right brush to encourage an individual to brush correctly is greater than ever because the consumer has more choices at better prices and more education on maintaining healthy teeth. The nexus of consumer education, partnerships, and gifting that encourages brushing and educates consumers on the importance of good oral health is discussed.

Overview.—The boom in cosmetic dentistry has spurred tremendous growth in the sales of over-the-counter whiteners, power toothbrushes, and portable oral care products. The challenge for manufacturers is to reach consumers with educational material regarding their products and oral health care. The approaches to this challenge taken by several manufacturers are highlighted. Partnerships between the dental profession and industry are also viewed as a way to educate consumers and keep them apprised of the latest advances in oral health care. Gifting is also being explored by many dental companies, and the spike in sales around Christmas time may be evidence of the potential for gifting as an avenue for increasing sales and further educating the consumer regarding good oral health.

Conclusions.—Dental companies have discovered that even the lowly toothbrush can be sexy, and their products have been transformed into a multibillion dollar industry. The ultimate beneficiaries of the increasing interest in oral health and the growth of the personal oral care industry are consumers, who now have more choices at better prices and more education regarding the proper techniques and benefits of caring for their teeth.

▶ These last 2 articles (Abstracts 10–34 and 10–35) are included to reinforce our view of the need for effective sources of information for patients who are under "self care." Although there are major campaigns to market oral health products, most self-care information comes from the dentist's office. The Surgeon General's Report emphasized the opportunity for education concerning self care as a tool to improve oral health. Product manufacturers, with their considerable advertising budgets, can also play a major role in this effort, as illustrated by these articles. Hopefully, these companies can be educated so that their products include approaches to prevention based on the latest information (eg, design of toothbrushes for infants that help close the window of infectivity).

S. Wotman, DDS

Professional Monopoly, Social Covenant, and Access to Oral Health Care in the United States

Benn DK (Univ of Florida, Gainesville)
J Dent Educ 67:1080-1090, 2003   10–36

Background.—The lack of access to health care, including oral health care, is a significant and growing problem in the United States. Approximately 32 million individuals in this country lack dental insurance and access to public dental services such as Medicaid or Medicare, and 7 million need dental care. The disparities in oral health care in the United States, the national health care expenditures for medicine and dentistry, the obligation of the dental profession to society, and methods for improving access to care in a socially responsible manner are addressed in this report.

Overview.—Compared with access to general health care, access to oral health care is poor. Among the general population, more than one third of the population lack dental insurance. In some high-risk populations, such as Native Americans, two thirds have unmet dental needs. Only 1% of Medicaid-eligible children have a dental examination before 12 months of age. The geographic maldistribution of dentists, the lack of knowledge among the population regarding the implications of disease in primary teeth, lower reimbursement rates, and excessive bureaucracy are some of the persistent factors barring access to care. It is the position of the American Dental Society (ADA) that the dental profession has a professional and social responsibility and obligation to find ways to deliver care to the needy. The ADA has proposed that most of the burden for funding access to care by the poor should come from increased public funding to bring fees up to existing private fee levels. Unfortunately, dentistry has not fared well in the public expenditure arena. Among the alternative methods for improving access to care described in this report are the Access to Baby and Child Dentistry (ABCD) program and the training and support of mothers and physicians as providers of primary prevention. New roles for allied dental personnel are advocated, including oral diagnosis and simpler treatments such as cutting cavities, filling teeth, and extracting primary teeth, as is currently allowed in the United Kingdom, Australia, New Zealand, and Canada. Finally, a number of practical steps for improving access are presented. These steps include an explicit social contract that 5% of the patient pool of private dentists consist of uninsured or public program patients; acceptance of indigent patients; expansion of the ABCD model of care; and independent education and state licensing for allied dental personnel.

Conclusions.—The current methods of providing oral health care in the United States are inefficient, expensive, and available only to those who can afford them. If access to care remains elusive for large segments of the population, legislative pressure to break the dentist monopoly on treatment may grow in states in which the public's oral health is substandard.

▶ The problem of how to provide oral health care to the entire population of the United States, thus assuring oral health, has been an ongoing challenge to the profession. Like most of the health professions, dentistry has been waiting for the public to provide funding so that the dentist can devote time to the care of these additional patients. We have learned that there is a difference between need and demand for oral health care through the experience of an increased number of dentists produced to meet the need in a system that is based on who seeks care and who can pay for it. The authors of this article suggest that, in an era of evidence-based dentistry, it is possible to improve the efficiency of dentists so that they can serve more patients. In addition, the suggestion is made that the responsibility for oral health in the United States belongs to the profession as a result of its contract with society, which provides a monopoly in exchange for social responsibility. The authors lay out an explicit program by which the profession can address the needs of the unserved and underserved populations without compromising individual dentists' need to realize a fair return for their professional efforts. This article deserves wide discussion whenever dentists meet, especially in a time when some dentists are able to reduce their hours and maintain their current income.

S. Wotman, DDS

11 Orthodontics

Introduction

The articles included in this chapter this year can be placed into 2 major topic areas: Diagnosis and Treatment Planning and Treatment Methodologies. The 2 topic sections represent a broad spectrum of items of potential interest for clinicians in the area of orthodontic care.

In the Diagnosis and Treatment Planning section, there are articles introducing clinicians to new clinical considerations and methods related to patient assessment regarding new technology, changing scope of orthodontic diagnosis, tooth-size–arch-size relationships, and informed consent. These articles were chosen because they are interesting and because they provide a comprehensive overview of selected subject matter often related to everyday clinical decision making.

Another group of articles involves Treatment Methodologies. This series of case reports and original articles includes a broad spectrum of clinical situations and practical solutions. Subjects include the utility of enamel reduction procedures and the predictable incremental expansion of the mandibular dentition with the lip bumper. Additionally, more complex subjects include rapid expansion of the palate and closure of anterior open bites using implant anchorage. And finally, we identify some unusual and novel articles that include management of a previously treated orthodontic case, the use of "periodontal ligament distraction" to move a tooth into an extraction site in an adult patient, and a comprehensive, multidisciplinary approach to managing an osseous defect utilizing guided bone regeneration.

The purpose of this cross-section of the current literature is to provide information and data for interesting topics that will hopefully stimulate your interest and serve as a catalyst for your further consideration of these articles and other related literature.

William K. Lobb, DDS, MS

Diagnosis and Treatment Planning

Orthodontic Diagnosis in Young Children: Beyond Dental Malocclusions
Jefferson Y (Mount Holly, NJ)
Gen Dent 51:104-111, 2003   11–1

Background.—All patients require comprehensive orthodontic evaluation, but this is especially critical for young children, who achieve 70% of their adult facial proportions by 5 years of age and nearly 100% by puberty. Early treatment can correct malocclusions and facial/skeletal disharmonies more easily and even reverse them by applying functional appliances. The key areas of orthodontic assessment were outlined.

Evaluation.—A good medical history should seek sources of potential problems with bleeding, underlying disorders possibly requiring medical clearance or consultation, allergies, and head and neck disorders. Nutritional factors are important, with bottle-fed babies more often having allergies, narrow mouths, malocclusions, and skeletal problems than breast-fed babies. Facial and oral trauma should also be noted along with the orthodontic history. Concerns the patient or parent may have should be described in writing. Reasons for referral are usually dental crowding and misalignment, but others include Class II or III malocclusions, crossbites, deep bites, and anterior open bites.

Identification of Problems.—Most orthodontic problems are related to facial/skeletal problems such as short, long, or narrow faces; Skeletal II and III malpositions; and facial asymmetry. Cephalometric analysis will identify facial/skeletal problems. To screen for TMJ dysfunction (TMD), an inner ear palpitation test provides a simple and inexpensive method. Crepitus, popping, and clicking may also signal TMD. When patients have a short face or Skeletal II malocclusion plus complaints of TMD, headaches, neck-shoulder-back pains, ear infections, hearing disorders, ringing in the ears, dizziness, or other medical problems, the use of removable orthotic appliances or functional appliance therapy may improve facial esthetics and profile, as well as relieve symptoms caused by compressed joints. A frequent cause of facial and dental abnormalities is upper airway obstruction, with mouth breathing producing abnormal facial and tongue muscle activities. Adenoids, swollen tonsils, and Skeletal III malocclusions can all lead to mouth breathing; correction can improve academic performance, increase weight and height, correct nocturnal enuresis, ameliorate psoriasis, avoid recurrent streptococcal pharyngotonsillitis, improve behavior, and alleviate attention-deficit/hyperactivity disorder. Upper airway obstruction of any cause should be corrected before orthodontic treatment is undertaken, and any persistent abnormal myofunctional habits should be addressed by a qualified myofunctional therapist after treatment is completed.

Conclusions.—Oral health consists of more than dental health and includes freedom from chronic conditions of the oral and facial area, absence of cancer in these locations, correction of orofacial birth defects, and freedom from other diseases and disorders that involve the craniofacial complex. It is common to limit orthodontic diagnosis to dental problems; however, it is the responsibility of the orthodontic professional to address the total health and well-being of the patient.

▶ Orthodontics involves more than the diagnosis and treatment of dental malocclusion. Indeed, comprehensive orthodontic management involves the diagnosis and treatment of a broad range of conditions involving dental, skeletal, and soft tissues interacting at rest and during function. This article provides an overview of the significance of early orthodontic assessment and diagnosis. The article also provides several clinical examples of orthodontic problems that need recognition and attention as early as possible in order to provide for the most effective and efficient treatment options. The relationship between orofacial health and general health is reiterated in this article.

W. K. Lobb, DDS, MS

Dynamic Smile Visualization and Quantification: Part 1. Evolution of the Concept and Dynamic Records for Smile Capture
Sarver DM, Ackerman MB (Univ of North Carolina, Chapel Hill; Univ of Pennsylvania, Philadelphia)
Am J Orthod Dentofacial Orthop 124:4-12, 2003   11–2

Introduction.—The "art of the smile" is linked to the clinician's ability to recognize the positive elements in each patient and to devise a strategy to enhance the attributes that fall outside the parameters of the prevailing esthetic concept. New technologies have enhanced the ability to observe patients more dynamically and have facilitated the quantification and communication of newer concepts of function and appearance. Clinical examination and record taking in the treatment of the smile were described.

Clinical Examination.—The first critical step in treatment of a smile is the clinical examination. The orthodontist works with 2 dynamics: (1) soft tissue repose and animation, including how the lips animate on smile, gingival display, crown length, and other attributes of the smile; and (2) the facial change throughout a patient's lifetime, including the impact of skeletal and soft tissue maturation and aging characteristics. The most important element in the clinical examination is the direct measurement of lip-tooth relationships, both dynamically and in repose.

Record Taking.—Record taking is the second step in treatment of a smile. Digital photography, digital videography, radiography, and plaster study cases are used to precisely record the dynamic and static attributes of a patient's smile. The records are obtained frontally and obliquely to provide a 3-dimensional description of smile characteristics.

Conclusion.—From a thorough clinical examination and record taking, smile analysis and treatment strategies involved in achieving optimal smile esthetics may be performed.

▶ This article introduces the reader to the esthetics of a smile and its importance to the diagnosis of dynamic facial esthetics in orthodontic patients, compared with the more traditional static frontal view that clinicians have focused on in the past. This article outlines the need for dynamic records and discusses a method to capture the dynamic recording of a smile and speech by using digital videography. Both the visualization and quantification of a dynamic smile involve clinical examination of lip-tooth relationships in action and at rest, and record taking with digital photography, digital videography, radiography, and plaster casts. The records are used to develop a 3-dimensional description of the smile that can be captured to form a database. From this database, a "smile analysis" can be completed for each individual patient. This article encourages the use of dynamic records and technology to expand the capability of orthodontics in treatment planning and diagnosis.

W. K. Lobb, DDS, MS

Dynamic Smile Visualization and Quantification: Part 2. Smile Analysis and Treatment Strategies
Sarver DM, Ackerman MB (Univ of North Carolina, Chapel Hill; Univ of Pennsylvania, Philadelphia)
Am J Orthod Dentofacial Orthop 124:116-127, 2003   11–3

Introduction.—In part 1 of this 2-part series on treatment of a smile, clinical examination and record taking were reviewed. In part 2, smile analysis and treatment strategies were discussed.

Smile Analysis.—Each dimension has an important role in smile composition. The social smile is a voluntary smile used in social settings or when posing for photographs. The social smile is used to analyze the smile in the frontal, oblique, sagittal, and time-specific dimensions. There are 3 transverse characteristics of the smile in the frontal dimension: the arch form, buccal corridor, and the transverse cant of the maxillary occlusal plane. The frontal smile is the only dimension that allows the orthodontist to visualize any tooth-associated or skeletal asymmetry transversely. The visualization of the complete smile arc provided by the oblique view expands the definition of the smile arc to include the molars and premolars. The 2 characteristics of the smile best observed in the sagittal dimension are overjet and incisor angulation. The dimension of time reveals the effect of maturation and aging on the soft tissue, including (1) lengthening of the resting philtrum and commissure heights, (2) reduction in turgor, (3) decrease in incisor display at rest, (4) reduction in incisor display during smile, and (5) reduction in gingival display during smiling.

Treatment Strategies.—In problem-oriented treatment planning, the problems that necessitate improvement or correction are addressed. The next fundamental component in treatment planning should include identifying and quantifying the positive aspects of the patient's esthetic arrangement.

Conclusion.—The focus on the lineaments of the smile represents a reemphasis of the importance of physical diagnosis and the appreciation of the soft tissues that both drive treatment planning and limit the treatment response. New technology enhances the ability to visualize patients more dynamically and facilitates the quantification and communication of newer concepts of function and appearance.

▶ The second of a 2-part series, this article focuses on the methodology for recording, assessing, and planning treatment of the patient's smile. This article provides a comprehensive overview of the diagnosis and evaluation of a smile involving the frontal, oblique, and saggital dimensions. The effects of growth, aging, and maturation are also considered and represent the fourth dimension of time. This article uses several clinical examples to illustrate the use of this methodology for treatment planning purposes. With available technology to factor in the dynamic and static dimensions of the smile, clinicians are strongly urged to reconsider the importance of physical diagnosis of orthodontic concerns, and to consider in more detail the soft tissues related to the dentition. The smile and its contributing elements all affect treatment planning and provide limitations to our treatment results. With enhanced patient evaluation by using technology such as this, we can consider these new concepts of esthetics and function.

W. K. Lobb, DDS, MS

Tooth Size-Arch Length Relationships in the Deciduous Dentition: A Comparison Between Contemporary and Historical Samples

Warren JJ, Bishara SE, Yonezu T (Univ of Iowa, Iowa City; Tokyo Dental College, Chiba City, Japan)
Am J Orthod Dentofacial Orthop 123:614-619, 2003   11–4

Background.—Crowding of the teeth is caused by a combination of small arch size and large teeth, and is assessed by determining the tooth size–arch length discrepancy (TSALD). Compared with a historical sample, contemporary children have been found to have significantly shorter maxillary and mandibular arch lengths in the deciduous dentition. A comparison was undertaken between tooth size and TSALD in the deciduous dentition from a contemporary sample of children born in the mid 1990s and those of similar children in a historical sample, born in the late 1940s.

Methods.—The 2 samples included white North American children and showed similarities in terms of geographic location, racial and ethnic background, and socioeconomic status. Both had a normal overjet (<4 mm) and anteroposterior molar relationship, no anterior open bite, and no crossbite; none had any permanent teeth that had erupted. Measurements included size of the mesiodistal teeth, arch lengths of the maxillary and mandibular arches, and TSALD.

Results.—Contemporary children had consistently larger mesiodistal teeth than the historical sample; the mean differences averaged about 0.1 mm per tooth, but the sums showed statistically significant differences in the mandibular arches. TSALDs were considerably smaller in the contemporary children than their historical counterparts, with all comparisons showing statistically significant differences. Both the mean and the median mandibular TSALDs were negative for contemporary children, illustrating that most children have a greater combined mesiodistal tooth size than arch length. Thirty-one percent of the boys and 41% of the girls showed at least 2 mm of negative TSALD, or crowding, of the mandibular arch.

Conclusions.—Measurement of the TSALD in contemporary children determined that crowding was common in the mandibular arch and was much more common and serious than in children 50 years ago. The combination of smaller arch lengths and slightly larger teeth in contemporary children resulted in a greater TSALD and indicated a greater prevalence of crowding in the deciduous dentition. Whether this persists in mixed and permanent dentition has yet to be established.

▶ It is interesting to consider the effect of time on interrelationships commonly used in orthodontic thinking. For example, this article considers the impact of time on the commonly used "tooth size–arch length discrepancy." The stated purpose of the study is to "describe secular changes that might have occurred in tooth sizes, and tooth size–arch length relationships" in the same cohorts of contemporary and historic samples of children in the deciduous dentition. The evidence presented in this study suggests that the tooth size is slightly larger in the more contemporary cohort, and that crowding was much more common and severe in the contemporary cohort of children, especially for the mandibular arch. The authors suggest that further study is necessary to determine whether this change will also be observed in the mixed and permanent dentitions, and to further establish these secular trends.

W. K. Lobb, DDS, MS

Evaluation of Antegonial Notch Depth for Growth Prediction
Kolodziej RP, Southard TE, Southard KA, et al (Univ of Iowa, Iowa City)
Am J Orthod Dentofacial Orthop 121:357-363, 2002   11–5

Background.—Orthodontic treatment planning would be greatly aided by some reliable technique of predicting facial growth. Some reports have suggested that the depth of the mandibular antegonial notch could be used for this purpose, but these studies have been based on subjects with extreme morphological characteristics. Longitudinal data from a random sample of young subjects were used to evaluate the predictive value of antegonial notch depth.

Methods.—The analysis included a random sample of 20 male and 20 female subjects from the longitudinal Iowa Facial Growth Study. As part of that study, the subjects underwent lateral cephalometric radiographs at 3 periods: prepubescence, around the age of 8.5 years; adolescence, age 12 years; and young adulthood, 17 years or older. Measurements of antegonial notch depth in prepubescence and adolescence were evaluated for their ability to predict vertical and horizontal growth of the jaws from childhood to adulthood.

Results.—There was a statistically significant negative correlation between antegonial notch depth in adolescence and horizontal growth of the maxilla and mandible from adolescence to adulthood. However, the absolute values for these correlations were below the threshold for clinical significance.

Discussion.—Antegonial notch depth in childhood did not predict future facial growth in a random sample of untreated young subjects. In patients with nonextreme morphological characteristics, antegonial notch depth is not a clinically useful predictor for orthodontic treatment planning.

▶ Some investigators have suggested that the morphology of the antegonial notch is a predictor of subsequent facial growth. This study tests this hypothesis in a sample of untreated patients who are more like what a clinician may encounter in practice in that they do not represent examples of extreme individual morphology. In this study, a statistically significant negative correlation was found between the antegonial notch depth and subsequent horizontal mandibular growth; conversely as the antegonial notch depth decreased, the amount of horizontal growth observed increased.

Despite the statistical relationship observed, the strength of the relationship was weak, and this study did not find any clinically significant correlation between the antegonial notch depth and the amount of horizontal growth. The clinical significance of any relationship is what is important. This study concludes that the depth of the antegonial notch "fails to provide sufficient indication of future facial growth to warrant its application as a growth predictor in a nonextreme population." So the clinical practice of palpation and estimating the depth of the antegonial notch and using this as a clinical predictor of facial growth for the majority of patients is contraindicated.

W. K. Lobb, DDS, MS

Congenitally Missing Mandibular Second Premolar: Treatment Outcome With Orthodontic Space Closure
Fines CD, Rebellato J, Saiar M (Univ of Minnesota, Minneapolis; Mayo Clinic and Mayo Found, Rochester, Minn)
Am J Orthod Dentofacial Orthop 123:676-682, 2003   11–6

Background.—Mandibular second premolars are congenitally missing in 2.5% to 4% of the population, with bilateral absence noted in 60% of these patients. Treatment options may be limited by the time the absence is discovered. A case demonstrated one of the treatment alternatives that can be chosen in these cases.

Case Report.—Girl, 11 years 5 months, was referred by the family dentist for a general orthodontic consultation, which revealed a Class I dental relationship with the mandibular dental midline deviated 1.0 mm to the right of the maxillary dental midline, a deep overbite with a 50% overlap of the maxillary incisors on the mandibular incisors, a tight overjet, and a Bolton discrepancy (1.4 mm of maxillary deficiency). Radiographs showed teeth 18, 28, and 35 (FDI numbers) were congenitally absent, and the mandibular left deciduous second molar had short roots. In the absence of a history of trauma and because the patient's father and younger brother also showed congenital lack of a second premolar, the etiology of the malocclusion was deemed genetic. Treatment was undertaken with the objectives of achieving a Class III molar relationship on the left and Class I on the right, alleviating the crowding, resolving the overbite, and retaining the widths between molars and canines while maintaining the patient's soft tissue profile. The choices for treatment included extraction of the deciduous molar and orthodontic closure of the space plus extraction of the deciduous molar and 3 other premolars; retention of the mandibular deciduous second molar; autotransplantation; implant replacement; and fixed partial denture replacement. Extraction of the deciduous molars and placement of 0.018-inch straightwire appliances were accomplished at age 11 years 6 months. On eruption, tooth 45 was rotated, mesial in and distal out, which was corrected by using a lingual elastomeric chain from 45 to 44. The archwires were changed and upper and lower elastomeric chains were placed as treatment progressed. Closure of the extraction space was achieved after 15 months, with appliances used to complete movement during the next 4 months. On cephalometric superimpositions, the orthodontic treatment had achieved a predominantly vertical growth pattern, resolution of the crowding, and a Class III molar relationship on the left, as well as bilateral canine guidance. A final midline discrepancy of about 1 mm caused by a weaker Class I canine relationship on the left was not addressed because of the cosmetic restorations that would have been needed. Panoramic radiographs taken at age 16 years 6 months revealed that tooth 38 was nearly fully erupted into occlusion with the maxillary second molar. Once tooth 48 erupts, it will likely be removed.

Conclusions.—Good patient cooperation enhanced the outcome for this case of congenitally missing tooth. The options for achieving orthodontic space closure in this adolescent were not as broad as for younger patients, but the result demonstrates that a good outcome can be achieved.

▶ The management of congenitally missing second premolar teeth is high-lighted and reviewed through this case report. In this case, a female patient aged 11 years 5 months is managed with orthodontic space closure for a unilaterally missing second premolar. The relative importance of timing of the diagnosis and treatment of this condition is discussed, as well as the various treatment alternatives available to manage this fairly common problem.

W. K. Lobb, DDS, MS

The Uninformed Orthodontic Patient and Parent: Treatment Outcomes
Baird JF, Kiyak HA (Univ of Washington, Seattle)
Am J Orthod Dentofacial Orthop 124:212-215, 2003   11–7

Background.—Informed consent involves the process of a health care provider educating a patient concerning a health condition and its possible treatments, as well as the risks and benefits of these treatments. The use of a document indicating that the patient has given informed consent is common, but the education of patients so that they are truly fully informed is lacking. With respect to dental settings, informed patients can be better consumers with more reasonable expectations for outcomes. A special emphasis is needed in orthodontic treatment, where long-term patient compliance can be critical and where patients are often children, requiring parents also be educated to ensure compliance. The degree of understanding shown by children and parents about the nature of the problem, the purpose of treatment, and the associated risks, as well as their roles in the orthodontic therapy process, were assessed to determine problems associated with obtaining informed consent. In addition, the educational level and verbal intelligence quotient of the child and parent were assessed for their impact on informed consent.

Methods.—Twenty-one children aged 7 to 12 years were studied, along with 1 parent or guardian, 71.4% of whom were mothers. Participants were asked open-ended questions about why treatment was being done, what risks were involved, and what their responsibilities were. The responses obtained were compared with information in the children's charts. The children had been in treatment for 1 to 24 months, with a mean of 7.84 months.

Results.—Both the children and their parents or guardians scored low on the vocabulary tests, with a mean parents' score of 46.10 and a mean children's score of 8.38 on the Wechsler Adult Intelligence Scale or Wechsler Intelligence Scale for Children. The reasons for treatment recorded on the charts included general malocclusion or crowding (primary reason), crossbite, Class II malocclusion, overbite, and overjet; those offered by parents or children were usually crooked teeth or crowding, but the diagnosis given by the orthodontist was recalled by only 75% of the parents and 58% of the children. Ten children said they didn't know why the treatment was being done; parents recalled an average of 2.1 reasons, but charts documented an average of 4.1 reasons (Table 1). Fifteen children had already had

TABLE 1.—Most Commonly Cited Reasons and Diagnoses for Treatment

Diagnosis	Chart	Parent	Child
Crooked teeth or crowding	13*	12* (9)†	12* (7)
Crossbite	12	2 (2)	1 (1)
Class II malocclusion	9	0	0
Overbite	7	7 (3)	4 (3)
Overjet	7	0	0
Upper and lower fit	4	4 (1)	0
Oral habits	4	1 (0)	1 (0)
Diastema	2	1 (0)	1 (0)
Don't know or no response	0	3	10

Note: n = 21 parent-child pairs.
*Total can be >21 because multiple responses allowed.
†Numbers in parentheses represent concurrence between chart and parent or chart and child responses.
(Reprinted by permission of the publisher from Baird JF, Kiyak HA: The uninformed orthodontic patient and parent: Treatment outcomes. *Am J Orthod Dentofacial Orthop* 124:212-215, 2003. Copyright 2003 by Elsevier.)

at least one problem during treatment, yet 12 children and 7 parents stated that no risks attended orthodontic treatment, and 5 children and 5 parents could not recall any risks. Problems encountered during the treatment and documented in the child's record were often not recalled (Table 2). A correlation was found between parents' recall of risks and the child's satisfaction with the information given by the orthodontist. Marginal correlations were identified between parents' educational level and number of risks recalled, and between scores on the Wechsler Adult Intelligence Scale vocabulary test and number of reasons for treatment recalled.

Conclusions.—Even when responses were given by the children and parents surveyed, they often did not reflect the actual diagnoses or reasons for treatment documented in the chart. Parents' vocabulary scores and number of reasons given for treatment were significantly correlated, whereas parental educational level was marginally linked to recall of treatment risks. Over-

TABLE 2.—Risks of Orthodontic Treatment Cited by Parent and Child Compared With Problems Actually Experienced

Problems or Risks	Chart*	Parent	Child
Broken wire or bracket	6*	2† (1)‡	2* (1)
Gingivitis or periodonitis	6	2 (0)	0
Lip or mouth trauma	2	0	0
Pain	2	3 (0)	1 (0)
Tooth decay	1	2 (1)	0
Staining or decalcification	1	1 (0)	2 (0)
Relapse	1	0	0
None	0	7	12

Note: n = 21 parent-child pairs.
*Problem experienced, per notation in patient chart.
†Total can be >21 because multiple responses allowed.
‡Numbers in parentheses represent concurrence between chart and parent or chart and child response.
(Reprinted by permission of the publisher from Baird JF, Kiyak HA: The uninformed orthodontic patient and parent: Treatment outcomes. *Am J Orthod Dentofacial Orthop* 124:212-215, 2003. Copyright 2003 by Elsevier.)

all, there was poor recall for the reasons for treatment or associated risks among the parents and children surveyed.

▶ Informed consent is a critical element of risk management that is important in orthodontic case presentations. It is possible that patients, parents, or both do not comprehend and retain information given to them during the case presentation visit. Indeed, the risk of treating a patient without informed consent is significant and should be considered. This article discusses this issue and presents data from a study that evaluates both the patient's and parents' understanding of the orthodontic treatment, specifically assessing the effect of vocabulary and educational level on the patient's and parents' comprehension. This study concludes that both the patients and their parents exhibited poor recall of the reasons for treatment, or associated risks. Although not a conclusion of this study, these data reinforce the need to provide a written version of the informed consent in order to provide a more informed patient/parent.

W. K. Lobb, DDS, MS

Unusual Orthodontic Retreatment
Janson G, Janson MR, Cruz KS, et al (Univ of São Paulo, Brazil)
Am J Orthod Dentofacial Orthop 123:468-475, 2003   11–8

Background.—Significant patient compliance and anchorage control are needed to achieve good results in the treatment of Class II malocclusions. The treatment generally involves the extraction of 4 first premolars to correct the anteroposterior discrepancy. A patient with a Class II malocclusion underwent the 4 extractions but did not achieve the desired improvement and was retreated.

Case Report.—Woman, 23, was undergoing orthodontic treatment with extraction of 4 first premolars to correct her Class II Division 1 malocclusion but had a persisting large overjet that was attributable to her lack of compliance in wearing the headgear needed to reinforce anchorage (Fig 2). She had abandoned treatment with the orthodontic appliances still in place but desired to resume treatment 1½ years later. Radiographs showed that her maxillary third molars were favorably placed functionally, but this was not true of the mandibular third molars, and the maxillary incisors had significant root resorption after the previous therapy. No active periodontal disease was present. Faced with the choices of combined surgery and orthodontic treatment, extraction of the maxillary second premolars and retraction of the anterior teeth, or extraction of the maxillary second premolars and chin augmentation to improve her profile, the patient chose to have the maxillary second premolars extracted and anterior teeth retracted, even though this involved more time and compliance on her part. Conventional 0.022-in slot edgewise appliances were

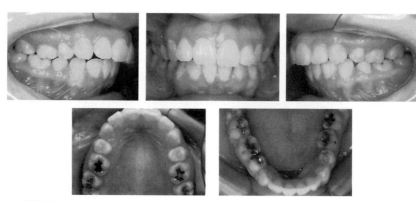

FIGURE 2.—Intraoral photographs after incomplete treatment that included removing 4 first premolars. (Reprinted by permission of the publisher from Janson G, Janson MR, Cruz KS, et al: Unusual orthodontic retreatment. *Am J Orthod Dentofacial Orthop* 123:468-475, 2003. Copyright 2003 by Elsevier.)

used, with a transpalatal arch soldered to the first premolars to reinforce anchorage. Cervical headgear was installed, with instructions that it be worn 18 hours a day; patient compliance was excellent. Anchorage was enhanced by banding the maxillary second molars. Retraction was accomplished with the use of stainless steel archwires, elastic chains, and Class II elastics. Extraction spaces were closed, the transpalatal arch was removed, and headgear was discontinued when the canines achieved a Class I relationship; finishing occlusal procedures were then done. Treatment required 35 months and yielded a satisfactory posttreatment profile both from a clinical viewpoint and from the patient's perspective. Reasonable Class I canine and Class II molar relationships were present on both sides, and the maxillary and mandibular third molars were in function. Retreatment was required for root resorption, and some degree of anchorage loss had occurred. Tooth contact was refined by means of occlusal equilibration.

Conclusions.—The occlusal and esthetic results achieved in this retreatment were satisfactory, although the approach was unusual and presented some risks. Thus, additional extractions of the maxillary second premolars can produce successful retreatment outcomes for poorly treated Class II cases with large and unpleasant overjets. The patient's compliance is a key factor in treatment success, so developing a sound plan and discussing it with the patient is essential.

▶ Retreatment of a previously treated case requires a careful analysis and assessment of the treatment outcomes and what might be possible to accomplish with further treatment. This case presentation discusses the retreatment of a Class II Division 1 case that was initially treated with 4-bicuspid extraction. The patient in this case presents for retreatment 1½ years after abandoning treatment with the orthodontic appliances still in place. Additionally, the main cause for lack of progress with the original treatment plan was lack of patient compliance with headgear wear. A new treatment plan was developed that included the extraction of the remaining upper bicuspids to correct the residual overjet and Class II canine relationships. Various other options including surgery were discussed as alternatives for this patient. The various indications and contraindications for retreatment of a case such as this are discussed in detail. A favorable albeit limited result was demonstrated with this retreatment.

W. K. Lobb, DDS, MS

Treatment Methodologies

Enamel Reduction Procedures in Orthodontic Treatment

Rossouw PE, Tortorella A (Baylor College of Dentistry, Dallas)
J Can Dent Assoc 69:378-383, 2003   11–9

Background.—Interdental stripping or interproximal enamel reduction is used during orthodontic treatment to achieve better tooth alignment and occlusion and to simplify the long-term maintenance of realigned teeth. The indications for and methods of performing enamel reduction procedures were outlined.

Methods.—A literature search was undertaken to identify the indications for enamel reduction and the methods that are proving most effective.

Results.—Enamel reduction is indicated in patients with good oral hygiene and (1) Class I arch length discrepancies with orthognathic profiles, (2) minor Class II dental malocclusions, or (3) Bolton tooth-size discrepancies. Enamel reduction gains space for the alignment of irregularly positioned teeth and can be accomplished by use of the air-rotor technique. About 50% of the interproximal enamel can be removed safely, with no evidence of increased susceptibility to caries or periodontal disease in healthy environments; however, patients with inflammation may be predisposed to a more rapid progression of periodontal disease. Applied to the premolars and molars, enamel reduction of 50% will yield 9.8 mm of additional space with which to realign the mandibular teeth. Tooth size analysis should be included in the treatment planning stage for tooth-size discrepancies. An index of the mesiodistal to faciolingual dimensions has been used to guide enamel reduction planning, with values of 88% to 92% for the mandibular central incisor and 90% to 95% for the mandibular lateral incisor serving as guidelines. Studies have confirmed that grinding of young teeth undertaken in orthodontic treatment causes no discomfort to the patient and produces minimal or no long-term clinical or radiographic reactions. Theoretically, potential adverse events associated with enamel reduction include increased frequency of caries, periodontal disease, and temperature sensitivity. However, the alignment procured by enamel reduction has promoted interproximal gingival health, and the incidence of caries has not been increased significantly. The use of a mechanical stripping procedure plus the chemical action of 37% phosphoric acid produced enamel surfaces that encouraged "self-healing." It is impossible to eliminate all the furrows left on the enamel by diamond burs and disks and 16-blade tungsten carbide burs, but well-polished surfaces can be achieved with a tungsten carbide bur with 8 straight blades.

Conclusions.—The use of enamel reduction carries many advantages in preventing and managing alignment problems. Its disadvantages are being addressed through the use of various techniques, including combined mechanical and chemical methods.

▶ The proximal reduction of enamel has become a common method to create space between teeth. This space is used to correct a variety of orthodontic problems, including alignment of teeth during treatment and alignment of teeth during retention. This article presents the indications for enamel reduction, the various related factors to the planning and use of this methodology, and the advantages and disadvantages of this treatment approach. A critical feature of this treatment approach, regardless of the method of enamel reduction used, is to finish the enamel surface to a smooth final form.

W. K. Lobb, DDS, MS

Rapid Palatal Expansion in the Young Adult: Time for a Paradigm Shift?
Stuart DA, Wiltshire WA (Univ of Manitoba, Winnipeg, Canada)
J Can Dent Assoc 69:374-377, 2003   11–10

Introduction.—Histologic and radiologic evidence suggests that the maxillary suture is not fused enough to inhibit the opening of the maxillary palatal suture in patients who are in their late teens or early 20s. A growing body of evidence is challenging the belief that palatal expansion without surgery is not possible in patients older than 15 to 16 years. The midpalatal suture may be closed when assessed radiographically, but it is not necessarily fused, as demonstrated by recent literature and the following case report.

Case Report.—Man, 19 years 7 months, was seen for orthodontic correction of a malocclusion. Clinical examination and orthodontic records showed a skeletal deficiency in the transverse dimension of the maxillary arch. Surgery was recommended and the patient refused. It was determined that nonsurgical rapid palatal expansion should be performed before placement of full-fixed orthodontic appliances. After a thorough clinical assessment and an anterior maxillary occlusal radiograph, a maxillary Hyrax appliance was designed for the patient. It had full acrylic coverage of the maxillary posterior teeth to maintain the vertical dimensions and prevent cuspal interference during the expansion procedure. He was instructed to turn the screw once daily (to loosen the structural junction). After 7 days, the expansion on the Hyrax appliance was about 1.5 mm at the expansion screw. There was no midline diastema, and he did not report any pain. He was instructed to continue turning the expansion screw twice daily for 5 days. The expansion 1 week later was 5 mm, and there was no midline diastema. He then turned the screw 3 times daily for 3 days, then once daily for 2 days. The expansion was 7 mm, and he had a midline diastema of 3 mm. A posttreatment maxillary anterior occlusal radiograph confirmed that the midpalatal suture had opened. A stainless steel ligature was positioned through the expansion screw to fixate its position. The midline diastema self-closed completely after about 6 weeks. At 6 months after rapid palatal expansion, an occlusal radiograph showed the presence of new bone formation in the midpalatal suture area.

Conclusion.—Nonsurgical rapid palatal expansion is a viable option for young adults well into their early 20s.

▶ The use of surgery as an adjunct to rapid palatal expansion in an adult patient is well documented as an accepted technique. There is also evidence that nonsurgical rapid palatal expansion is possible and feasible in adult patients as an alternative to a surgically assisted technique. The authors of this article suggest that given the clinical outcomes reviewed, "it is time for a paradigm shift" with respect to the clinical management of rapid palatal expansion in patients into their early 20s. The authors review a case of a male patient, aged 19 years 7 months, treated with nonsurgical rapid palatal expansion.

W. K. Lobb, DDS, MS

Dental Distraction for an Adult Patient
Bilodeau JE (Springfield, Va)
Am J Orthod Dentofacial Orthop 123:683-689, 2003   11–11

Introduction.—The latest advancement in the distraction armamentarium is the periodontal ligament distraction technique reported by Liou and Huang, which involves a canine distraction procedure for moving a canine into a first premolar extraction site in less than 1 month. This technique requires no posterior anchorage and no extraoral force, and thus has significant clinical application when anchorage requirements are crucial.

Case Report.—Man, 37, had a Class I malocclusion with a mild anterior crossbite, with his mandible deviated to the left. He was seen for concerns about crooked teeth, biting his cheeks, and his upper midline not being in the center of his face. He had a straight face profile and a Class III appearance, with the chin deviated to the left. He was able to close his lips without mentalis strain. Dental casts revealed that the maxilla was constricted and the posterior teeth were in a crossbite. He had a 2-mm open bite on the left, and the maxillary right canine was missing. A panoramic radiograph revealed that the maxillary right lateral incisor and first premolar were tipped toward each other into the canine extraction space. There was some localized bone loss, and the right central and lateral incisors were disto-axially inclined. Skeletal cephalometric measurements were within the normal range, so orthognathic surgery was not appropriate. The mandibular first premolars were extracted. The remaining mandibular teeth, including the third molars, were banded or bonded sequentially by using the 10-2 system of Merrifield, and distraction osteogenesis was performed. Posttreatment dental casts showed a Class I occlusion with normal overjet and overbite and no crossbite. He had good canine and incisional guidance on the right. The premolar functioned as a canine. A posttreatment panoramic radiograph revealed that no additional bone loss occurred. Some clinically insignificant blunting of the mandibular third molar and maxillary anterior tooth roots was seen. The root of the distracted canine was not affected. A posttreatment cephalometric radiograph and its tracing showed that the desired changes were achieved with treatment.

Conclusion.—Treatment goals were achieved through distraction osteogenesis in a patient with a problematic crossbite.

▶ This case report includes treatment of an orthodontic problem utilizing dental distraction as a means to rapidly retract a canine in a bicuspid extraction space without any significant need for anchorage. This case is treated using a "periodontal ligament distraction technique," whereby the tooth and interseptal bone are rapidly moved into the extraction site. In a short period (approximately 15 days), the bone distal to the canine and mesial to the second premolar is brought into close proximity. New bone is formed on the mesial of the distracted canine, thereby maintaining integrity of the osseous tissues surrounding the tooth being moved. The author points out that a critical feature of this technique is the surgical preparation of the extraction site to facilitate the bodily movement of the canine. This technique has significant potential to manage cases with critical anchorage requirements, like the case outlined in this report.

W. K. Lobb, DDS, MS

Comparison of Skeletal and Dental Changes Between 2-Point and 4-Point Rapid Palatal Expanders
Lamparski DG, Rinchuse DJ, Close JM, et al (Natrona Heights, Pa; Univ of Pittsburgh, Pa)
Am J Orthod Dentofacial Orthop 123:321-328, 2003   11–12

Background.—Expansion therapy became increasingly popular in the early 20th century because of the belief that it improved nasal breathing and enhanced general vitality. Its popularity decreased at midcentury with the advent of extraction-oriented treatment plans. More recently, there has been a resurgence of interest in palatal expansion as orthodontists try to use more dentally conservative approaches and limit dental extraction. The use of rapid palatal expansion therapy produces physical separation of the bony palate and premaxilla; its goals are to maximize orthopedic movements and minimize orthodontic movements of the teeth. Four teeth are generally included in the appliance, but with more teeth there are more problems in construction and insertion of the expander. A 2-point expander between only the first molars can be constructed by removing the 2 anterior wires from a 4-point hyrax expander. Whether there is a significant difference in the outcomes achieved with a 2-point versus a 4-point palatal expander was investigated.

Methods.—Thirty patients aged 6 to 16 years were randomly assigned to treatment with 2-point or 4-point expanders. Dental and radiographic landmarks were compared, with measures including midpalatal suture separation and dental expansion. In the 4-point expansion appliance, a hyrax expansion screw had bands cemented to the maxillary first permanent molars and either the maxillary first premolars or the maxillary deciduous first molars (Fig 1). The jackscrew on the 2-point appliance was similar to that of the 4-point expander, but banding was only done to the maxillary first permanent molars (Fig 2).

Results.—The range of appliance separation was 4.490 to 8.620 mm, with a mean of 5.790 mm. The 15 patients in the 2-point group had a mean age of 10.8 years (range, 6.58-14.58 years) and evidenced a mean amount of appliance separation of 5.986 mm (range, 4.520-8.620 mm). The 15 patients in the 4-point group had a mean age of 11.33 years (range, 7.75-13.92 years) and achieved a mean amount of appliance separation of 5.594 mm (range, 4.490-7.260 mm). There were no significant differences found between the 2 groups with respect to total molar cusp width, molar gingival width, canine cusp width, canine gingival width, or diastema width. Some differences were noted, however, with the 4-point appliance creating more expansion, an overall greater increase in the maxillary perimeter, and better retention of the changes than the 2-point appliance. The effects on the midpalatal suture and dentition were similar between the 2 appliances.

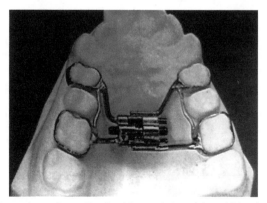

FIGURE 1.—Four-point appliance. (Reprinted by permission of the publisher from Lamparski DG, Rinchuse DJ, Close JM, et al: Comparison of skeletal and dental changes between 2-point and 4-point rapid palatal expanders. *Am J Orthod Dentofacial Orthop* 123:321-328, 2003. Copyright 2003 by Elsevier.)

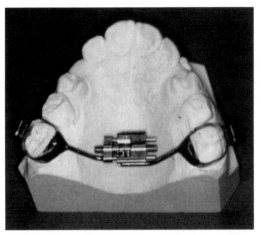

FIGURE 2.—Two-point appliance. (Reprinted by permission of the publisher from Lamparski DG, Rinchuse DJ, Close JM, et al: Comparison of skeletal and dental changes between 2-point and 4-point rapid palatal expanders. *Am J Orthod Dentofacial Orthop* 123:321-328, 2003. Copyright 2003 by Elsevier.)

Conclusions.—No statistically significant differences in outcome were noted between the 2 groups. The 2-point appliance affected the midpalatal suture and dentition in much the same way as the 4-point appliance. Therefore, the 2-point appliance could be used to achieve skeletal and dental expansion comparable to that obtained with the currently more popular 4-point appliance.

▶ Rapid palatal expansion is an effective technique to alter the bucco-lingual dimension of the maxillary arch. Usually, clinicians seek to maximize the orthopedic effects of the appliance while minimizing the orthodontic movement of teeth with these appliances. In this article, the authors compare 2 appliances designed to expand the palate. They compare an appliance that engages 4 points (teeth) in its design, with an appliance that engages 2 points (teeth) in its design. The study concludes that for most of the parameters measured, there were no significant differences between the 4-point and 2-point appliances. Some suggestions are made for further study of these 2 appliance types, including comparing (1) the results of these 2 appliances several months or years after treatment; (2) the differences with respect to relative orthopedic versus dental changes; and (3) the effects of these appliance types on periodontal and pulpal tissue responses during treatment. I would also add that it would be beneficial in future studies to consider any differences in patient comfort and acceptance of the 2 appliance types.

W. K. Lobb, DDS, MS

A Longitudinal Study of Incremental Expansion Using a Mandibular Lip Bumper

Murphy CC, Magness WB, English JD, et al (Univ of Texas, Houston)
Angle Orthod 73:396-400, 2003   11–13

Background.—Nonextraction therapy is being chosen more often for orthodontic treatment, with greater focus on developing the arches through expansion therapy in the management of crowded teeth. The lower arch can be developed by using the mandibular lip bumper, which allows for expansion of the mandibular arch both anteroposteriorly and transversely. Studies have documented the degree of change accomplished by using the mandibular lip bumper, but an analysis has not previously established when arch expansion occurs, which would guide the clinician in making decisions regarding the use of fixed appliances for definitive correction.

Methods.—The mandibular lip bumper was used in 44 adolescent patients, with measures taken to determine whether the expansion occurs evenly between appointments or is attenuated with time. Arch width and arch length were documented with dental cast measurements. The lip bumper was fixed in place 24 hours a day with ligature wire, power chains, or elastic separators. Adjustments were made at appointments every 4 to 6 weeks, when mandibular alginate impressions were taken and immediately poured into diagnostic study models.

Results.—Approximately equal time segments between times when measurements were obtained were determined (Table 1). All patients had a treatment period that extended through the first 2 time segments at least. The greatest median expansion increase (4.4 mm) was noted in arch length expansion, whereas the least (2.0 mm) was noted in width expansion between the canines. For each dimension measured, the expansion was greatest during the first 100 days of treatment, with the percentage of total expansion declining between segments with continued treatment, and minimal expansion noted in the final 2 time segments. Ninety percent of the increased space was achieved in the first 300 days. An expansion of 59.5% was achieved during the first time segment between the second premolars, whereas only 5%

TABLE 1.—Average Number of Days Included in Each Time Segment for All Patients

Time Segment	Number of Days
1	105.4
2	104.6
3	97.4
4	77.5
5	85.8
6	51.7

(Courtesy of Murphy CC, Magness WB, English JD, et al: A longitudinal study of incremental expansion using a mandibular lip bumper. *Angle Orthod* 73:396-400, 2003.)

occurred in the last 2 time segments between the canines. No significant differences in the amounts of expansion were linked to the type of tooth being analyzed.

Conclusions.—Lip bumper therapy was able to effectively increase the space and alleviate crowding of the mandibular arch in the patients studied. This expansion was not evenly distributed across the course of treatment, but the majority of the change occurred during the first 100 days of treatment, with 90% of the change achieved within 300 days. Only minimal expansion occurs after that point, so use of the mandibular lip bumper longer than that appears unnecessary.

▶ The mandibular lip bumper can serve as a useful adjunct to nonextraction orthodontic therapy. It allows for expansion of the mandibular dental arch in the anteroposterior as well as transverse dimensions. This retrospective study reviews the incremental expansion occurring over a defined period. Specifically, the study determines whether the changes that take place in the dental arch occur evenly between measurements or whether the expansion attenuates with treatment time. The results of this study indicate that the majority of the expansion occurs during the first 300 days and that using the appliance beyond 300 days does not result in additional expansion. This article presents a stimulating consideration of the most effective way to use a lip bumper as an adjunctive appliance in nonextraction therapy.

W. K. Lobb, DDS, MS

Closing Anterior Open Bites by Intruding Molars With Titanium Miniplate Anchorage
Sherwood KH, Burch JG, Thompson WJ (Nova Southeastern Univ, Fort Lauderdale, Fla)
Am J Orthod Dentofacial Orthop 122:593-600, 2002   11–14

Background.—The treatment of anterior open bites in adult patients must take into account these patients' possible tendency to develop root resorption with orthodontic manipulation, the possibility that incisor extrusion may be destructive in this compromised area of the dentition, and the potential effects on esthetics. Posterior maxillary dentoalveolar excess may be present in or responsible for the open bite, usually requiring orthognathic surgery; however, other methods that are less invasive have been proposed. The use of titanium miniplates to serve as anchorage to intrude maxillary posterior teeth and close anterior open-bite malocclusions was investigated. In addition, the true intrusion of molars in adult patients were definitively measured, and the skeletal and dental changes that accompany open-bite closure were documented.

Methods.—The 4 patients evaluated had long-standing open bites without any habit history and had refused orthognathic surgery, opting instead for the less-invasive miniplate-assisted orthodontic treatment. All had true

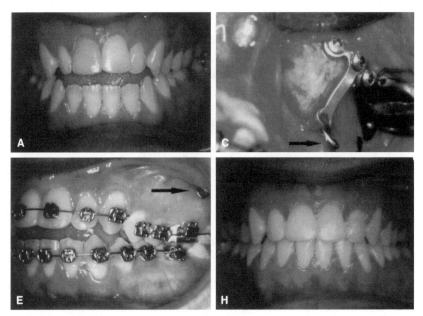

FIGURE 4.—Clinical pictures: **A,** Pretreatment frontal view. **C,** Insertion of miniplate on maxillary strut (*arrow* points to loop on miniplate that will project through vestibule). **E,** Preintrusion lateral view (*arrow* points to miniplate loop). **H,** Six months after appliance removal. (Reprinted by permission of the publisher from Sherwood KH, Burch JG, Thompson WJ: Closing anterior open bites by intruding molars with titanium miniplate anchorage. *Am J Orthod Dentofacial Orthop* 122:593-600, 2002. Copyright 2002 by Elsevier.)

intrusion of the maxillary molars, with a mean of 1.99 mm and a range of 1.45 to 3.32 mm.

Results.—Open-bite closure was accomplished for all 4 patients, with a mean closure at the incisors of 3.62 mm and a range of 3.0 to 4.5 mm (Fig 4, A, C, E, and H). Reductions were achieved in the mandibular, occlusal, and Y-axis plane angle. All patients had declines in their anterior facial heights accompanied by increases in SNB angles. Neither clinical nor radiographic evidence of movement of any miniplate was present, and patients tolerated the plates well.

Conclusions.—Open bites can be closed by using miniplates as skeletal anchorage to achieve intrusion of the posterior teeth in adults. With the intrusion, the occlusal plane angle of open-bite patients shows corresponding changes. The intrusion of the posterior teeth in the patients studied achieved closure of the anterior open bites, reduced the anterior vertical facial height, decreased the mandibular plane angle, and produced counterclockwise rotation of the mandible.

▶ The use of osseous implants as adjunctive anchorage units in the treatment of orthodontic problems has become commonplace. This study reviews a challenging clinical approach to manage anterior open bites through intrusion of molar teeth. Placement of titanium miniplates in conjunction with intrusion mechanics in the cases included in this study demonstrates the potential for intrusion of molars and correction of anterior open bite malocclusion. It appears that a clinically successful use of miniplate anchorage to significantly reduce anterior open bites is possible and presents a viable alternative to orthognathic surgery designed to intrude the maxillary buccal segments as an adjunctive procedure in managing anterior open bites.

W. K. Lobb, DDS, MS

Guided Bone Regeneration to Repair an Osseous Defect
Carvalho RS, Nelson D, Kelderman H, et al (Boston Univ; Harvard School of Dental Medicine, Boston; Amsterdam)
Am J Orthod Dentofacial Orthop 123:455-467, 2003   11–15

Background.—More adults are seeking orthodontic corrections and present periodontal problems ranging from localized single-tooth lesions to advanced generalized disease. To address these periodontal issues in anticipation of orthodontic correction, multidisciplinary approaches are needed, including techniques to regenerate lost periodontal structures such as guided tissue regeneration or guided bone regeneration (GBR). When bony defects were treated with bone grafts, it was noted that some firmly attached tissue exhibited the consistency of bone without the accompanying histologic characteristics. The use of bone analogs, principally decalcified freeze-dried bone allografts (DFDBA), allowed significant new bone formation at periodontal defect sites. A case was described in which GBR and DFDBA were used to repair an osseous defect caused by extracting a premolar before orthodontic tooth movement in an adult.

Case Report.—Man, 37, was concerned because his teeth were moving, and he wanted them to be straight. He had sustained trauma to his maxillary right central incisor with discoloration of the facial enamel that had been treated endodontically. He also had generalized gingival recessions in the maxillary and mandibular teeth as well as poorly adapted amalgam restorations in the posterior teeth. The diagnosis included a convex profile with slight mandibular retrognathism, a Class II molar relationship with proclined maxillary incisors, retroclined mandibular incisors, a deep curve of Spee, an 8-mm overjet, a 4-mm overbite, and moderate crowding in both arches. Treatment goals focused on eliminating crowding of the arches, reducing overbite and overjet, producing a more stable dental arch form, and obtaining a functional and flatter curve of Spee. The orthodontic treatment plan included the extraction of 2 maxillary first premolars and achieving maximum anchorage in the maxillary arch by using a palatal bar. Proclination of the incisors would gain some space in the mandibular arch. Placement of full banded and bonded maxillary and mandibular appliances was undertaken, but in the midst, a porcelain crown was placed on the maxillary right central incisor by the patient's general dentist. The apical third of the

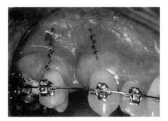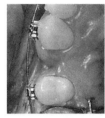

FIGURE 5.—**A**, Buccal and **B**, occlusal views of alveolar bone defect after extraction of remaining root fragment. Note complete absence of buccal plate on area correspondent to maxillary right first premolar. (Reprinted by permission of the publisher from Carvalho RS, Nelson D, Kelderman H, et al: Guided bone regeneration to repair an osseous defect. *Am J Orthod Dentofacial Orthop* 123:455-467, 2003. Copyright 2003 by Elsevier.)

maxillary right first premolar fractured while extracting the maxillary premolars, remaining in the bone; the entire buccal plate of bone fractured when attempting to remove the apex, producing a significant alveolar bone defect (Fig 5) and changing the focus of orthodontic therapy. Periodontal treatment was needed before tooth movement began. Because of the buccal bone fracture, a DFDBA was

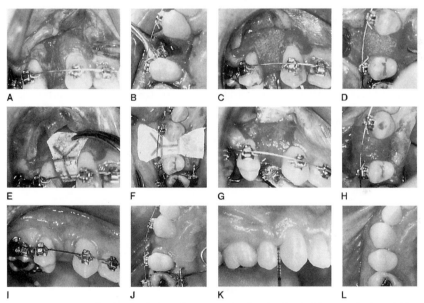

FIGURE 6.—Buccal and occlusal views of extraction site. **A** and **B**, Surgical flap exposing buccal ridge defect. Bone height at canine was at 1 mm to CEJ before distal movement. Periosteum was removed over ridge defect, and bone was decorticated before DFDBA. Note extent of osseous damage in extraction site. **C** and **D**, DFDBA to rebuilt buccal plate. **E** and **F**, Placement of membrane with titanium reenforcement for GBR. **G** and **H**, Removal of GBR membrane 2 months postoperative showing regenerate. **I** and **J**, Two weeks healing after membrane removal. **K** and **L**, One month after debonding. Note bone level on buccodistal surface of canine as shown by periodontal probe. *Abbreviations: CEJ*, Cementoenamel junction; *DFDBA*, decalcified freeze-dried bone allografts; *GBR*, guided bone regeneration. (Reprinted by permission of the publisher from Carvalho RS, Nelson D, Kelderman H, et al: Guided bone regeneration to repair an osseous defect. *Am J Orthod Dentofacial Orthop* 123:455-467, 2003. Copyright 2003 by Elsevier.)

placed in conjunction with a GBR protocol by using a nonresorbable polytetrafluoroethylene membrane combined with titanium to prevent further buccal alveolar bone loss (Fig 6). At a check 18 months after GBR surgery, the buccal bone height was 2 mm from the cementoenamel junction of the canine. Crowding was relieved without excessive incisor proclination or disruption of the soft tissue esthetics. Orthodontic treatment achieved a more stable arch form for the maxillary and mandibular dentitions, a stable Class II molar relationship with a canine neutroclusion in both sides, and an improved overbite and overjet to within cephalometric norms. Neither balancing interferences nor evidence of temporomandibular dysfunction was seen after the 37-month treatment period.

Conclusions.—Dental and occlusal relationships were improved for this patient through the use of both orthodontic and periodontal procedures. Regenerative therapy regained alveolar bone and prevented further attachment loss as a result of orthodontic movement.

▶ The significance of the multidisciplinary management of periodontally involved dentitions requiring orthodontic treatment is illustrated and discussed in this case report. Specifically, this report discusses the management of an osseous defect created during the removal of the maxillary premolars as a preparatory step in the orthodontic treatment plan for an adult patient. As the orthodontic treatment plan included retraction of the anterior segment distally into the created extraction space, the osseous defect created a new clinical challenge. A periodontal treatment plan involved GBR to prevent further loss of bone as the canine was retracted into the site of the buccal ridge defect. This report provides a good overview of the multidisciplinary treatment planning and decision making necessary to effectively and efficiently manage a patient problem that includes osseous defects.

W. K. Lobb, DDS, MS

12 Dental Laboratory Science

Introduction

The odontologic landscape is changing at an accelerating pace, driven by rapid advances in technology and improved communication methods to satisfy the ever-increasing expectations of an Internet-savvy population.

The contemporary practitioner is confronted with making choices on a daily basis from an ever-growing gamut of restorative materials and has to increasingly rely on laboratory technicians to assist in material selection and treatment planning.

Among the areas of greater innovative activity, we see the following trends: a continued emphasis on high-strength all-ceramic restorations; a refinement in existing indirect modalities such as physically and optically improved porcelain and composite systems; timely improvements in implant esthetics and implant component streamlining; and a growing awareness of the value of dentist-technician communication and collaboration in the successful outcome of indirect cases.

Now more than ever, the contemporary dental professionals must arm themselves with objective information and make critical choices from an expanding constellation of products and techniques. We should remind ourselves to gather the necessary information from unbiased and comprehensive sources such as this YEAR BOOK OF DENTISTRY. And we should do so at the onset of treatment planning, lest we be drawn by the siren songs of new, exciting—and yet unproven—technology, at our patients' expense.

Charles Moreno, CDT, MDT

Indirect Restorative Modalities

Probability of Failure of Veneered Glass Fiber–Reinforced Composites and Glass-Infiltrated Alumina With or Without Zirconia Reinforcement
Chong K-H, Chai J (Univ of Michigan, Ann Arbor)
Int J Prosthodont 16:487-492, 2003   12–1

Background.—Metal-free restorations have been shown to have the capacity to provide esthetic results that cannot be matched by conventional metal-ceramic restorations. Leucite-reinforced and glass-infiltrated alumina all-ceramic single restorations are the metal-free restorations that have shown acceptable clinical success. However, data on the clinical reliability of all-ceramic fixed partial dentures (FPD) have only recently been collected, and the studies of these FPDs were relatively short. The probability of failure under flexural load of veneered specimens of a unidirectional glass fiber-reinforced composite, a bidirectional glass fiber-reinforced composite, a glass-infiltrated alumina, and a zirconia-reinforced glass-infiltrated alumina was determined.

Methods.—A metal-ceramic system was used as a control system in this experiment. Ten uniform beams of the veneered core materials were fabricated for each system and subjected to a 3-point bending test. Data were analyzed with the Weibull method, and the failure load of specimens at a 10% probability of failure was compared. The mode of failure was also analyzed.

Results.—The 10% probability of failure load of these systems was not significantly different from that of the metal-ceramic control system. The 10% probability of failure load for the unidirectional glass fiber-reinforced composite was much higher than that of the other 3 systems, which were similar to one another.

Conclusions.—The unidirectional glass fiber-reinforced composite was found to be much less likely to fracture under a flexural load than a bidirectional glass fiber-reinforced composite, a glass-infiltrated alumina, and a zirconia-reinforced glass-infiltrated alumina.

▶ This study compares the load failure probability of 4 contemporary indirect metal-free restorative products (2 composite-based and 2 ceramic-based) against a traditional ceramic-to-noble alloy system.

The compressive strength of alumina oxide or zirconium oxide are inherently greater than that of glass or composite and are often touted as the superior feature to the restorative systems of which they are a component.

In this and other studies, the probability of load failure (B10) of a glass fiber and composite system (Fiberkor/Sculpture) was comparable to that of the ceramometal system, and less than that of the other composite and ceramic systems tested.

These results suggest to clinicians and dental technicians that the presence of a high-strength particle in a restorative material is not a de facto assurance of greater physical properties of the entire system and that the selection of metal-free modalities as restorative solutions should therefore be based more on the aggregate properties of the entire system than the isolated physical properties of 1 of its elements.

C. Moreno, CDT, MDT

Clinical and Laboratory Considerations for the Use of CAD/CAM Y-TZP– Based Restorations

Raigrodski AJ (Louisiana State Univ, New Orleans)

Prac Proced Aesthet Dent 15:469-476, 2003   12–2

Background.—Prospective studies evaluating the long-term success of yt-trium-tetragonal zirconia polycrystal (Y-TZP)–based materials are currently underway. Y-TZP–based infrastructures for crowns and fixed partial dentures (FPDs) have demonstrated favorable physical, mechanical, and optical properties. Computer-assisted design/computer-assisted manufacturing (CAD/CAM) technology is used in some Y-TZP–based restorative systems. However, technicians should be able to use traditional concepts of infrastructure design for both crowns and FPDs when using Y-TZP–based restorative systems. The properties of Y-TZP–based materials as a restorative infrastructure were described, and the use of traditional concepts of framework design with CAD/CAM technology was reviewed.

Overview.—Yttrium oxide is a stabilizing oxide that is added to zirconium oxide to generate a multiphase material known as partially stabilized zirconia, or Y-TZP. A number of Y-TZP–based restorative systems for crowns and FDPs have been described in the scientific literature. The Lava Y-TZP–based infrastructure is highlighted in this report.

Different methods are used to design the various restorative systems, yet all of the Y-TZP–based systems share the characteristics of high strength and longevity, good biocompatibility, metal-like radiopacity, and low thermal conductivity. Other advantages of these Y-TZP–based restorative systems include favorable marginal placement and the ability to use conventional cementation procedures, as these materials do not require adhesive cementation. In comparison with other all-ceramic systems for FPDs, the Y-TZP–based system presents a relatively small connector surface area.

In terms of esthetics, many of these systems present a white, opaque infrastructure that may limit the restoration's esthetic potential. The Lava Y-TZP infrastracture can be colored into 1 of 8 shades before the final sintering procedures. Limitations of the Lava Y-TZP–based infrastructures are related primarily to the use of the system for FPDs and include restricted interocclusal distance, heavily stressed connectors and bruxism, restricted infrastructure design, and limited clinical data on the survival of the restorations.

Conclusion.—Y-TZP–based materials are emerging as all-ceramic restorative materials in dentistry as a result of their mechanical properties and biocompatibility, and the initial results of ongoing clinical studies evaluating FPDs utilization of these restorative systems are encouraging. This article presented a comprehensive review of the various fabrication approaches of these infrastructures.

▶ Zirconium oxide and, more exactly, yttrium stabilized zirconia, is here to stay. As the physical and optical properties of this material are more clearly understood, so are its applications as a restorative material. This article gives a comprehensive overview of the various fabrication approaches of Y-TZP infrastructures. Dental technicians working with zirconium frames were originally faced with fighting a stark-white, opaque substructure. New systems can produce well-fitting, adequately shaded frameworks that promise acceptable strength as long as preparation, design, and fabrication protocols are respected. It behooves the contemporary dental professional to become familiar with these preparative protocols.

C. Moreno, CDT, MDT

Adhesion of Porcelain to Titanium and a Titanium Alloy
Suansuwan N, Swain MV (Khon Kaen Univ, Thailand; Univ of Sydney, Eveleigh, Australia)
J Dent 31:509-518, 2003   12-3

Background.—The study of titanium as an alternative for use in medical and dental alloys has been prompted by biological concern regarding existing metals and metal alloys currently in use. Dental implants fabricated from titanium have been shown to have excellent biocompatibility and an acceptable long-term success rate in the past decade. However, the bonding of porcelain to titanium for porcelain fused to metal crowns has remained a problem for the current use of metal-ceramic restorations. Goals of this study were to determine the adhesion at the titanium-porcelain interface through a fracture mechanics approach and to investigate the bonding mechanism by scanning electron microscopy and x-ray microanalysis.

Methods.—Specimens of 4 titanium-porcelain bonding systems were prepared in a rectangular shape for a 4-point bending test on a universal testing machine. A limited number of load and partial unload cycles were performed on the precracked specimen, and the strain energy release rate or interfacial toughness (G_C value) was calculated for each system. The interface was examined with a scanning electron microscope, which also facilitated quantitative x-ray microanalysis. The interface was also compared with a simulation of an atomically sharp interface to determine whether diffusion bonding occurred.

Results.—The highest G_C value was demonstrated by the titanium/Titankeramik with GoldBonder bonding system, while the titanium/Duceratin system provided the lowest G_C value. At 48.9 ± 12.4 J/m^2, the titanium/Titankeramik with GoldBonder system was significantly higher than that of the nickel-chromium/porcelain (40.3 ± 4.8 J/m^2), which is a clinically acceptable bonding system. X-ray microanalysis indicated that diffusion of some elements may have occurred at the interface.

Conclusions.—Of the 4 bonding systems utilizing titanium and titanium alloy for adhesion to porcelain, the titanium/Titankeramik with GoldBonder system was found to have the highest strain energy release rate. There was some evidence of diffusion of some elements on x-ray microanalysis, particularly of the porcelain into the metal. This diffusion may facilitate the bonding during the firing.

▶ Porcelain-to-titanium metal-ceramic restorations have not gained the popularity that may have been surmised, in spite of the potential benefits this system may have. Fusing our most esthetic and stable dental material, porcelain, to one of the most biostable, inexpensive and tough alloys, titanium (usually TiAl6V4), would give us many benefits—including strength, cost, and biocompatibility—over base metal and noble alloy porcelain fused to metal systems. While the conclusions of in vitro research point to strong bonds of ceramics to titanium, the processing difficulties—and hence elevated cost—of casting or machining titanium and the painfully technical sensitivity of the ceramic application have kept porcelain bonded to titanium restorations from gaining wide acceptance as a practical modality.

C. Moreno, CDT, MDT

Relative Wear of Enamel Opposing Low-Fusing Dental Porcelain
Clelland NL, Agarwala V, Knobloch LA, et al (Ohio State Univ, Columbus)
J Prosthodont 12:168-175, 2003   12–4

Background.—The loss of enamel opposing conventional dental porcelains has been an ongoing concern. In vitro wear studies have shown porcelain to be more abrasive than gold, amalgam, composite, or enamel. As a result, the use of porcelain was avoided by many clinicians in the replacement of functional tooth surfaces; however, alternative restorations were not always esthetically acceptable to patients. The development of new esthetic restorative materials has been spurred by demands from the public as well as the dental profession.

Several low-fusing ceramics have been introduced as being less abrasive to opposing natural dentitions than conventional porcelains. However, there have been conflicting results in studies of various low-fusing porcelains; these variations in experimental results may be attributable in part to the different porcelains selected for each study. This study evaluated the wear of enamel against several low-fusing porcelains and investigated the effects of ceramic firing temperature and enamel wear variability. In addition, the repeatability of the test method was evaluated.

Methods.—Five low-fusing dental porcelains (Finesse, Rhapsody, IPS d.Sign, Omega 900, and Duceram LFC) and 1 traditional feldspathic porcelain (VMK 68) were formed into 10 disks and used as a substrate for the wear test. Enamel was harvested from extracted human molars and machined into 60 cusps with a 5-mm spherical radius. An oral wear simulator was used to simulate chewing, and the size of the resulting enamel wear facets was evaluated after a specified number of chewing cycles. A portion of the experiment was then duplicated to assess the repeatability of the data and to determine the effects of overfiring on enamel wear. Scanning electron microscopy was used to evaluate representative ceramic samples from each group after testing.

Results.—None of the low-firing ceramics provided significantly less wear than the traditional feldspathic control porcelain. In contrast, 3 of the low-fusing porcelains (Omega 900, Rhapsody, and Duceram LFC) resulted in significantly greater enamel wear than the traditional control porcelain. The increased ceramic firing temperature had no significant effect on enamel wear. The wear data were repeatable, with no significant differences between the enamel wear from 2 separate experiments. Both experiments showed that ceramic material significantly affected enamel wear.

Conclusion.—It is suggested that variations in ceramic composition and microstructure may affect the opposing enamel wear but that low-fusing temperatures are not a guarantee of low enamel wear. The clinical relevance of the testing apparatus used in this study may be questioned, but the testing method was repeatable.

▶ We are often presented with new low-fusing dental ceramics that promise to reduce antagonist wear. These kinder, gentler ceramics often claim to derive these beneficial abrasive properties from their reduced maturing temperatures and/or modified crystalline structure. This interesting study reveals that several of these so-touted low-wear ceramics are not necessarily any kinder than traditional feldspathic porcelains. So again, don't let the marketing claims of a manufacturer (or a laboratory technician who is repeating them) replace good sound research. And don't let the promise of a new material steer you away from in-depth treatment planning and sound occlusion management.

C. Moreno, CDT, MDT

Changes in Translucency and Color of Particulate Filler Composite Resins
Nakamura T, Saito O, Mizuno M, et al (Osaka Univ, Japan)
Int J Prosthodont 15:494-499, 2002   12–5

Background.—All-ceramic crowns are superior in terms of permeability to light, so no light-blocking metal is needed in their fabrication. This quality makes the all-ceramic crown particularly effective in providing natural-appearing dental restorations. However, all-ceramic crowns are so hard and brittle that they may fracture with use or abrade the opposing teeth. Particulate filler composite resins with improved strength and wear resistance have recently been introduced, and crowns composed entirely of composite resin are now in clinical use.

These composite resin crowns are reported to provide good fit and fracture resistance in addition to the natural-looking qualities of all-ceramic crowns. However, they can change color when used in the oral environment for prolonged periods. Particulate filler composite resins have a higher content of inorganic filler and an improved resin matrix, so it is thought that these resins would provide superior strength and color stability in comparison with composite resin crowns. Changes in translucency and color of particulate filler composite resins that can be fabricated into metal-free crowns were evaluated.

Methods.—Five types of particulate filler composite resins (Artglass, BelleGlass, Estenia, Gradia, and Targis), 2 conventional composite resins

(Herculite XRV and Solidex), and 1 control ceramic material (Empress) were used in this study. Disks with a thickness of 1 mm were fabricated from each material and subjected to an accelerated test by immersion in 60°C distilled water for up to 8 weeks. Color measurements were made before and after immersion. Translucency changes were assessed by determining the contrast ratio, and color changes were evaluated by determining the color difference.

Results.—Targis and Solidex showed a significant increase (6% to 7%) in contrast ratio and a decrease in translucency after water immersion. A visually perceptive color difference of more than 2.0 was found for Targis, Gradia, and Solidex. However, the maximum color difference was 3.0, which would have been considered clinically acceptable.

Conclusion.—This study found stability in both color and translucency in the particulate filler composite resins.

▶ Filled composites have subtle optical properties that make them an excellent choice as a restorative material, be it in direct or indirect applications. It has been universally observed that original composites would discolor and stain in the oral environment. Indirect composites—because of their additional heat, pressure, or modified atmosphere processing—obtained greater levels of polymerization and promised not only improved physical properties but greater color stability. In spite of this, indirect composites seem to have this discoloration stigma attached to them. This study tries to determine the color stability of several current composite materials, and its observations may lead you to give some of these materials a greater role as a restorative modality.

C. Moreno, CDT, MDT

Biological Compatibility of Prosthodontic Materials
Campbell SD (Univ of Illinois at Chicago)
Int J Prosthodont 16(suppl):52-54, 2003   12–6

Background.—Traditionally, the biocompatibility of dental materials has focused on the identification of direct toxic effects, which are usually measured by cellular death or histologic changes in the adjacent tissues. This knowledge, combined with clinical observation and case reports, has been the basis of outcome measures of biocompatibility. However, it has been shown that many biological effects occur within cells below the classically defined toxic levels. Thus, there is the possibility of host biological changes beyond those considered part of conventional biocompatibility. A review of the current understanding of the biological compatibility of prosthodontic materials was reviewed, and areas in which greater understanding is needed were highlighted.

Overview.—Biocompatibility is not an absolute property; the manner in which the material is used is an important factor in determining biocompatibility of prosthodontic materials. Thus, the decision to use these materials should be based on a consideration of both the biological risks and the potential clinical benefits. Much has been learned regarding biocompatibility in recent years with the increase in understanding of cellular mechanics and biological systems, but much remains to be learned. Neither patient populations nor professional populations with elevated occupational exposure—such as dental technicians and dental office personnel—have been studied sufficiently to make certain that all currently used materials are free of biological consequences. Exposure and concentrations of many of these agents have not been measured in biologic systems.

Among the materials for which more research in biocompatibility is needed are restorative composites, resins, and dental bonding agents; dental luting agents; dental alloys; dental ceramics; denture acrylic resins; and dental bleaching agents. In addition, more research is needed on the environmental impact of dental material waste and the potential for direct toxic effects on cells and biological systems from high doses of prosthodontic materials.

Conclusion.—Dental materials are largely biocompatible, but little information is available regarding the consequences of low-dose exposure to these materials. There is a need for more research into the effects of low-dose exposure on patients, as well as introduction of the current knowledge base into the dental curriculum.

▶ New and improved restorative products are added each year to the spectrum of prosthetic materials. As our materials and techniques multiply, evolve, and improve, so must our knowledge of their effects on human cells and biological systems. Some notorious offenders have recently been pulled off the market after many years of use (ie, beryllium). However, other questionable substances remain in circulation, due in part to the lack of conclusive evidence on either side of the debate. This article effectively raises the question as to whether the apparent safety of a prosthodontic material may be determined as much by the results of insufficiently sensitive and/or extended biocompatibility tests as by the inherent, and yet immeasurable, effects on its host, and warrants that we all keep an open mind, eye, and ear to our everyday practice.

C. Moreno, CDT, MDT

Communication and Collaboration

Diagnostic and Technical Approach to Esthetic Rehabilitations
Romeo G, Bresciano M (Torino, Italy; Univ of Torino, Italy)
J Esthet Restor Dent 15:204-216, 2003   12–7

Background.—The functional and esthetic outcomes of an oral rehabilitation are determined by the clinician's understanding of the patient's needs and by effective communication among the entire dental team. It is particularly important to involve the patient in the decision-making process when there are esthetic considerations, and the entire treatment team should have a thorough understanding of the patient's requirements and expectations. The technical steps required to achieve an optimal esthetic result that will meet the patient's expectations are described.

Overview.—In addition to being involved in the decision-making process, the patient should be made aware of the limitations of restorative therapy. The involvement of the dental technician from the beginning of the treatment plan is an excellent way to ensure good cooperation because the technician will have direct contact with the patient. This increases the chances of obtaining a correct and straightforward fabrication of the prosthesis and avoids the problems that can develop during complex prosthetic treatments. The logically sequenced procedures in oral rehabilitation of esthetic areas are the construction of the diagnostic wax-up, fabrication of the provisional stratified resin restorations, and fabrication of the final ceramic restorations—all of which are illustrated.

Conclusions.—Optimal results in oral rehabilitation involving esthetic areas are dependent on excellent communication among the dental team and between the team and the patient. The technical execution of the restoration should follow a series of logically sequenced steps and checks. It is important that the diagnostic wax-up receive adequate attention so that the steps that follow will proceed in a straightforward manner.

▶ The predictable achievement of esthetic success in dental reconstruction hinges more than ever on the effective collaboration of the dental triad—the patient, the dentist and their team, and the dental technicians involved with the case. This comprehensive report details a practical protocol for the development of esthetically critical cases, which can be applied or adapted to most scenarios involving the esthetic zone. While a single esthetically-pleasing result may be fortuitously produced by any practitioner and any technician, it is my belief and also the belief of all the clinicians with whom I collaborate that to achieve consistent and predictable excellence, one must follow a systematic protocol similar to the one reported in this and countless other articles. In addition, one must follow this protocol regularly to develop and refine the dental team's quality of communication. The routine practice of a systematic approach to esthetic dentistry by the entire dental team has proven to be the most effective and repeatable assurance of satisfaction.

C. Moreno, CDT, MDT

Color Measurements as Quality Criteria for Clinical Shade Matching of Porcelain Crowns

Dancy WMK, Yaman P, Dennison JB, et al (Atlanta, Ga; Univ of Michigan, Ann Arbor)

J Esthet Restor Dent 15:114-122, 2003   12–8

Background.—Selection and communication of an optimal shade match for porcelain crowns may be one of the most important aspects of cosmetic restorative dentistry. The most widely used technique in clinical shade matching involves the use of shade guide tabs. However, these shade tabs are usually thicker and are fabricated from a different porcelain than the restoration, which makes it nearly impossible to properly match porcelain restorations with these shade tabs. The use of instrumental color measurement in clinical shade matching to porcelain-fused-to-metal (PFM) and all-porcelain crowns was investigated, and the relative effects of clinical and laboratory factors related to shade matching for PFM and all-porcelain crowns were determined.

Methods.—The study included 40 patients whose treatment plans involved the use of PFM or all-porcelain crowns. The patients were randomly assigned to 1 of 2 groups for shade selection: group 1 underwent conventional visual assessment, and group 2 underwent photocolorimetric analysis. A photograph was taken of the target tooth and of 4 shade guide tabs selected by 2 visual observers. The crown was fabricated either by visual selection or by the lowest E* values determined from the photographs and from a spectrophotometer. The E* values were calculated according to the Commission International d'Eclairage (CIE) Lab system. All 40 restorations were fabricated at the same laboratory. At the cementation appointment, clinical criteria were used to evaluate anatomy and contour, surface texture, and the amount of glaze as it related to color perception before cementation.

Results.—The mean E* between the reference tooth before preparation and the crown before cementation in the visual assessment group was 10.49, and the mean E* in the photocolorimetric group was 8.99. The observers and the colorimetric technique were found to be perfect in 41% of cases and to vary in 59% of cases. No significant difference or correlation was observed between shade selection methods and the clinical criteria used in evaluation.

Conclusions.—No significant difference was noted in shade selection using the conventional visual assessment by 2 experienced clinicians or the photocolorimetric technique.

▶ The fact that this study concludes that shade communication with a spectrocolorimeter was just as effective to relate shade to the laboratory technician as a visual measurement points to the advantages and limitations of using electronic color measuring devices. The colorimeter can provide a fairly consistent determination of the shade, regardless of the level of experience of the operator. Colorimetric measurements are valuable if used as an adjunct in color communication, but are insufficient on their own as they do not relate the characterizations and subtle nuances that make an anterior restoration lifelike. A high-resolution photograph, be it analog or digital, must be made available to the dental technician, as some electronic shade-taking systems do also provide. In addition, translucent all-ceramic restorations cannot be easily measured in the laboratory since the final shade is influenced by the substrate to which they will adhere. And most importantly, the technicians must have the skills necessary to reproduce what they see, regardless of the recording system used.

C. Moreno, CDT, MDT

Repeatable Alignment—Part II: Consistent Photographic Alignment Accuracy

Snow SR (Univ of California, Los Angeles)
Prac Proced Aesthet Dent 15:551-557, 2003   12–9

Background.—The attainment of predictable esthetic results requires the use of a variety of dental principles for tooth display, alignment, and relative proportion. Visual information regarding violations of these tooth arrangement principles must be clearly documented with dental photography to ensure accurate communication. Thus, accuracy in the alignment of photographs is crucial for effective treatment planning and evaluation. Several common alignment complications that may occur during the capture of diagnostic photography were discussed, and a technique for repeatable alignment accuracy was proposed.

Overview.—Photographing a full face allows the clinician to use the patient's upright head posture to aid in alignment of the image. The sides of the patient's head or the horizon may be used as references for balanced image alignment. However, the use of the higher magnifications appropriate for dental photography eliminates many useful peripheral landmarks from view.

Horizontal landmark irregularities include canting of the interpupillary line or occlusal plane, but midline discrepancies may occur when the nose or chin does not coincide with the facial midline or when the dental midline does not align with the facial midline. Vertical discrepancies are manifest when the facial midline is not perpendicular in relation to the horizontal plane. Thus, facial landmarks are unpredictable and irregular, and these variations must be ignored to obtain repeatable and diagnostic photographs.

A standardized protocol for photographic alignment is necessary. The Frankfurt horizontal guideline is a standardized alignment guideline that is used in orthodontic analysis as a primary reference plane for evaluation of osseous proportions and dental alignment.

Conclusion.—A systematic protocol must be used to obtain repeatable diagnostic dental photographs. Solutions to the most common complications that may arise during the capture of diagnostic photography were presented in this report.

▶ The value of clinical photography as an archival, diagnostic, and communication tool is well understood. From a dentist-technician collaboration standpoint, facial, oral, and intraoral views are marginally—if at all—useful for esthetic reconstruction purposes if they are not taken in proper and consistent alignment. A systematic protocol is detailed here to achieve the repeatable perspectives necessary to make your clinical photographs— digital or analog—of most clinical value to you and your dental technician. This is a must-read for all dental photographers.

C. Moreno, CDT, MDT

Guidelines for Digital Scientific Presentations

Marchack CB (Univ of Southern California, Los Angeles)
J Prosthet Dent 88:649-653, 2002   12–10

Background.—Digital media are in common use for communication in many fields. These media have afforded speakers presenting information more options for the delivery of their material, and speakers are now able to use these new digital media to facilitate and enhance their presentations. With the increasing number of presenters using video projectors and computers, a discussion of factors that influence the quality of a digital video projection presentation would seem warranted. Factors that may improve the quality of a scientific presentation by use of digital media were discussed.

Overview.—An effective and dynamic presentation is dependent on a combination of content, design, and delivery. In addition to the many design and layout factors of a slide, continuity is an essential component in the design of an effective presentation. Recommendations for optimal composition of text slides are presented here. The addition of photographs to a presentation can be accomplished though scanning or digital creation. However, the quality of the output of the video projector is a limiting factor in the use of scanning procedures and digital camera technology. Digital photographs may be easily cropped, aligned, and color corrected with several types of photo-editing software, allowing the presenter to precisely show the subject while providing the best composition.

The equipment used in a presentation also has a significant effect on the quality of the presentation. Because a multitude of equipment may be used, the presenter should be familiar with equipment compatibility at the outset. The choice of projector is also an important consideration, as is the setup of the room in which the presentation will be delivered.

Conclusion.—There are many advantages to the use of digital presentations. However, the speaker may lose the message if these presentations are not carefully planned. Guidelines for the presenter of scientific presentations using digital media are provided here.

▶ Digital presentations are the present, and photographic slides are suddenly obsolescent. Even the Kodak Corporation will be phasing out the celluloid-based technology that they so brilliantly developed. Every form of imaging has gone from the digital x-ray systems to the professional-grade megapixel single-lens reflex cameras that are now astoundingly powerful and affordable. And fast Internet connections have become a necessity more than a luxury in any actualized dental office or laboratory. So just as we once familiarized ourselves with carousels, slide projectors, and dissolve units, so must we all now master this new, exciting, and ubiquitous digital educational vehicle. This piece will give you a good foundation to share your digital information through effective computer-driven presentations.

C. Moreno, CDT, MDT

Implants

In Vivo Fracture Resistance of Implant-Supported All-Ceramic Restorations

Yildirim M, Fischer H, Marx R, et al (Univ of Aachen, Germany)
J Prosthet Dent 90:325-331, 2003   12–11

Background.—All-ceramic dental implant abutments have been shown to have several advantages over metal implant abutments in increased surface hardness, toothlike color, and the facilitation of an individually designed emergence profile. However, the mechanical shortcomings of ceramics include a sensitivity to tensile forces resulting from the inherent brittleness of ceramic restorations. The fracture will begin at a single location, such as a flaw or micropore. Under stress, such as occurs in mastication, a crack will then form from a defect site and proceed for some time as a subcritical flaw propagation. An absolute failure can occur when the flaw penetrates the ceramic. In recent years, advances have been reported in the fabrication of high-strength all-ceramic abutments for anterior implants. The fracture loads of implant-supported Al_2O_3 and ZrO_2 abutments restored with glass-ceramic crowns were quantified.

Methods.—Ten Al_2O_3 abutments and 10 ZrO_2 abutments were placed on Brånemark dental implants and prepared for restoration with glass-ceramic crowns. After fabrication according to manufacturer guidelines, the crowns were bonded to the all-ceramic abutments with a dual-polymerizing resin luting agent. The fracture loads (N) were determined by force application at an angle of 30° by use of a computer-controlled universal testing device. The data were analyzed with the unpaired *t* test.

Results.—Significant differences were seen on statistical analysis between the 2 groups, with a mean fracture load value of 280.1 N for the Al_2O_3 abutments and 737.6 N for the ZrO_2 abutments.

Conclusions.—Both types of all-ceramic abutments were found to exceed the established values for maximum incisal forces reported in the literature (90-370 N). The ZrO_2 abutments were found to be more than twice as resistant to fracture at the Al_2O_3 abutments.

▶ Now that the viability of osseointegrated dental implants has been unquestionably established, our attention has turned toward improving the esthetic results of these types of reconstructions. ZrO_2, or more precisely yttrium-stabilized ZrO_2, is emerging as an esthetically improved substitute to metal that might appear to possess the physical properties necessary to withstand the biomechanical forces of the oral environment. In the foreseeable future, I believe we can expect an increased use of ZrO_2, such as in abutment components, substrates for crowns, and fixed partial dentures. Could there be a ZrO_2 implant on the horizon?

C. Moreno, CDT, MDT

All-Ceramic Restorative System for Esthetic Implant-Supported Crowns: In Vitro Evaluations and Clinical Case Report
Castellon P, Potiket N, Soltys JL, et al (LSU, New Orleans, La; Victor, NY; Centerpulse Dental, Inc, Carlsbad, Calif)
Compend Contin Educ Dent 24:673-683, 2003   12–12

Background.—Ceramometal crowns have been widely used for successful restoration of tooth form and function on dental implants. However, they have been less successful in meeting the demands of patients for natural-looking restorations. The prosthesis can have a dull appearance next to adjacent natural dentition when a thin porcelain veneer covers the underlying metal framework, and porcelain degradation from toothbrushing can intensify this disparity in appearance over time. All-ceramic restorative systems have been developed in response to the demand for improved esthetics, but material strength and restorative costs have presented clinical challenges. These problems have been addressed in the development of a new restorative system with tooth-shaped ceramic coping for the anterior and premolar jaw regions. The results of in vitro evaluations of this new system and a case report on the clinical use of this system are discussed.

Methods.—Fatigue and 17° compression tests were performed in vitro to evaluate the mechanical strength of the 6 tooth-shaped copings and several luting agents of the system. In the case report, the system was used for a functional and esthetic restoration in a 48-year-old woman who presented with a missing mandibular left canine.

Results.—In the in vitro tests, all 6 tooth-shaped copings far exceeded the range of forces associated with restoration in the anterior jaw, with crown-endurance limits for fatigue and 17° compression proving to be 70% higher and 46% higher, respectively, than the established minimum fatigue endurance limits for these categories. In the clinical case evaluation, the ceramic restorative system performed well and provided excellent results.

Conclusions.—The all-ceramic restorative system presented in this report, with tooth-shaped ceramic copings for the anterior and premolar jaw regions, performed well in fatigue and compression tests and provided excellent clinical results.

▶ One of the many challenges the dental technician faces when fabricating metal-free implant-supported restorations is the complexity of creating a fully contoured prosthesis that will be adequately contoured. This must be accomplished despite the insufficiently wide implant platform, and still maintain sufficient structural support for the external and weaker porcelain. New and more practical solutions are needed to make the fabrication of implant-supported all-ceramic crowns simpler and less labor intensive. The system described here brings many appealing solutions to these dilemmas and warrants a closer look as an elegant alternative to computer-aided design/computer aided-manufactured custom-milled abutments, excessively thin copings, and ever-expanding component selections. I hope that more systems such as this one will continue to be introduced.

C. Moreno, CDT, MDT

Esthetic Considerations

A Review of Esthetic Pontic Design Options
Edelhoff D, Spiekermann H, Yildirim M (Univ of Aachen, Germany)
Quintessence Int 33:736-746, 2002   12–13

Background.—The restoration of anterior edentulous areas with fixed partial dentures represents a challenge for the clinician. Conventional fixed partial dentures are the most popular treatment measure in use today because of their ease of use and favorable long-term results. In these restorations, the pontic must fulfill the complex role of replacing the function of the lost tooth—providing a desirable esthetic appearance, enabling adequate oral hygiene, and preventing irritation of the tissue. The pontic must also meet certain structural requirements to ensure the mechanical stability of the restoration.

There have been many proposals advanced for the selection of pontics, some of which involve contradictory design options. Clinical and technical options available for the fabrication of esthetic pontics were reviewed, and practical procedures were illustrated.

Overview.—Options for pontic design include conical, hygienic, and saddle designs. The conical pontic was used to prevent collapse of the extraction site after removal of a tooth and to imitate the natural emergence profile of the tooth. However, the adjacent soft tissue tended to become inflamed after extended periods of service, and the alveolar bone resorbed. It is likely that these reactions occurred because the pontic did not allow adequate oral hygiene.

A modified application of the conical pontic—the immediate pontic—is still used to maintain the topography of the alveolar ridge after tooth extraction. The hygienic pontic allows maintenance of a healthy periodontium. However, the gap between the pontic and the alveolar ridge is large enough to trap food particles and to allow the tongue to enter. The functional, esthetic, and phonetic drawbacks limit use of the hygienic pontic to the posterior region of the mandible.

The saddle pontic provides highly esthetic results, assuming that the alveolar ridges are free of defects. There is no palatal gap, and trapping of food particles is not expected because the pontic adapts itself to the alveolar ridge. However, it is generally agreed that this technique should not be used.

Conclusion.—The pontic design in the maxillary anterior region is primarily influenced by esthetic and phonetic considerations. Restorative measures are often complicated by local defects of the alveolar ridge. Solutions proposed for this problem involve the modification of the pontic design and pretreatment of the recipient site. A variety of clinical and technical options for the design of esthetic and functional pontics for the anterior region were presented in this report.

▶ The optimal integration of an undetectable pontic in an anterior fixed partial denture remains one of the greatest challenges in prosthetic dentistry and is often the prize of good teamwork. A satisfactory outcome may involve complex soft and hard tissue plastic reconstruction, guided regeneration, exact pontic and connector design, and—of course—a mastery of dental ceramics. The achievement of excellence in these cases also demands a comprehensive understanding of the physiologic characteristics of periodontal tissue by the technician as much as the clinician. If the pontics on your bridges don't look as though they are naturally growing out of the gums, share this article with your technician, your dentist, and your specialist, and take on the challenge of the invisible pontic as a team.

C. Moreno, CDT, MDT

13 Evidence-Based Dentistry

Introduction

Each year, I find that the evidence-based dentistry literature is fascinating reading. So often, when all of the scientific literature on a specific topic is considered, the evidence is amazingly inconclusive and contradicts the assumptions about effectiveness that so many of us hold. It appears that easily the most frequently missing data are controlled clinical trials research data.

Let me give you an example from my discipline of endodontics. We have considerable "bench top" research data on such topics as root canal preparation and obturation. We have innumerable comparisons between various techniques, instruments, and materials but with very little data from real clinical trials. On the basis of our in vitro research, we assume one technique, instrument, or material is superior to another and will give better clinical results. First of all, we don't know that the same results would be obtained in actual clinical treatment, and secondly, even if the results were the same, would the differences observed actually be clinically significant? As we scan the evidence-based dentistry literature, we see that the scenario I have raised above is duplicated over and over.

That being said, the emphasis today on evidence-based dentistry has spurred very significant activity in this area, and more solid evidence for clinical decision making is being generated. This chapter addresses many different topics, but let me highlight a few of them for you. While there is considerable interest in the associations between oral diseases and systemic diseases, one systematic review article did not find evidence indicating that oral associations with cardiovascular disease call for tooth extractions. Another article found evidence that combining fluoride and chlorhexidine was effective in preventing the progression of caries root surface lesions. Still another article addressed the effectiveness of scaling and root planing in reducing pocket depth and increasing attachment levels.

A very interesting article that used computer modeling looked at the application of evidence-based dentistry to caries management in practice. Another process article looked at the place of observational studies in evidence-based dentistry, in contrast with the "purist" viewpoint favoring controlled clinical trials. The author did a beautiful job of making the case that observational studies have a proper place, and in fact are necessary as we develop our evidence base for what we do.

Kenneth L. Zakariasen, DDS, MS, MS(ODA), PhD

Clinical Science

Oral and Cardiovascular Disease Associations Do Not Call for Extraction of Teeth

Joshipura KJ, Douglass CW (Harvard School of Public Health, Boston)
J Evid Base Dent Pract 2:261-266, 2002   13–1

Background.—There have been reports in the press of a potential link between periodontal disease and systemic diseases such as cardiovascular disease. However, a causal relationship has not yet been established. The existing evidence for a relationship among periodontal disease, tooth loss, and cardiovascular disease was reviewed to determine whether the risk of cardiovascular disease is reduced with the extraction of teeth.

Methods.—Articles evaluating both periodontal disease and tooth loss as risk factors for cardiovascular disease were included in the review. The literature search yielded 105 articles; after further evaluation, 9 eligible cohort studies were identified. From these 9 articles, 6 longitudinal studies that evaluated both periodontal disease and tooth loss as risk factors for coronary heart disease were included in the final analysis.

Results.—Tooth loss may be associated with a similar or greater risk for coronary heart disease in comparison with periodontal disease (Table 1). The association between periodontal disease and coronary heart disease ranged from a relative risk of 1.01 in 1 study to 1.37 in another, after controlling for common risk factors—that is, there was a 1% to 37% increased risk of coronary heart disease among people with periodontal disease compared with those without.

In comparison, the relative risk for tooth loss and coronary heart disease ranged from 1.01 to 1.90 across the studies, or a 1% to 90% increase. The association between periodontal disease and stroke ranged from 1.07 to 1.63 across studies, while the relative risk for tooth loss and stroke ranged from 1.07 to 1.63 across studies (Table 2).

Conclusion.—This review of the literature found modest and similar associations between risk of coronary heart disease and both periodontal disease and tooth loss. The evidence in the literature thus far regarding the association of both periodontal disease and tooth loss with coronary heart disease and stroke does not support the removal of teeth that have periodontal disease as a method for reduction of cardiovascular disease risk. This is because tooth loss showed a similar association with cardiovascular disease.

▶ One of the primary strengths of the commitment to practice evidence-based dentistry is the obligation to look at all of the available evidence regarding a particular question, not simply accepting 1 article as the definitive answer to a clinical question you may have. This article illustrates this concept. Where

TABLE 1.—Associations Between Periodontal Disease, Tooth Loss, and Incidence of Coronary Heart Disease

Longitudinal Studies (First Author)	Publication Year	Number of Subjects	Population	Years of Follow-up	Exposure	Outcome	RR*	95% Confidence Intervals**
DeStefano	1993	5041	NHANES I	14	Perio disease vs no gingivitis/perio	CHD	1.25*	(1.06, 1.48)
DeStefano	1993	5398	NHANES I	14	0 teeth vs no gingivitis/perio		1.23*	(1.05, 1.44)
Joshipura	1996	43,316	Health profess	6	Perio disease vs no perio	CHD	1.04	(0.86, 1.25)
Joshipura	1996	38,354	Health profess	6	0-10 teeth vs 25+		1.32	(0.98, 1.77)
Hujoel	2000	5611	NHANES I	21	Perio disease vs no gingivitis/perio	CHD	1.14	(0.96, 1.36)
Hujoel	2000	4027	NHANES I	21	0 teeth vs dentate	CHD	1.16	
Howell	2001	22,037	Physicians	12.3	Perio disease vs no perio	Nonfatal CHD	1.01	(0.82, 1.24)
Howell	2001	22,037	Physicians	12.3	Tooth loss	Nonfatal CHD	1.01	(0.87, 1.17)
Morrison	2000	1441	Canadian	23	Perio disease vs no gingivitis/perio	Fatal CHD	1.37	(0.80, 2.35)
Morrison	2000	4285	Canadian	23	0 teeth vs no gingivitis/perio	Fatal CHD	1.90*	(1.17, 3.10)

*Relative risk adjusting for factors common to both oral conditions (periodontal disease and/or tooth loss) and cardiovascular disease. Factors include age, sex, smoking, obesity, exercise, alcohol, diabetes; specific factors included vary across studies. The adjusted associations mean that they cannot be explained by the fact that smoking (and/or other factors) increases the risk for both oral conditions and stroke.

Abbreviations: NHANES, National Health and Nutrition Examination Survey; *RR*, relative risk.

(Courtesy of Joshipura KJ, Douglass CW: Oral and cardiovascular disease associations do not call for extraction of teeth. *J Evid Base Dent Pract* 2:261-266, 2002.)

TABLE 2.—Associations Between Periodontal Disease, Tooth Loss, and Incidence of Stroke

Longitudinal Studies (First Author)	Publication Year	Number of Subjects	Population	Years of Follow-up	Exposure	Outcome	RR*	95% Confidence Intervals**
Morrison	2000	1441	Canadian	23	Perio disease vs no gingivitis/perio	Fatal stroke	1.63	(0.72, 3.67)
Morrison	2000	4285	Canadian	23	0 teeth	Fatal stroke	1.63	(0.77, 3.42)
Howell	2001	22,037	Physicians	12.3	Perio disease vs no perio	Nonfatal stroke	1.01	(0.81, 1.27)
Howell	2001	22,037	Physicians	12.3	Tooth loss	Nonfatal stroke	1.07	(0.91, 1.27)
Wu	2000	5,434	NHANES I	21	Perio disease vs no gingivitis/perio	Ischemic stroke	2.11*	(1.30, 3.42)
Wu	2000	5,816	NHANES I	21	0 teeth vs no gingivitis/perio	Ischemic stroke	1.41	(0.96, 2.06)

*Relative risk adjusting for factors common to both oral conditions (periodontal disease and/or tooth loss) and cardiovascular disease. Factors include age, sex, smoking, obesity, exercise, alcohol, diabetes; specific factors included vary across studies. The adjusted associations mean that they cannot be explained by the fact that smoking (and/or other factors) increases the risk for both oral conditions and stroke.

(Courtesy of Joshipura KJ, Douglass CW: Oral and cardiovascular disease associations do not call for extraction of teeth. *J Evid Base Dent Pract* 2:261-266, 2002.)

1 article—particularly one that does not compare other possible factors associated with a disease—may seem to indicate a strong association, surveying all of the available research indicates that the association is not strong enough to mandate a major change in treatment, and indeed indicates that the change in treatment you may pursue has just as strong association with the disease, ie, tooth loss.

A second strength of the commitment to practice evidence-based dentistry is the rapid realization that uncovering definitive causal relationships is a very complex business to pursue and that no quick and easy answers are usually available. Hence, the need for experts, such as the authors of this article, who can ask the proper questions and seek the appropriate data from all of the available articles to provide a status report and an interpretation as to where we are currently on a given clinical question.

K. L. Zakariasen, DDS, MS, MS(ODA), PhD

The Effectiveness of Routine Dental Checks: A Systematic Review of the Evidence Base
Davenport CF, Elley KM, Fry-Smith A, et al (Univ of Birmingham, England; Consultant in Dental Public Health Rowley Regis and Tipton PCT, West Bromwich, England; Consultant in Dental Public Health, Stoke on Trent, England)
Br Dent J 195:87-98, 2003   13–2

Background.—There has been a significant improvement in recent years in general oral health in the United Kingdom (UK). Dental checkups at 6-month intervals have been customary in the UK since the inception of the National Health Service. With the general improvement in oral heath in the UK have come questions as to whether dental checkup recall intervals should be adjusted to reflect current oral health needs more closely and optimize the clinical and cost effectiveness of dental checkups. The effectiveness of routine dental checkups of different recall frequencies for adults and children was systematically reviewed.

Methods.—The resources searched for this study included electronic databases up to March 2001, relevant Internet sites, citation checking, and contact with experts and professional dental bodies (Fig 1). The inclusion criteria were study design (any); deciduous, mixed, and permanent dentition; and routine dental checks consisting of clinical examination, advice, charting (including monitoring of periodontal status), and report. The comparator was no routine dental check or routine dental checks of a different recall frequency. The primary outcome measures were caries, periodontal disease, quality of life, and oral cancer.

Results.—A total of 28 studies were identified for review. The studies were poorly reported and clinical heterogeneous, conditions that restricted comparison between studies as well as generalizability to the situation in the UK. No consistency was evident across multiple studies in regard to the direction of the effect of different dental check frequencies on measures of caries in deciduous mixed or permanent dentition, periodontal disease, or oral cancer

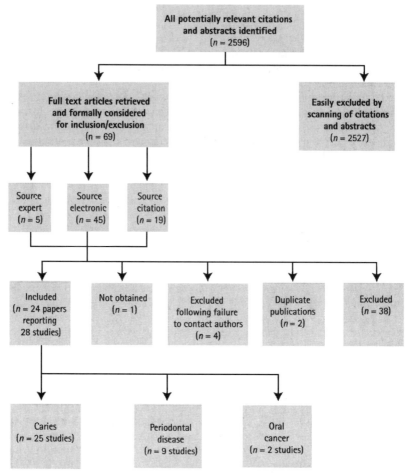

FIGURE 1.—Summary of study inclusion and exclusion process. (Courtesy of Davenport CF, Elley KM, Fry-Smith A, et al: The effectiveness of routine dental checks: A systematic review of the evidence base. *Br Dent J* 195:87-98, 2003.)

in permanent dentition. None of the studies included in this review were found to link empirical measures of quality of life associated with oral health and frequency of dental checks.

Conclusion.—This review was unable to identify any high-quality evidence to either support or refute the practice of encouraging dental checkups at 6-month intervals for adults and children.

▶ As practitioners, we know that there is an incredible range in the occurrence of dental diseases among our patients. For example, some of our patients have no or little dental decay and/or periodontal disease. Others have significant experience with both diseases. However, conventional thinking and practice are to recall patients approximately every 6 months, which probably means that some patients are recalled more often than needed while others are recalled less often than needed.

This article discusses how the National Health Service program in Great Britain remunerates dentists for 6-month recall appointments, yet does not have sufficient "high-quality evidence to support or refute the practice of encouraging 6-monthly dental checks in adults and children." Once again, a generally accepted concept looks questionable when analyzed from the evidence viewpoint.

The concept of regular checkups certainly seems sound logically, but it would also seem logical to plan the intervals for regular checkups on the basis of the individual patient's oral health indicators. This article, like the previous article (Abstract 13–1), illustrates the complexity of oral health care research needed to answer what would at first glance seem to be a relatively straightforward question.

K. L. Zakariasen, DDS, MS, MS(ODA), PhD

The Effects of the Combination of Chlorhexidine/Thymol- and Fluoride-Containing Varnishes on the Severity of Root Caries Lesions in Frail Institutionalised Elderly People

Brailsford SR, Fiske J, Gilbert S, et al (GKT Dental Inst, London)
J Dent 30:319-324, 2002   13–3

Introduction.—As the general population in industrialized countries grows older and a greater proportion of elderly persons retains all or most of their natural teeth, the importance of good and appropriate oral health is paramount, particularly for the more vulnerable institutionalized elderly population. The clinical effects of a fluoride-containing varnish (Fluor-Protector) in combination with a chlorhexidine-containing varnish (Cervitec) on existing root caries lesions were assessed in a group of frail elderly adults in a randomized, double-blind, longitudinal investigation.

Methods.—All leathery and soft root caries lesions in 102 elderly institutionalized adults were coated with Fluor-Protector. Participants randomly assigned to the test group also had their teeth coated with Cervitec, and those in the placebo group also had their teeth coated with a placebo varnish. These treatments were repeated 5 times during a 12-month period. Participants were followed up for clinical parameters linked with root caries, measurements of individual lesions, and salivary levels of caries-associated bacteria.

Results.—The clinical severity of the lesions in the test group did not change significantly during the 12-month evaluation period. The mean lesion width and lesion height and length of the exposed root increased significantly and the lesions were markedly closer to the gingival margin in the placebo group. No significant changes in salivary levels of caries-associated microorganisms after 12 months were observed, although there was an initial significant drop in the salivary levels of mutans streptococci in both treatment groups.

Conclusion.—The combined application of Fluor-Protector and Cervitec is a useful, easy, quick, and noninvasive method for controlling and managing existing root caries lesions. This procedure can be performed by a dental hygienist and may be beneficially applied in other high-risk groups, including persons with Parkinson disease, debilitating neuromuscular conditions, and dry mouth from any cause.

▶ This article and related articles showing similar results are important as we contemplate dealing with dental caries in an aging population. This will be a continuously growing problem. The baby boomers are aging. They are the largest generational age cohort that has occurred. At the same time, people today are living longer and are remaining dentate. That does not mean they are escaping the sequelae of acute and chronic diseases. As pointed out by this article, many older individuals become frail and institutionalized, and this number will grow substantially as the baby boomers age. Frail individuals have difficulty caring for themselves, are difficult for caregivers to monitor and provide oral health care for, and often suffer continuous significant dental disease and degeneration. Preventive regimens that are easily applied and effective will be incredibly important in keeping the aging population healthy with regard to oral diseases. The combination therapy described here appears to be effective in stopping the progression of root surface lesions in the institutionalized elderly. Other literature points out that 2 other clinical studies support these findings. In this case, the addition of the chlorhexidine appears to result in a considerable advantage, undoubtedly because of its ability to kill microorganisms locally that are responsible for the progression of the caries process. It is interesting to note that there is also currently considerable interest in the effectiveness of chlorhexidine in reducing microbial levels during root canal therapy. Certainly, more controlled clinical trials of broader scope are needed to more fully elucidate how these types of preventive, or disease-arresting, measures can be utilized to their most effective extent.

K. L. Zakariasen, DDS, MS, MS(ODA), PhD

Reported Bruxism and Stress Experience

Ahlberg J, Rantala M, Savolainen A, et al (Helsinki Univ Central Hosp; Univ of Helsinki; Riihimäki District Hosp, Finland; et al)
Community Dent Oral Epidemiol 30:405-408, 2002   13–4

Introduction.—Bruxism has often been linked with temporomandibular disorders and is more common among persons who are better educated and among females, particularly in their reproductive years. Stress has increasingly been considered as an initiating, predisposing, and perpetuating factor for bruxism, although an implicit relationship is not understood. A standardized questionnaire was used to evaluate whether perceived bruxism is linked with stress experience, age, gender, work role, and occupational health care use among a nonpatient multiprofessional population.

Methods.—A total of 1784 employees of the Finnish Broadcasting Company, aged 30 to 55 years, were mailed a self-administered questionnaire addressing demographics, perceived bruxism, total stress experience, and use of health care services provided by the company.

Results.—Of 1339 respondents (75%), 51% were male, and the mean age for all respondents was 46 years. No significant differences were observed in demographic status by age or gender. Bruxism and stress experiences did not differ significantly with regard to work category. Bruxism was more common in females than males ($P < .05$). In all work categories (management, journalists, production, planning, maintenance, and administration), frequent bruxers reported more stress, and the perceptions were significantly differently polarized between the groups ($P < .001$). During the preceding 12 months, females had 4.4 and males had 3.5 visits to a physician ($P < .01$), and 2.4 and 1.6 visits to a dentist ($P < .01$), respectively. Females reported more bruxism ($P < .001$) and stress ($P < .05$) than did males, regardless of age. Frequent bruxism was significantly positively associated with severe stress experience (odds ratio, 5.00; 95% confidence interval, 2.84-8.82) and was slightly negatively associated with increasing age and work in administration ($P < .05$).

Conclusion.—Frequent bruxism may be associated with ongoing multifactorial stress in normal life and work. Clinicians need to be aware that bruxism may be indicative of more complex stress disorders.

▶ What I find particularly interesting here is the consideration of both the dental problem, and the connection of the dental problem to a possibly very significant systemic problem. As dentists, we know that extensive bruxism can lead to damage of oral structures, and we want to reduce or eliminate bruxism for that reason. However, complex stress disorders are systemic problems whose possibility may be "red flagged" by the observation that bruxism is occurring. As clinicians, we focus on the oral environment and surrounding structures, but we must be ever vigilant in recognizing that general systemic conditions can affect or manifest themselves in the oral environment, and that oral conditions can be local indicators of significant general systemic conditions.

K. L. Zakariasen, DDS, MS, MS(ODA), PhD

Tobacco Smoking Is Strongly Associated With Periodontal Disease

Bergström J (Karolinska Inst, Huddinge, Sweden)
J Evid Base Dent Pract 3:92-93, 2003   13–5

Introduction.—The relationship between tobacco smoking and periodontal disease has not been established and was thus examined in 120 persons with "established periodontitis" and 120 age-, gender-, and plaque-matched controls.

Methods.—Fifty-percent of participants were women. The primary outcome measure was pocket probing depth, which may be considered a surrogate end point for periodontal disease.

Results.—Cigarette smoking was significantly linked with pocket probing depth (odds ratio, 2.7), especially among men (odds ratio, 6.4). Pocket probing depth was sensitive to increasing levels of exposure, heavy exposure being linked with more severe depth of periodontal pockets versus light exposure. Gingival bleeding was significantly less pronounced in smokers than in nonsmokers.

Conclusion.—The effects of smoking depend on the level of exposure (ie, number of cigarettes smoked per day and duration of smoking). Smoking behavior of periodontal patients must be considered in the treatment plan. Treatment of the smoking patient with periodontal disease that does not include counseling and advice on smoking cessation is both incomplete and unprofessional.

▶ While this case-control study, as the reviewer points out, is not conclusive in itself in establishing smoking as a risk factor in periodontitis, the results add to the accumulating evidence that smoking is indeed a risk factor. The reviewer makes a very interesting point that smoking behavior of periodontal patients must be taken into account in treatment planning and that not including counseling and advice on smoking cessation where appropriate is both unscientific and unethical, and thus unprofessional. This same reasoning will also hold true in relation to smoking and oral pathology.

I believe that, for too long, we as dental professionals have often simply accepted smoking as something a patient chooses or chooses not to do and that we have not considered it as a significant risk factor which we should address with the patient as one of our professional responsibilities. The scientific evidence says that it is indeed a risk factor, and we have a professional obligation to work with patients in eliminating risk factors. Dental schools are beginning to work with dental students on how to provide smoking cessation counseling to patients, not something that is easy to do effectively without training in this area.

K. L. Zakariasen, DDS, MS, MS(ODA), PhD

The Psychosocial Impact of Orthognathic Surgery: A Systematic Review
Hunt OT, Johnston CD, Hepper PG, et al (Queen's Univ, Belfast, Northern Ireland)
Am J Orthod Dentofacial Orthop 120:490-497, 2001   13–6

Introduction.—Most patients who seek surgical-orthodontic treatment do so out of a desire to improve their facial and dental appearance and not because of concerns regarding occlusal function. The major potential benefits of surgical-orthodontic treatment are probably less social embarrassment and improved self-esteem and self-confidence. Yet modern health care demands a higher level of evidence, especially for lengthy and expensive interventions linked with well-recognized risks. A systemic literature review was performed to examine the reported psychosocial benefits of orthognathic surgery.

Methods.—Literature searches were performed by using MEDLINE (1966 to December 2000), Web of Science (1981 to December 2000), and reference sections of identified articles. Key orthodontic, oral surgery, and psychology journals were also hand searched. Randomized controlled trials, other controlled clinical trials, prospective trials with or without controls, and retrospective trials with or without controls were reviewed for inclusion. Two reviewers extracted data and independently evaluated the quality of the trials.

Results.—Twenty-nine trials were considered relevant and included a number of prospective and retrospective trials. Data indicated that patients who undergo orthognathic procedures experience psychosocial benefits, including improved self-confidence, body and facial image, and social adjustment. There were wide variations in study designs and a lack of uniformity in measurement of psychosocial constructs. This made it difficult to quantify the degree and duration of psychosocial benefits.

Conclusion.—The psychosocial benefits of undergoing orthognathic surgery have not been clearly defined in a meaningful scientific manner. Well-controlled longitudinal investigations that monitor patients from before their orthognathic treatment to 5, 10, and 15 years after treatment are urgently needed. In addition, properly validated psychological assessment methods that are more specific to orthognathic patients need to be developed.

▶ This extensive systematic review of the literature regarding the psychosocial impact of orthognathic surgery is excellent in its thorough analysis of the literature. One important finding is that while most studies report positive psychosocial impacts, precise definitions of what is meant by psychosocial impact are difficult to pin down and are inconsistent between studies. In addition, well-controlled longitudinal studies are badly needed to draw definitive conclusions. Thus, the authors conclude that the scientific evidence is not strong to support conclusions regarding the beneficial psychosocial effects of orthognathic surgery. This may indeed be true, but it will certainly leave the clinician wondering what direction to pursue in practicing evidence-based dentistry. Again, let me refer you to an article (Abstract 13–11) on observational studies. It is clear that substantial observational data are available that can help us to some understanding of this clinical question and thus provide some basis for making recommendations to patients. As clinicians, I repeat that I believe we must use the best evidence available in making clinical decisions and recommendations. However, the best evidence available may not be as good as we would like, such as from randomized controlled trials, but we do have to work with what we have, and we still have to make clinical decisions and recommendations. As reviews of evidence regarding clinical questions are formulated, it is helpful to know whether something is "proven," but in the absence of that, it is very helpful to have some idea of which way the available evidence is pointing. This clinical question is a case in point.

K. L. Zakariasen, DDS, MS, MS(ODA), PhD

Meta-analysis of the Effect of Scaling and Root Planing, Surgical Treatment and Antibiotic Therapies on Periodontal Probing Depth and Attachment Loss

Hung H-C, Douglass CW (Harvard School of Dental Medicine, Boston)
J Clin Periodontol 29:975-986, 2002   13–7

Background.—The effect of scaling and root planing on periodontal probing depth and attachment loss was investigated in a meta-analysis. Evidence was presented relating to the reduction of periodontal probing depth and gain of attachment level after scaling and root planing, after scaling and root planing compared with surgical treatment, and when compared or combined with the treatment effect of 3 specific local antibiotic regimens.

Methods.—The meta-analysis provided a statistical analysis combining the results of several studies and yielded increased power to identify trends quantitatively. Although a meta-analysis usually weights the inverse of standard errors, approximately half the studies did not offer the standard errors, so sample size was used to weight the relative contributions of the studies; larger studies were given more weight than smaller studies. In the evaluation of antibiotic therapy, the 3 locally delivered antibiotics were tetracycline, metronidazole, and minocycline.

Results.—Scaling and root planing produced reductions of 0.15 to 0.62 mm for shallow initial pockets, 0.40 to 1.70 mm for medium initial pockets, and 0.99 to 2.80 mm for deep initial pockets. The gain of attachment was −0.50 to 0.29 mm, −0.10 to 1.09 mm, and 0.32 to 2.00 mm, respectively. The effect of scaling and root planing on periodontal probing depth was not significant for patients with shallow initial probing depths, but as initial depth increased the effect grew more significant. Gain of attachment level also depended on the initial periodontal probing depth. Compared with these nonsurgical techniques, surgical treatment was favored in reducing periodontal probing depth for medium and deep initial pockets. Nonsurgical methods are favored over surgical treatment for gain of attachment level in shallow and medium initial periodontal probing depths, but surgical results were better for deep initial pockets. The meta-analysis evaluating the results of scaling and root planing with local antibiotic applications found a consistent advantage in reducing periodontal probing depth and gain of attachment level when antibiotics were used. Adjunctive antibiotic therapy offered the additional benefits of a 0.23 to 0.61 mm reduction of periodontal probing depth and a 0.13 to 0.24 gain of attachment. Using the antibiotics alone provided no better or worse improvement than scaling and root planing alone.

Conclusions.—Scaling and root planing proved not to produce significant reductions in periodontal probing depth when the initial depth was shallow, but significant reductions were achieved when the initial pockets were medium or deep. Regarding gain of attachment level, scaling and root planing appear to produce a slight loss for shallow pockets but significant gains with medium or deep initial probing depths. Thus, initial probing depth significantly influences the outcome of scaling and root planing. Surgical results were better than those with nonsurgical techniques for the initial medium or deep probing depths, but the results with shallow initial depths favored the use of nonsurgical techniques. Antibiotic therapy produced results similar to those achieved with scaling and root planing. A consistent improvement in both parameters was noted when local antibiotic therapy was combined with root planing and scaling.

▶ The research discussed here provides significant findings, some of which will be controversial when compared with traditional therapies utilizing the surgical approach. However, the potential advantages of scaling plus antibiotics at this point in time should be considered only that—potential advantages. More research is certainly needed in this area before definitive answers can be given. As one reviewer of this article has pointed out, while scaling plus antibiotics appears statistically to be better than scaling alone, the differences were not clinically significant—an important distinction. Perhaps further research will determine which combination of treatment regimens will give consistent clinically significant positive differences, the kind of differences that lead to a clearly improved periodontal health status. It looks promising.

K. L. Zakariasen, DDS, MS, MS(ODA), PhD

Evaluation of the Effectiveness of a Pre-brushing Rinse in Plaque Removal: A Meta-analysis
Angelillo IF, Nobile CGA, Pavia M (Univ of Catanzaro "Magna Græcia," Italy)
J Clin Periodontol 29:301-309, 2002   13–8

Background.—The clinical trials testing the effectiveness of the prebrushing rinse PLAX have produced controversial results, with some finding that PLAX improves the removal of dental plaque over toothbrushing alone and others demonstrating no benefit. A meta-analysis was performed to review the results, identify similarities and differences among the studies, and identify patterns to permit an overall estimate of the outcome. Data were pooled from various studies on the effectiveness of PLAX as an adjunct to oral hygiene and oral health maintenance.

Methods.—Nineteen studies came from MEDLINE or other sources and were combined according to whether long-term or short-term treatment with PLAX was examined. One-day studies focused on the effect of PLAX after rinsing and after rinsing and brushing; longitudinal studies assessed the effect at various follow-up points.

Results.—Ten of the studies were 1-day studies and 15 were longitudinal. In the 1-day studies, plaque level was documented at 3 stages (after abstaining from oral hygiene at baseline; after a supervised timed rinse with PLAX, water, placebo, or nothing; and after supervised brushing) and compared to determine how effective PLAX was. PLAX was noted to reduce plaque levels significantly compared with placebo and rinsing only; no difference was found with brushing. Brushing alone after rinsing with PLAX was found to be superior to the use of placebo; brushing with toothpaste after rinsing with

PLAX showed no difference from use of the placebo. For longitudinal studies, subjects received either PLAX or placebo to use before brushing at home for a period of 1 to 52 weeks; a baseline and postbrushing plaque score was assigned, along with a gingivitis score. Plaque removal in the longitudinal studies was improved at first and then with the increased duration of PLAX treatment; no significant difference was noted at 6 weeks, but it was present at 1 to 2 weeks, 12 weeks, and 24 weeks. In a few studies, when triclosan/copolymer was used, PLAX performed less well than the placebo. When sodium benzoate was used, a significant reduction in plaque levels was present after 3 to 4 weeks but not at 6, 12, or 24 weeks. Meta-analysis of studies supported by companies producing PLAX and other prebrushing rinse companies did not change the results, but meta-analysis of studies not supported or supported by independent institutions noted the plaque index to be significantly reduced by PLAX in 1-day postbrushing studies. With rinsing and after 1 to 2 and 4 weeks the effect was the same as with placebo. After 12 and 24 weeks, 3 studies that evaluated gingivitis found a significant reduction in inflammation with the use of PLAX.

Conclusions.—PLAX significantly reduced plaque levels after rinsing, but brushing did not improve plaque removal. It was determined that the effectiveness of PLAX can be masked by the presence of toothpaste; brushing without toothpaste after rinsing with PLAX removed more plaque than brushing with toothpaste. Longitudinal studies found the effect of PLAX in removing plaque to be more pronounced than in 1-day studies. Longer follow-up documented a greater degree of plaque removal than short-term analysis. A significant reduction in inflammation was achieved with PLAX rinsing after 12 and 24 weeks, but overall the effect of PLAX on oral health was minimal.

▶ When a clinician reviews one article, it may appear that there is a clear answer to a clinical question. However, it is difficult to find comparability between research studies in the ways that they are done, and it is also difficult to find consistency in the findings between studies. This can happen easily when there are differences in research design, shortcomings in research design, difficulties in control of variables and study protocols, differences in the groups studied in the various research projects, and a host of other factors. The bottom line is that when all the pertinent research data on a particular topic are considered, it is sometimes very difficult to arrive at a clear-cut answer to a clinical question. Such appears to be the case here. Isn't it interesting that, while the authors conclude that the magnitude of the beneficial effects discussed here appear likely to be small, such products are undoubtedly used in very significant quantities.

K. L. Zakariasen, DDS, MS, MS(ODA), PhD

The Effect of Chlorhexidine Acetate/Xylitol Chewing Gum on the Plaque and Gingival Indices of Elderly Occupants in Residential Homes: A 1-Year Clinical Trial

Simons D, Brailsford S, Kidd EAM, et al (Guy's, King's and St Thomas's Dental Inst, London)

J Clin Periodontol 28:1010-1015, 2001   13–9

Introduction.—It is challenging to maintain good oral hygiene among elderly nursing home residents. Even oral hygiene provided by caregivers has been found to be inadequate. Chlorhexidine acetate/xylitol (ACHX) chewing gum was evaluated as a chemical aid to improving plaque control in institutionalized elderly.

Methods.—The study included 111 elderly residents of 21 homes in one British district. After baseline plaque and gingival indices were assessed, the residents were randomly assigned to receive ACHX gum, gum containing xylitol only, or no gum. Residents in the gum groups were to chew 2 pellets for 15 minutes twice daily. After 1 year, plaque and gingiva indices were assessed again. A survey was performed to assess the residents' opinions about the chewing gum.

Results.—Patients assigned to ACHX gum had significant reductions in plaque and gingival indices during the year of the study (Table 3). Among patients assigned to xylitol gum, the plaque index decreased, but the gingival index was unchanged; neither score changed significantly in the no-gum control group. The residents accepted gum-chewing well, but those assigned to ACHX gum felt it was more likely to keep their mouths healthy.

Discussion.—Chewing ACHX gum can reduce plaque and gingival indices in elderly nursing home residents. Long-term use may enhance oral hygiene in a dependent elderly population.

▶ The results of this study are very encouraging . . . a simple and apparently effective technique for improving oral hygiene in a group where traditional oral hygiene practices can be difficult to administer and follow. However, more research is needed to verify and more fully elucidate the potential positive effects for the elderly. While some research may seem only abstractly connected to the real clinical world, it is clear that research such as this directly addresses the very real clinical problems faced by clinicians and patients. However, even though the clinical questions may seem quite straightforward,

---

TABLE 3.—Plaque and Gingival Indices at 12 Months

	ACHX ($n = 43$)	X ($n = 37$)	N ($n = 31$)
PI	$0.8\pm0.8^*$	$1.6\pm1.0^*$	$2.6\pm0.6^*$
GI	$0.5\pm0.7^*$	$1.2\pm1.0^*$	$2.2\pm1.0^*$

$^*p<0.001$ (all significantly different from each other).

(Courtesy of Simons D, Brailsford S, Kidd EAM, et al: The effect of chlorhexidine acetate/xylitol chewing gum on the plaque and gingival indices of elderly occupants in residential homes: A 1-year clinical trial. *J Clin Periodontol* 28:1010-1015, 2001. Reprinted by permission of Blackwell Publishing.)

the research study complexity, in attempting to arrive at firm answers, can easily be seen. Research, in any form, is seldom an uncomplicated pursuit.

K. L. Zakariasen, DDS, MS, MS(ODA), PhD

Process

Applying Evidence-Based Dentistry to Caries Management in Dental Practice: A Computerized Approach
Benn DK (Univ of Florida, Gainesville)
J Am Dent Assoc 133:1543-1548, 2002   13–10

Background.—A supplement from the *Journal of the American Dental Association* in 1995 suggested that dentists should consider managing the treatment of their patients on the basis of risk of caries developing, as determined by scientific findings. According to the supplement, people could be classified into low-, medium-, and high-risk categories, with management varying by classification. This is an example of the application of evidence-based dentistry to caries management. This study evaluated the barriers to adoption of evidence-based dentistry and suggested possible outcomes for dentists and patients that may result from the adoption of evidence-based dentistry for caries management.

Methods.—The complexity of adopting evidence-based dentistry for a general dentist was estimated by means of flowchart analysis. The ease of collecting comprehensive patient screening data, identifying risk factors, and classifying risk were considered in the analysis. The adequacy of conventional caries charting for representing different stages and behavior of carious lesions was examined, as was the difficulty in producing treatment plans according to different levels of caries risk. The possible financial and organizational results of application of evidence-based dentistry caries management methods and an increase in the use of hygienists were also assessed.

Results.—Only 1 flowchart page was required for traditional caries management strategies, while evidence-based strategies required 16 flowchart pages (Table 1). Under the evidence-based approach, 2 full-time hygienists and 25% of a dentist's time, managing only patients at low risk of developing caries, could generate the equivalent gross income of 1 full-time dentist working conventionally. The addition of a third hygienist and devotion of 75% of a dentist's time to management of the remaining patients would gross a similar amount again (Table 2).

Conclusion.—The change from traditional to risk-based management of caries requires complex decision making that is unlikely to occur with paper chart methods. Computers are ideal tools for use in collection of patient screening data and automation of the treatment planning process to reduce the complexity of clinical management. However, conventional methods of charting caries are not applicable to caries management using evidence-based dentistry.

▶ This interesting article looks at the concept of actually applying evidence-based dentistry in the real world of clinical practice through managing treat-

TABLE 1.—Management of Patients With Caries Risk: Comparison of Traditional Management With Use of Evidence-Based Dentistry

Variable	Traditional Management of Patients With Caries Risk	Risk-Based Management of Patients With Caries Risk*				Change From Traditional to New (%)
		Low Risk	Medium Risk	High Risk	Total†	
Percentage of Dentist's Time Spent With Patients	100	25	25	50	100	N/A*
Office Gross per Year of Dentist in Solo Practice†	$390,790	$429,333	$175,886	$252,442	$857,662	119
No. of Unique Patients Seen per Year	1,123	4,667	198	226	5,090	353
No. of Patient Visits per Year‡	2.4	1	2	4	N/A‡	N/A
Annual Gross per Patient‡	$348	$109	$445	$1,117	N/A	N/A
Total No. of Dentist Hours per Year‡	1,581	399	395	791	1,585	N/A
Mean Dentist Hourly Rate	$247	$1,076	$445	$319	N/A	N/A
Mean No. of Dentist Hours per Patient per Year	1.41	0.08	2.00	3.25	1.13	N/A
Total No. of Hygienist Hours per Year	1,750	3,500	600	1,150	5,250	N/A
Mean No. of Hygienist Hours per Patient per Year	1.56	0.75	3.00	5.00	N/A	N/A

*Based on identification of groups at risk for developing caries by 1 dentist who employs 3 hygienists.
†Total number of different patients seen per year, not number of patient visits.
‡Source: American Dental Association.
Abbreviation: N/A, Not applicable.
(Courtesy of Benn DK: Applying evidence-based dentistry to caries management in dental practice: A computerized approach. *J Am Dent Assoc* 133:1543-1548, 2003. Copyright 2003 American Dental Association. Reprinted by permission of ADA Publishing, a division of ADA Business Enterprises, Inc.)

TABLE 2.—Illustration of Different Management Strategies and Cost Differences According to a Patient's Caries Risk Assessment Classification

Patient's Caries Risk Level	Annual Frequency of Dental Visits*	Procedure	Cost of Procedure ($)†	Total Annual Charges ($)
Low	1	Oral examination	25	25
	1	Prophylaxis	50	50
	1	Four bite-wing radiographs	34	34
Subtotal			109	109
Medium	2	Oral examination	25	50
	2	Prophylaxis	50	100
	1	Bite-wing and intraoral radiographs	95	95
	4	Fluoride or sealant treatment	25	100
	1	Restorative procedure	100	100
Subtotal			295	445
High	4	Oral examination	24	96
	4	Prophylaxis	50	200
	1	Complete radiograph series	151	151
	8	Fluoride/chlorhexidine/sealant treatment	25	200
	2	Restorative procedures	200	400
	1	Periodontic treatment	70	70
Subtotal			520	1,117

*Source: American Dental Association Council on Access, Prevention, and Interprofessional Relations: Caries diagnosis and risk assessment: A review of preventive strategies and management. *J Am Dent Assoc* 126:1S-24S, 1995.

†Source: Pelehach L: Patients hit with higher treatment costs. Dental Practice Reports 8:18-27, 2000. Median national procedure fees used.

(Courtesy of Benn DK: Applying evidence-based dentistry to caries management in dental practice: A computerized approach. *J Am Dent Assoc* 133:1543-1548, 2003. Copyright 2003 American Dental Association. Reprinted by permission of ADA Publishing, a division of ADA Business Enterprises, Inc.)

ment according to the patient's risk of developing dental decay. This makes logical sense because we would be monitoring and addressing the patients' oral health based on data that indicate their risks of developing disease, rather than on the basis of arbitrary time intervals—in essence, diagnosis and treatment customized to the patients' real needs. Not surprisingly, the decision making necessary to do this is relatively complex, and can best be done with a computerized system.

The author proposes such a system that they are ready to implement in their dental school. This seems to me to have tremendous potential, and it will be interesting to see the outcomes as this concept is implemented. I have no doubt that we will proceed in this direction in dentistry and in all other areas of health in the future.

K. L. Zakariasen, DDS, MS. MS(ODA), PhD

Observational Studies and Evidence-Based Practice: Can't Live With Them, Can't Live Without Them

Coulter ID (University of California, Los Angeles)
J Evid Base Dent Pract 3:1-4, 2003   13–11

Background.—The major limitation in the use of observational studies in systematic evidence reviews is their lack of randomization, precluding true analysis of efficacy. Pooling of observational data can be done only with caution. At the same time, observational studies may seem to be more relevant to the actual clinical setting. The types and appropriate use of observational studies in evidence-based practice are discussed.

Strengths and Weaknesses of Observational Studies.—Some observational studies seek to overcome the lack of controls by various approaches to "building in" comparison groups. For example, cohort studies compare 2 groups with a single difference in treatment or exposure, whereas case-control studies compare cases with a disease to control subjects who do not have the disease. Other types of observational studies include case reports, case series, and cross-sectional surveys. The first problem is to determine whether the 2 groups in an observational study are comparable before the intervention or exposure is studied. Matching may attempt to overcome this limitation, but perfect matching is usually impossible. Issues of group membership, such as diagnostic criteria, and confounding variables are also important limitations. Observational studies can show correlations between outcomes and events, yet they cannot demonstrate causation.

Observational studies still play a wide range of important roles, such as describing unexpected results, providing evidence about new treatments, and reporting on variable treatment responses. They can also address questions that cannot ethically or practically be studied in a randomized trial. In addition, because they may more closely reflect actual clinical situations, observational studies may be more persuasive to health care providers.

Comparison With Randomized Trials.—Increasingly, the literature on a given clinical problem will include both randomized and observational studies. Recent comparisons suggest that the results of randomized and nonrandomized studies of the same treatment correlate well. Some authors have pointed out that observational studies have less variability in their point estimates, questioning the place of randomized controlled trials at the top of the research hierarchy. Individual randomized trials can have discrepant results, questioning whether a single trial should be considered the gold standard for treatment decision making. The gap between randomized and observational studies is not as wide when the comparison is with cohort and case-control studies rather than with observational studies of all types.

Discussion.—Observational studies continue to have an important role to play in evaluating health care research. At least for the stronger types of observational studies, the results appear no more misleading than those of randomized trials.

▶ I really like this article! It reflects a realistic, practical view of research and clinical practice. While the randomized controlled trial has been viewed as the gold standard in clinical research, as is appropriate in most cases, the reality is that far more information is available from observational studies than from randomized controlled trials. As you have seen from the previous articles in this chapter, oftentimes few or no randomized controlled trials are available to shed light on a significant clinical question. As I discussed in the previous article (Abstract 13–10), from a practical standpoint we must utilize the best evidence available in formulating clinical directions even when randomized controlled trial evidence is not available. It was particularly encouraging to read the author's section on controlled trials versus observational studies, referring to the relatively recent publications that have certainly enhanced the credibility of observational studies. I believe the author makes a very good case for the important role that observational studies have to play.

K. L. Zakariasen, DDS, MS, MS(ODA), PhD

14 Practice Management

Introduction

This year's chapter begins with a timely and important topic—homeland security, and the significant role that dentists, individual dental offices, and the profession as a whole can play in responding to bioterrorism and mass catastrophes. Read these articles for information on how to prepare your office. Also included in this chapter are articles regarding strategies for building successful partnerships, methods to increase office productivity, the state of malpractice coverage for dentists, trends in dental visits and private dental insurance coverage, and a variety of information related to occupational risks.

Kristin A. Zakariasen Victoroff, DDS

Bioterrorism and Catastrophe Response: A Quick-Reference Guide to Resources
Han SZ, Alfano MC, Psoter WJ, et al (Harvard School of Dental Medicine, Boston; New York Univ)
J Am Dent Assoc 134:745-752, 2003   14–1

Introduction.—The dentist's response to catastrophe has been redefined by bioterrorism, which can be explosive, chemical, biological, radiologic, or nuclear in nature. An informed response to terrorist attacks necessitates accurate information regarding agents and diseases that have the potential to be used as weapons. Information concerning the most probable bioterrorist weapons was reviewed to provide an easy-to-use guide for dental practitioners to use in a quick evaluation of quality information about bioterrorism and catastrophe response.

Methods.—Data from the Center for Disease Control was reviewed to create a quick-reference guide to bioterrorism and catastrophe response resources that can be accessed from the World Wide Web and print journals. These data were condensed into a resource list that is current, relevant to dentistry, and noncommercial. The Web sites cited include those endorsed by federal agencies, academic institutions, and professional organizations. The articles included those that were published in English within the past 6 years in referred journals available in most institutions of higher education.

Results.—A table was created that acts as a quick-reference guide to resources, describing agents and diseases with the greatest potential for use as weapons, including anthrax, botulism, plague, smallpox, tularemia, and viral hemorrhagic fevers. Within the body of the table are Web site and journal citations for background and patient-oriented information, signs and symptoms, and prophylactic measures and treatment for each of the agents and diseases. The table facilitates easy access to this information, particularly in an emergency.

Conclusion.—Fast, accurate diagnosis limits the spread of the contagious diseases of bioterrorism. Information concerning biological weapons can allow the dentist to provide faster diagnosis, inform patients regarding risks, prophylaxis, or treatment, and define the dental role in terrorism response.

Homeland Security: Five Ways to Protect Your Family, Your Practice and Your Community
Diogo S (AGD Impact)
AGD Impact August/September:10-15, 2003   14–2

Background.—The focus of this article is on the protection of the dentist and his or her practice from bioterrorism and the services the dental profession can provide to the community in response to a bioterrorist attack or other mass catastrophe.

Overview.—A report of a consensus workshop of the American Dental Association listed the services that dentists could provide in case of bioterrorist attack or mass catastrophe in the form of education, risk communication, diagnosis, surveillance and notification, distribution of medications, treatment, decontamination, sample collection, and forensic dentistry. Included in this report was a call on local dental societies to develop an integrated response to bioterrorist attack as part of a community mass disaster response plan and for educational programs to prepare dentists to provide services that they may be asked to perform in an emergency. On an individual level, it is important for dentists to be able to recognize the symptoms of a variety of bioagents.

A concise description of these agents and their effects is provided, along with a list of Web-based resources. The 5 steps to preparing dentists to respond to a national and local catastrophe are acceptance of involvement; organization; being informed; connection with existing and evolving sources of information; and attentiveness.

Conclusion.—There is an important role for dentists in the preparation for and response to a bioterrorist attack or mass catastrophe on a local or national level. In terms of disaster prevention, surveillance is one of the most crucial roles for dentists. They are unlikely to see patients in the late stages of an anthrax or smallpox infection, but dentists and dental offices are well positioned to pick up on trends and to identify unusual clusters of symptoms or odd cancellation episodes. Dentists are urged to watch for an increase in flu-like symptoms (but without runny noses) and any neurologic symptoms.

Most importantly, dentists need to act now to determine their level of involvement and to prepare to act on that level.

▶ These 2 articles focus our attention on a timely and important issue: the role of dentists in responding to bioterrorism and other catastrophes. On a day-to-day basis, our attention is focused on dental treatment of individuals in our own offices. However, this article reminds us that because we possess unique health care training and skills, we are a resource for the nation. It is our responsibility to use our training as needed during a public health emergency. The first article (Abstract 14–1) provides a good discussion of the role the dental profession might play in responding to the results of an act of bioterrorism, and provides straightforward and concrete steps individual dentists can take now in order to be prepared should an emergency arise. The second article (Abstract 14–2) identifies a variety of information resources, both Web-based and in print. Both are vitally informative reading.

K. A. Zakariasen Victoroff, DDS

ADA Members Weigh in on Critical Issues
Burgess K, Ruesch JD, Mikkelsen MC, et al (American Dental Association, Chicago)
J Am Dent Assoc 134:103-107, 2003   14–3

Background.—Dental practitioners are confronted with many new challenges in the areas of science, new technology, patient care, dental reimbursement, and government regulation. How these challenges are affecting current private practitioners was determined.

Methods.—A questionnaire was sent to 6310 members of the American Dental Association (ADA) in January 2000. Follow-up mailings were sent in February, March, and April of that year. Data collection was completed in July 2000. Included in the survey were questions about critical performance issues and perceptions of the ADA and its priorities. Members were asked to rate the identified issues' importance to them. A total of 3558 completed surveys were received, which yielded an adjusted response rate of 59.5%.

Results.—The top 3 issues included "maintaining my ability to recommend the treatment option I feel is most appropriate for my patients," "receiving fair reimbursement for the dental services I provide," and "protecting myself, my staff, and my patients from communicable diseases." In comparison with the overall membership, new dentists found items other than these top 3 to be more significant. New dentists were found to be more concerned than the overall membership with securing funds for their practice and paying off debt. Among minority dentists, greater levels of concern were expressed about other issues, such as providing care to underserved populations and the intrusion of medicine into dental treatment.

Conclusions.—The membership of the ADA as a whole expressed similar views on many significant issues facing dentistry and the ADA's priorities; however, there were important differences with regard to some issues. The

ADA should continue to consider the relative rankings of professional issues among its membership and to note those issues of special interest to select member subgroups in the planning and implementation of Association activities.

▶ This article highlights issues important to ADA member dentists. Readers will likely see some of their own concerns reflected in the results. As dentists progress through various career and life stages, the relative importance of various issues can and usually does change. Hence, the contributions of dentists at all stages are vital if the variety of challenges and issues of concern to the profession are to be addressed.

K. A. Zakariasen Victoroff, DDS

Partnership Is a Three-Step Process
Bass AP III (Fortune Management, Tullahoma, Tenn)
J Am Dent Assoc 134:1114-1117, 2003   14–4

Introduction.—Many dentists consider bringing in a future partner and yet are reluctant to do so for a variety of reasons. Described is a 3-step process for achieving a successful partnership.

Three Phases to Partnership.—Bringing in an associate can be considered when the dentist has all the work he or she wants to do or can possibly do. During phase 1, the associate is introduced to and integrated into the practice. Phase 2 is the at-risk associate phase in which the new dentist starts to assume financial responsibility for his or her portion of the practice. This is the time to formulate a set of operating principles to address any potential problems. Phase 3 is the partnership phase in which the partner takes on his/ her full function within the team. Two separate corporations should be formed: 1 for the senior dentist and 1 for the junior dentist. The needs of each dentist vary dramatically, and a single corporation cannot serve either party well. There are many ways to split a partnership's profits, and options should be discussed before a partnership is formed.

Conclusion.—Even after a partnership is formed, there will be challenges. Regular meetings, division of responsibility, and open, nonjudgmental communication will diffuse the problems experienced in day-to-day practice and will help the partners enjoy a rewarding association for the duration of the partnership.

▶ Many dentists say that bringing an associate and potential future partner into their practice is one of the most challenging aspects of managing their practice. Anyone who has observed a dysfunctional associate-owner or partner-partner relationship knows that discord between partners can affect the practice in a profoundly negative way. However, it does not have to be this way. This article provides helpful guidance about the process of incorporating an associate/future partner into the practice.

While the article stresses the nuts and bolts of the process (advance planning of time frames, compensation formulas, financing), there are 2 less tangible aspects of associateship/partnership that shoud be taken very seriously. First, are the values of the 2 dentists involved aligned? Do they have similar practice philosophies and values about patient care standards, professionalism and ethics, work ethic, work and family balance, the role of continuing education and lifelong learning, and how employees should be managed and treated? Very divergent value sets will lead to significant problems and should not be ignored.

Second, have the 2 dentists established open and functional lines of communication? Not all issues can be anticipated in advance, and legal agreements can only outline courses of action related to major issues, not the finer points of day-to-day interaction. There should be evidence that an effective working relationship can be achieved.

K. A. Zakariasen Victoroff, DDS

Malpractice Reform
Schlossberg M
AGD Impact July:10-15, 2003

14–5

Introduction.—In December 2001, The St Paul Companies, Inc, the largest writer of medical malpractice policies in the United States at the time, discontinued its 65-year involvement in the health care market. This left 114,000 health care providers, including physicians and dentists, without malpractice protection. Safeco, Frontier, and AIG have since dropped health care malpractice coverage. In March 2003, the American Medical Association named 18 states in which medical liability has reached crisis proportions. Dentists are not immune from large awards. In 2002, a North Carolina jury awarded $5 million to a plaintiff who sued his dentist. Tips for reducing the chances of being sued are discussed.

Cutting Lawsuit Risk.—Fifty-nine percent of all claims filed against dentists are for improper performance. The fact that very few patients win a judgment indicates that some patients may have an unrealistic expectation of some procedures. Many cases are due to a communications breakdown between dentist and patient, not bad dentistry. The following are suggestions for decreasing the chances of being sued: Keep accurate records, writing down exactly what the patient was told in the layman's terms used to communicate with the patient; thoroughly explain all procedures, treatments, fees, and projected outcomes; learn about risk management from books and seminars; for dentists with a paperless office, give the practice's attorney an electronic back-up of records on a monthly or quarterly basis; don't step outside your skill level; make sure that dental staff members understand and perform risk management in their daily work.

Conclusion.—Dentists with a history of multiple claims or a single high-cost claim may have difficulty finding a policy. The risk of being sued can be greatly reduced in offices that practice risk management in their communication with patients and in their daily work regimen.

▶ Most of us are aware that our physician colleagues are facing a crisis in availability and cost of malpractice insurance, but we may feel that what's going on with physicians will not affect dentists. This article provides an informative discussion of the current crisis and points out ways in which dentists have been or may be affected. Although we may not currently face a crisis, our profession needs to closely monitor the current situation in order to prevent problems down the road. We cannot assume that we will not be affected.

K. A. Zakariasen Victoroff, DDS

Five More Ways to Add $200,000 or More to Your Practice
Levin RP (Levin Group)
Compend Contin Educ Dent 24:562-567, 2003   14–6

Background.—The Levin Group has specialized in the implementation of business systems in dental practices. Studies by the Levin Group have shown that most dental practices can increase their production by 30% without increasing working hours. There are many systems available to help a dental practice grow. Five strategies that have been found to be effective in adding $200,000 or more to a dental practice were presented.

Overview.—The first strategy is to examine the service mix of the practice, or the manner in which a practice combines all the types of services. It has been shown that over 81% of dental appointments still involve only single-tooth treatment. In fact, many patients would benefit from more comprehensive dentistry and preventive dentistry, which are not being addressed by many practices. In addition to the many new services now available in dentistry, cosmetic dentistry adds another array of procedures that can be offered. A practice should have a clear formula regarding which procedures it will provide and how many of these procedures it will perform per week, per month, and per year, as well as in what parts of the schedule they will be placed.

The second strategy involves upgrading of services. Patients appreciate having a wide range of options and, in many cases, will select the higher end or more productive options because they believe them to be in their best interest.

The third strategy is to focus on selling skills, which is defined by the Levin Group as "education plus motivation." This should include training in case presentation, with emphasis on the best use of dialogue scripting to enhance communication with the patient, thereby increasing the patient's motivation to accept the recommended treatment.

The fourth strategy sresses that new technology must have a return on investment. Dentists should be seeking technology that provides improvement in 4 attributes—quality, speed, efficiency, and production. Technologies that do not provide improvements in at least 2 of these areas should not be purchased as they will be difficult to profitably incorporate into the practice.

The fifth and final strategy involves development of a competitive advantage. The author is a believer in high-end, boutique-oriented practices. Reputation remains an important component of a dental practice as most patients like to have some familiarity with the reputation of a specific practice.

Conclusion.—Increasing the revenue of a practice by $200,000 or more is not as difficult as it may first appear. The advanced strategies presented in this article point to specific components of a practice that can be examined and improved.

▶ This article underscores 2 important points about practice management. First, managing a practice does not have to be only a reactive process in which you respond to your circumstances as best you can. This author stresses that a proactive approach can be taken. Conscious choices can be made that will impact the direction in which the practice is going. To be proactive, you need to have accurate practice data in hand and you need to be able to make changes— to not do tomorrow exactly what you did today. In addition to emphasizing a proactive approach, the author's concept of competitive advantage is very useful. What is or will be unique about your office? What do you want the differentiating factor between your office and others to be?

Second, we are reminded that good communication with patients is still a vital part of successful dental practice. The author focuses on "education plus motivation." Patient education and motivation skills can be learned and improved. Again, be proactive and take steps to enhance your communication skills. Although many dentists believe that these skills are innate (you either have them or you don't), there is significant evidence to show that communication skills can be improved. There are many resources available—books, lectures, videotapes, and continuing education courses.

K. A. Zakariasen Victoroff, DDS

Recent Trends in Dental Visits and Private Dental Insurance, 1989 and 1999
Wall TP, Brown LJ (American Dental Assoc, Chicago)
J Am Dent Assoc 134:621-627, 2003   14–7

Introduction.—Until the 1970s, more than 95% of the cost of dental care was paid for directly by patients. Today, 50.6%, 43.4%, and 5.6% of total expenditures for dental care involve private dental insurance, out-of-pocket expenditures, and government-financed care, respectively. In 1980, 56% of full-time employees of medium and large private businesses participated in an employer-provided dental care plan. Participation rose to 77% in 1984 and then dropped to 57% in 1995. This rate was 32% in 1999. Recent reductions in the percentages of employees with private dental insurance may have a negative effect on the percentage of the population who receive oral health care. Recent National Health Interview Survey (NHIS) findings concerning private dental insurance and dental visits are reported.

Methods.—The NHIS is a multipurpose survey conducted by the National Center for Health Statistics, Centers for Disease Control and Prevention, and is the primary source of information concerning the health of the civilian, noninstitutionalized, household population of the United States. Most data concerning oral health in the NHIS are gathered for all persons 2 years of age or older. Data are reported annually. The interview samples for 1989 and 1999, respectively, were composed of 45,711 (116,929 persons) and 37,573 (97,059) households. Data concerning each household member were collected. Two subsamples were used to obtain data concerning dental visits and private dental health insurance.

Results.—The percentage of the population with a dental visit during the evaluation year rose from 57.2% in 1989 to 64.1% in 1999. The percentage of persons with private dental insurance dropped from 40.5% to 35.2%.

Conclusion.—A higher percentage of persons with private dental insurance reported having a dental visit compared with persons without private dental insurance. The increase between 1989 and 1999 in the percentage of persons with a visit was greater among uninsured persons. If this trend continues, a smaller portion of dental patients will be insured. This may have an impact on the demand for services and front office operations.

▶ This article points out that there are relationships between the percentage of the population with a dental visit, the percentage of the population with private dental insurance, and national economic trends. It is encouraging that the percentage of the US population with a dental visit rose between 1989 and 1999 (from 57.2% to 64.1%). At the same time, the percentage with private dental insurance fell from 40.5% to 35% and access to care issues appear to persist, with those who are not privately insured having fewer visits, particularly at lower income levels.

For private practitioners, this kind of information is helpful because it allows the individual to make practice management decisions for his or her practice in the context of national trends. It also indicates that dentists must be flexible and continually prepared to adapt to changing patient visit and reimbursement patterns.

K. A. Zakariasen Victoroff, DDS

Canadian Dentists' View of the Utility and Accessibility of Dental Research
Allison PJ, Bedos C (McGill Univ, Montreal)
J Dent Educ 67:533-541, 2003   14–8

Introduction.—One of the most important factors driving the evidence-based health care movement is the perception that a large proportion of treatments currently provided in all fields of health care is not supported by strong scientific evidence regarding their effectiveness. Even when information is accessible, it does not necessarily result in a behavior change. It can take up to 15 years for physicians to change their practices when presented with sound scientific information. The views of Canadian dentists concerning the utility and accessibility of the results of dental research were evaluated with use of a cross-sectional design to determine change within the context of a major reorganization of health care research in Canada.

Methods.—A postal questionnaire was mailed with the December 2001 issue of the *Journal of the Canadian Dental Association* to all registered Canadian dentists. There was no second mailing.

Results.—Of 17,648 questionnaires mailed, 2797 were returned (response rate, 15.8%). Of these, 64.3% of the dentists found research findings easily available, 88.8% found them useful, and 95.8% had already changed 1 or more aspects of their clinical practices as a result of research findings. Significant differences in preferred means of learning the results of research and preferred formats for written reports of research findings were obvious between generalists/clinicians and specialist/researchers.

Conclusion.—Responding dentists indicated interest in the results of research and reported applying them to their practices. Two main groups have different needs for learning the results of research: the generalists/clinicians and the specialists/researchers.

▶ Although the results of this study must be interpreted with caution due to the low (15%) response rate, this article does focus attention on an important issue: translation of research findings to clinical practice. With the current emphasis on evidence-based dentistry, 2 questions arise. First, are the amount and type of research being done sufficient to enable truly evidence-based dentistry? Second, are the results of research (the evidence) readily accessible to clinicians in practice? These questions are important for the profession, and clinicians need to be vocal about their needs. Are innovative approaches needed in order to generate and disseminate new knowledge in dental research?

In medicine, clinicians in private practice have responded to unanswered clinical research questions by forming practitioner research networks, most notably in family practice. The advantage of the networks is that some clinical research questions are best answered in the community office setting, with the population of patients seen in that setting. Perhaps practice research networks are needed in dentistry as well to generate the type of knowledge clinicians in private practice need.

K. A. Zakariasen Victoroff, DDS

The Technologically Well-Equipped Dental Office
Schleyer TKL, Spallek H, Bartling WC, et al (Univ of Pittsburgh, Pa)
J Am Dent Assoc 134:30-41, 2003   14–9

Introduction.—The pace of change for dentists has accelerated, requiring them to frequently evaluate, adopt, implement, troubleshoot, and maintain information technology (IT) in their daily practice. More than 85% of dentists use computers in their offices. An integrative view of a technologically well-equipped office is presented.

Well-Equipped Office.—The computing applications for dental practice usually are separated into administrative and clinical categories. Most systems have focused on administrative functions, including patient registration, accounts receiving, billing and insurance processing, recall reminders, and inventory management. Clinical applications include processing dental and medical health histories, charting digital imaging, diagnostic and treatment applications, and decisions-support, the latter of which can vary in their extent or maturity. The Internet has opened up possibilities never before available, including scheduling, electronic claims or submissions, online supply ordering, practice Web-site, e-mail-based recall, e-mail communications with patients, computer-based professional development, patient access to individual records, and remote consultations. Even the operatory can be equipped with a variety of computing devices, including an intraoral camera with a monitor for patient viewing, a computer that can be used for a variety of data entry and retrieval purposes (treatment planning, scheduling, charting, and accessing Internet resources), direct digital radiology sensors in various sizes, and a personal digital assistant that can be used to download selective information and act as a pocket-sized reference on drugs and other clinical topics. At the front desk, a device that combines the functions of a laser printer, fax machine, scanner, and copier can be used to save space. In the waiting area, a computer can be used for patient registration, including complete health and dental histories.

Conclusion.—Dental practitioners should develop a comprehensive plan for implementing or updating the IT infrastructure in their offices. Usability, integration, work flow support, cost-benefit analysis, and compliance with standards are important considerations in purchasing technology.

▶ This article provides an excellent overview of the numerous applications of technology in the dental office. The strength of the article is that the authors stress the need for a comprehensive strategic plan when determining the technology to be incorporated into an office. Identify and prioritize goals first, then choose technology to meet these goals.

K. A. Zakariasen Victoroff, DDS

▶ What does it mean to be "technologically well-equipped" and how do you get there? There is no magic formula or set of criteria for attaining this status when it comes to technology. Instead, being well equipped means finding out what options are available, examining your own unique setting, and applying the tools and methods that will make your office run better within a budget you can handle. This article begins with a categorization of technology applications and their utility in the dental office, an overview of "what's out there." It is not meant to be all-inclusive but delineates what might be considered "must-haves" for the typical office versus applications with less appeal, because they are not required for the office functioning or have a limited audience. Two things are evident from this portion of the article:

1. There are certain technology applications that are essential to managing nearly any office, so most practitioners can benefit from computer technologies.
2. Office technology applications have grown to the point where they can attract smaller audiences with specialized needs, giving some practitioners customized solutions to data management and office workflow.

If you have ever wondered what the state-of-the-art dental office could look like, this article offers a glimpse. IT is a part of the initial construction infrastructure, rather than an add-on "as an afterthought," the author states. This means that a state-of-art office will probably require either a new construction or significant remodeling. There are dental offices that have managed to incorporate a significant degree of technology into their office designs with these methods. This is doable with the right team of contractors, architects, and a technology consultant or expert who understands your needs and can translate them into workable solutions that fit with the rest of the team. Nonetheless, some of the items mentioned in this dream office, such as chairside computing and intraoral cameras, can indeed be added into an existing office and, with proper use, can have a considerable impact.

Once you have been "wowed" with all the technological possibilities, the article concludes with some very important guidelines for technology acquisition. This brings me back to my definition of being "well equipped." Examining your needs, you will need to plan for technology implementation. Exploring your options, you will need to select what is usable, fits your office work flow, and will integrate with existing systems. Finally, there is cost. It is often difficult to calculate the cost-benefit ratio because we forget about things like missed opportunities. For an intraoral camera, for example, try to think about how much more attractive treatment options will seem to a patient who can visualize the problem. The process for deciding the value of technology is a detailed one but worth the effort, given the potential.

M. A. Robinson DMD, MA

Safety Net Tightened: 2002 Health Care Law Pushes Clinics Over Increased Medicaid Reimbursement
Diogo SJ (Acad Gen Dentistry)
AGD Impact 31(2):20-22, 2003   14–10

Introduction.—The 107th Congress, which ended in December 2002, considered various legislative attempts to address access to oral health care for an estimated 3.6 million children with no insurance coverage. The Health Care Safety Net Amendments Act, which was signed by President Bush in October 2002, emphasizes improving access to oral health care for low-income children through strategies that include more public health clinics, implementing teledentistry programs, and encouraging dentists to work in areas where their skills are in short supply. Issues concerning dental care legislation are discussed.

2002 Health Care Law.—The Health Care Safety Net Amendments Act does not address the need for adequate funding of state Medicaid and State Children's Health Insurance Programs. Cynthia E. Sherwood, DDS, Chair of the Academy of General Dentistry (AGD) Council on Legislative and Governmental Affairs, praises the law's innovative provisions yet states that it fails to address the realities of the access problem in the United States. In June of 2002, the AGD presented senators with figures showing that about one third of all eligible children are not enrolled in Medicaids' Early and Periodic Screening, Diagnostic and Treatment, or State Children's Health Insurance Programs. In 2002, only 15% of AGD members treated Medicaid patients. The AGD also stated that "if reimbursement rates worsen, the already low participation of dentists in the Medicaid program is sure to further decrease." The Safety Net law establishes the Healthy Communities Access Program, which coordinates all available services for the uninsured and underinsured. This program includes private health care providers and private hospitals, which cover more than 60% of the costs of uncompensated care and private health care providers, who provide more than 75% of care for uninsured patients with Medicaid coverage. It provides $1.3 billion for the Consolidated Health Care Center Program, which served more than 9 million indigent, uninsured, and immigrant patients through community health centers, migrant health centers, health centers for the homeless, and for residents of public housing. It also strives to boost recruitment and retention of health care professionals to serve in underserved areas and improve the integration of health services among community providers.

Conclusion.—Legislative progress is being made, but access to dental oral care for underserved populations continues to be a public health care challenge.

Evaluation of a Dental Society–Based ABCD Program in Washington State

Nagahama SI, Fuhriman SE, Moore CS, et al (Univ of Washington, Seattle; Yakima Valley Dental Society, Wash; Med Assistance Administration, Olympia, Wash)
J Am Dent Assoc 133:1251-1257, 2002   14–11

Background.—Children of low-income families have difficulty gaining access to dental care, and the consequences of this decreased access to care are serious. For most of these children, access to care is limited by dentist participation in the Medicaid program. Low reimbursement is the most-cited reason for poor participation in the program. However, it is unlikely that raising fees will boost dentist participation: additional measures are also needed. The findings of a 2-year evaluation of a dental society–managed dental care program in the state of Washington are presented. The Mom & Me program, a variation of the Access to Baby and Child Dentistry (ABCD) program, was initiated in that state to increase access to dental care for Medicaid-enrolled children younger than 6 years in Yakima County.

Methods.—Included in this evaluation were enrollment and visit data, first- and second-year cost data, and results of a survey of dental society members. The main outcome measures were awareness of the dental needs of low-income children, the effect of the program within the community, and the level of support for the ABCD concept within the dental society.

Results.—An increase was seen of more than double the number of dentists treating Medicaid-enrolled children on a regular basis: from 15 to 38 general dentists. A total of 4705 children were enrolled in the first 2 years of the program, and approximately 51% of these children visited a dentist. In terms of the impact of the program on the community, 79% of participating dentists and 43% of nonparticipating dentists reported that the program somewhat or greatly improved awareness of the need for dental care among patients in the community. In addition, 81.6% of dentists surveyed indicated that they believed the Mom & Me program was somewhat or very helpful in improving the image of the dental society. It was reported that the backing of the dental society encouraged more dentists to open their doors to low-income children.

Conclusions.—The positive survey responses and support among dentists for a dental society–managed program under the ABCD program umbrella are indications that such a program can be an effective strategy for improving access to dental care among Medicaid clients.

▶ Both of these articles (Abstracts 14–10 and 14–11) address the access to care issue that has received considerable attention in the past few years. The first article (Abstract 14–10) reviews recent federal legislative developments and gives a discussion of some of the ways organized dentistry has been involved in trying to influence policy. The article underscores the position that a mechanism for provision of adequate funding for the delivery of dental services to the underserved will be vital in solving the access to care issue. The second article (Abstract 14–11) presents a description of a specific program designed to address a specific access to care problem in Washington state. This article serves as a reminder that access to care issues are complex and multifactorial. Given the different barriers to care that exist in different areas and among different populations, it is not likely that one universal solution will be discovered. For example, in this article, a variety of issues related to access—language barriers, lack of program awareness among those eligible, high appointment no-show rates—needed to be addressed. Each local area probably requires a slightly different approach. Innovative collaboration between local dental societies and practitioners, the local academic community, government, private foundations, and those with community outreach expertise, as demonstrated in this article, may be the most promising approach. This is food for thought to all practitioners who are waiting for an answer to the access to care issue: local involvement could be fruitful.

K. A. Zakariasen Victoroff, DDS

Managing Silver and Lead Waste in Dental Offices
ADA Council on Scientific Affairs (American Dental Assoc, Chicago)
J Am Dent Assoc 134:1095-1096, 2003   14–12

Introduction.—Organized dentistry's heightened awareness regarding environmental issues has led the American Dental Association Council on Scientific Affairs to develop recommendations for the proper management of silver and lead wastes. The management of both waste products is reported.

Silver Waste.—Silver is present in used fixer solution and is in the form of silver thiosulfate complexes, which are extremely stable and have very low dissociation constants. There are many options for disposing of used fixer solution. One of the following is recommended: an in-office silver recovery unit, a pickup-and-recycle service, drop-off at a designated silver waste drop-off facility, sending used fixer solution to a medical radiology laboratory or a commercial photographic processing laboratory, use of the "takeback" policy for used fixer solutions provided by some manufacturers or distributors of the fixer solution.

Lead Waste.—Lead foil in intraoral film packets should be recycled through a licensed facility. Lead aprons and lead collars that are no longer used should be disposed by a recycler licensed to handle lead waste.

Conclusion.—These recommendations for silver and lead disposal are intended to guide practitioners to ensure responsible disposal of wastes produced by dental offices and to minimize the release of potential pollutants into the environment.

▶ Concern for the environment continues to be an important aspect of professional responsibility. This article is helpful in providing guidance on appropriate management of silver and lead waste.

K. A. Zakariasen Victoroff, DDS

Allergic Contact Dermatitis in Dental Professionals: Effective Diagnosis and Treatment
Hamann CP, Rodgers PA, Sullivan K (SmartPractice, Phoenix, Ariz)
J Am Dent Assoc 134:185-194, 2003   14–13

Introduction.—Many allergenic chemicals are used in the dental profession, including bonding agents, disinfectants, preservatives, and processing chemicals that are added to rubber products. Repeated exposure can produce allergic contact dermatitis (ACD) in dental professionals. An orthodontic assistant had severe skin disease secondary to workplace exposure to allergens.

Case Report.—Woman, 48, an orthodontic assistant, had an 11-year history of severe skin problems, including redness, itching, and pustules on both hands, along with cracked and fissured fingertips.

These lesions were refractory to treatment with over-the-counter creams and medications. A dermatologist who did no skin testing attributed the symptoms to latex allergy. The use of nonlatex gloves did not relieve symptoms. While the patient was on disability leave, the skin on her hands healed completely. The symptoms recurred and intensified when she returned to work. She had a history of childhood fever and eczema. Her hyperkeratotic fingertips were scaly, dry, thickened, and deeply fissured, and the skin on the back of her hands and wrists was mottled with red, edematous patches. The skin was leathery, indurated, and thickened near the metacarpal joints; the skin closer to her wrists appeared thin. Patch and skin-prick testing were positive for ACD in reaction to several chemicals, including 3 major groups of processing chemicals often found in synthetic and natural vulcanized rubber products: carba mix, thiuram mix, and mercapto mix. Topical treatment with 0.1% tacrolimus was prescribed. It was recommended that the patient wear medical gloves made of PVC, polyurethane, or styrene-based thermoplastics. Because she used methacrylates daily, she was strongly encouraged to develop a "no-touch" technique. Some symptoms persisted, and it was recommended that she no longer handle uncured adhesives. At 3- and 10-month follow-up, her hands were completely healed and she was able to continue working.

Conclusion.—Not all skin reactions are associated with glove or natural rubber latex. Dental practitioners need to be aware of common chemical allergens, symptoms of ACD, and appropriate treatment for occupational skin disease.

The Air Turbine and Hearing Loss: Are Dentists at Risk?
Hyson JM Jr (Univ of Maryland, Baltimore)
J Am Dent Assoc 133:1639-1642, 2002   14–14

Introduction.—Damage to dentists' ears from use of the air turbine is of concern, but there is no conclusive proof that the turbine poses a health risk for dentists. A literature review was performed to assess hearing loss among dentists.

Literature Review.—A review of the literature revealed conflicting findings; none reported conclusive results. The Occupational Safety and Health Act (OSHA) allows 8 hours of exposure to a 90-dB sound pressure level stimulus. Noise levels of 100 dB have been reported with air turbines, particularly older drills, yet the daily cumulative drill noise duration of 12 to 45 minutes falls within the recommended OSHA guidelines. Recommendations for preventing hearing loss include the use of ear protection and periodic audiometry.

Conclusion.—Earlier reports are inconclusive concerning hearing loss due to use of the air turbine drill among dental students, faculty members, practicing dentists, and other dental staff members who use air turbine handpieces. Further investigation is necessary to determine whether there is a correlation between the use of the air turbine and hearing loss.

Use of HIV Postexposure Prophylaxis by Dental Health Care Personnel: An Overview and Updated Recommendations

Cleveland JL, and the National Surveillance System for Health Care Workers Group of the Centers for Disease Control and Prevention (Ctrs for Disease Control and Prevention, Chamblee, Ga)

J Am Dent Assoc 133:1619-1626, 2002   14–15

Background.—In 2001, the US Public Health Service published updated guidelines for postexposure prophylaxis (PEP) for health care workers exposed to HIV. Few studies of the use of PEP by dental health care workers have been published. Surveillance data were used to analyze the use of PEP by dental health care personnel exposed to HIV.

Methods and Findings.—The analysis included exposures to dental workers reported to the Centers for Disease Control and Prevention's National Surveillance System for Health Care Workers from 1995 to 2001. A total of 208 exposures were reported, including 199 percutaneous injuries, 6 mucous membrane exposures, and 3 skin exposures. The most common cause of percutaneous injuries was small-bore, hollow needles (one-third of cases). Two thirds of the injuries were moderate in depth, while most of the rest were superficial. About half of the devices involved in these injuries showed visible blood. Thirty-nine percent of the exposures occurred during oral surgery procedures, 21% during restorative procedures, and 15% during oral hygiene procedures.

Based on US Public Health Service criteria, about half of the injuries were classified as less severe. Of 186 source patients identified, 13% were HIV-positive. Of these, 58% had HIV-related symptoms or a high viral load. Three-drug PEP was indicated for three fourths of dental health care workers with exposure from an HIV-positive source. About one fourth of workers exposed to a source who later proved HIV negative started PEP, including several who took prolonged courses of PEP. None of the reported exposures led to HIV infection.

Discussion.—These surveillance data support previous studies showing a low risk of occupational HIV transmission to dental health care professionals. The absolute number of exposed workers is small, yet about three fourths of those with exposure to HIV-positive sources are candidates for 3-drug PEP. Rapid follow-up testing of sources and counseling could reduce unnecessary use of PEP.

▶ As dentists, we work very hard to enhance the health of our patients. At the same time, we must remember to safeguard our own health and the health of our employees. Protecting oneself and one's employees from occupational risks is an important aspect of practice management. All 3 of these articles

(Abstracts 14–13 to 14–15) provide needed information about potential occupational risks.

In one article (Abstract 14–14), while the results of the authors' literature review on hearing loss among dentists are inconclusive, the article does highlight a potential risk that many practitioners may not have been aware of. The best advice may be to monitor one's health—including hearing—carefully. Another article (Abstract 14–15) addresses HIV postexposure prophylaxis. Recommendations continue to evolve, and this article highlights the need to update our knowledge periodically. And another article (Abstract 14–13) addresses allergic contact dermatitis.

K. A. Zakariasen Victoroff, DDS

15 Dental Informatics

Introduction

The field of dental informatics is relatively new to most dentists, but it continues to grow in significance as computer and communications applications assume a more prominent role in dental care. Simply put, the objective of informatics is the use of available tools to bring about the fusion of data and knowledge in such a way as to expedite the tasks we perform as dentists. Tasks that involve a great deal of data, such as decision-making, are particularly amenable to improvement with informatics.

In this section, we focus on the foremost topics for 2003. Computing in the office and going "paperless" has become an intriguing option with several pros and cons. Understanding at least a little about a computer network is essential to this process, and a case study is included in this article set. The second topic area, computer-aided design/computer-aided manufacturing (CAD/CAM), uses computer algorithms and applies also to esthetic dentistry. Digital imaging, the third topic area, is well covered in several non–peer-reviewed journals. The articles selected here focus on research comparing image resolution of 2 systems and optimal image presentation for caries detection. Modeling is an important tool for informatics that allows us to create digital representations of objects. In the fourth topic area, we acquire a glimpse of how technologies similar to CT scans are being used to generate highly specific electronic jaw models that can facilitate implantology, maxillofacial prosthodontics, and orthodontic measurement. Finally, informatics can and should be an integral part of the educational process. The last topic set demonstrates computer-assisted instruction methodologies and the impact of teledentistry.

Literature in dental informatics is currently not as expansive as some other fields in dentistry. However, the level of interest appears high, and the far-reaching impact that informatics can have in so many areas holds promise for the future.

Michelle A. Robinson, DMD, MA

Office Computing and Networks

The Office Technology Backbone

Ulrich B (Auburn, Calif)
Am J Orthod Dentofacial Orthop 123:703-706, 2003   15–1

Background.—In redesigning his office to meet the changing needs of patients, a private practice dentist integrated technology used every day to achieve convenience and ease of access to the information and communication tools needed and to anticipate future needs. The use of an office technology backbone (OTB) was the method chosen.

Considerations and Planning.—A hardwired OTB was chosen for increased speed, security, and reliability with the acknowledgment that this required careful planning of cable routes and intense labor for installation. The elements of the OTB were a telephone punch block for telephone communication (wired to each telephone jack in the office), a video block patch panel for video transmission, and a data block patch panel for data transmission. To accommodate the possible 24 peripheral computer stations, complex cables from the OTB to the rough destinations were installed while the subfloor was being laid. Each peripheral site was designed to support up to 2 computers, various phones, and television output or camera input, which could include security or other uses, as well as a network hub for additional computer stations and linkage to the main network. During the planning stage, the total wattage needed for the equipment and computers on each circuit was estimated. When the ceiling and walls were framed, a nonverbal communication lighting system, 6 mounted security cameras without voice capability, several 2-stage motion and heat sensors as well as smoke detectors, and 3 security alarm keypads with voice capability were placed and wired.

Communications, Data, and Video Provisions.—Incoming call lines were provided by the local telephone company; the lines entered a 25-pair box and were linked to the OTB with the use of the Altigen block to the inside telephone punch board and to the telephone jacks, which made available either a regular analog telephone line or an Altigen digital line. Separate analog lines were provided for the various calling options (ie, private outgoing calls, fax, credit card, optional Internet dial out, and burglar and fire alarms). Computer cables for data and those for video were chosen with future technology in mind. The main server houses practice management data and permits the computers on the network to access patient information; the other computers acts as data servers, storing digital x-ray films, patient file folders with photographs, and interactive patient-education files. The same keyboard, mouse, and video monitor can be shared by several computers with the use of generic switches, so a single station can access various computers with various functions. Specialized computers are not used as work stations but serve their dedicated functions only. The power supply for the computers is an uninterruptible source that filters and regulates voltage from the outlet and allows 20 minutes of emergency battery power.

Conclusions.—The life span of technology is often brief, but an understanding of how devices work can sometimes extend useful life and permit repair or return to the manufacturer or warranty holder for repair. The dental office that has been planned with technology in place, particularly with the use of a planned OTB, can permit peripheral devices to be upgraded without halting office operations. The example offered was planned to accomplish this objective.

▶ This article describes a specific implementation of office computerization with the use of an OTB in a new construction office design. The author states that computers have been his hobby for 20 years. Novices or those not as interested in knowing the nuts and bolts of office networking may choose to work with a group of vendors or consultants who can assist in planning for such an implementation. The design presented here is a good snapshot of the current technologies that are being designed into a networked dental office. It includes high-speed Internet and both analog and digital telephone lines, a hard-wired (as opposed to wireless) data cabling system to network the office computers, and video cable for high definition television. Although there are articles that tout the advantages of wireless systems (see Abstract 15–2), the author notes that, for this undertaking, the wired system provides added security, speed, and reliability that wireless could not. Similar to the article included in the previous section (see Abstract 14–9) on the technologically well-equipped office, this article affirms the importance of careful planning up front and paying close attention to integration issues.

M. A. Robinson, DMD, MA

No Strings Attached: Wireless Networks Are a Better Way to Bring Office Computers Together
Akseizer S (Syosset, NY)
AGD Impact March:18-19, 2003   15–2

Introduction.—The use of computer networks is one of the fastest growing technology trends in dentistry. These systems bring the entire dental office together. Their use in bringing office computers together was discussed.

Wireless Networks.—The problem with computer networks is the numerous wires and cables needed to connect computers to one another. Network and Internet access are available by means of wireless networks. The newer systems use radio waves to provide high-speed connectivity over long distances. Wireless networks provide greater mobility, permitting both patients and practitioners to directly enter or review data and update medical histories from any computer in the system. The new mobility, along with touch-screen table personal computers, will transform the way general practitioners record and review patient data.

The wireless network usually involves a centrally located access point and a separate network receiver card for each connected device. The preeminent wireless network standard is 802.11b (wireless fidelity, or "Wi-Fi"). Currently, 802.11b access points cost between $100 and $300. The receivers may be placed directly into the computer as network cards or may be connected through Personal Computer Memory Card International Association or Universal Serial Bus ports, costing between $50 and $100.

The wireless network speeds cannot at this time approximate the speeds of traditional wired networks. Speed of a newer 802.11a is up to 54 Mbps at up to 68 ft. Newer models will increase both speed and distance. The wireless networks can be used to manage most of the currently available dental software. The wireless systems have built-in data encryption and password security.

Conclusion.—Wireless networks can help run a more efficient dental office without being costly or further complicating a technology driven practice.

▶ If your office contains 2 or more computers and associated peripherals that can be linked to share communications equipment such as printing and Internet access, then a network may be for you. With the advent of wireless networking, you can now enjoy the benefits of a network (ie, centralizing information storage and access to computerized software, services, and data) sans the wires and cables that can be problematic to install and work around. Wireless has become more mainstream, with several options to choose from and costs below $1000 for small offices where network distances would be less than 300 feet. Home users have taken advantage of the lower costs, setting up networks when there are several computers in the home and the flexibility of Internet connectivity from multiple locations is desired.

Other than cost, another barrier to wireless implementation has been security concerns. Earlier iterations of wireless were thought to be vulnerable to data interception and lacked the robustness of wired systems. Although the technology continues to improve, the appropriate steps must be taken to try to safeguard these networks from known security risks. *Network Magazine* has published several articles accessible from their web site on the status of wireless security. (http://www.networkmagazine.com; enter "wireless" in the site search field).

M. A. Robinson, DMD, MA

Virtual Records—Infallible?
Engar RC (Professional Insurance Exchange)
AGD Impact May:19, 2003   15–3

Background.—Many of today's dentists are seeking ways to achieve a paperless office, taking only digital radiographs and digital extraoral and intraoral photographs and keeping all patient records on the computer. But certain caveats apply. Dentists can protect themselves by following a few simple steps.

Data Storage.—The office must back up records at least twice a day and keep a copy of the files off-site. With respect to informed consent forms, electronic signatures are not yet mainstream and verifiable, so hard copy informed consent forms remain the best way to document the patient's acknowledgment of the risks involved with care. Test cases to determine the legal acceptability of virtual signatures have not yet arisen. To prove that the computer does not allow dated records to be altered, a date-marking system must be used that will stand up to the scrutiny of plaintiffs' attorneys, who may accuse dentists of making changes.

Digital Imaging.—Because of the potential for alteration, digital radiographs and digital photography can also be suspect. Any enhancement should be used judiciously.

Conclusion.—Record-keeping has been enhanced by computer technology and the role of imaging and its flexibility for applications in treatment greatly expanded. Accompanying pitfalls include how to prove that these digital records have not been altered and therefore represent legally acceptable proof in the court system. Backing up information, keeping separate file storage, obtaining written informed consent, using a date-marking system, and handling digital images judiciously will help protect dentists.

▶ Virtual records are, of course, not infallible. However, with each passing year, technological advancements and adherence to certain standards improve the reliability of digital record data. Important keys stressed in this article include backing up data, providing informed consent through digital signatures, and use of a computer log for auditing and tracking records.

To be completely paperless requires digital imaging. Concerns regarding alteration of digital images are being addressed through an imaging standard known as DICOM (Digital Images and Communications in Medicine) and the incorporation of tracking tools in the feature set of several of the software applications. Other standards that address the textual content of the record are also being considered. These standards are used extensively in medical electronic records to make them more reliable and portable. The same will one day be true for dentistry.

M. A. Robinson, DMD, MA

Computer-Aided Design/Computer-Aided Manufacturing (CAD/CAM)

CAD/CAM Ceramic Restorations in the Operatory and Laboratory
Fasbinder DJ (Univ of Michigan, Ann Arbor)
Compend Contin Educ Dent 24:595-604, 2003   15–4

Background.—Computer-assisted design/computer-assisted machining (CAD/CAM) technology has been used for more than 20 years to fabricate ceramic restorations and has evolved. The performance of current systems and their applications were outlined.

System Descriptions.—The dental operatory CEREC 3 system includes an acquisition unit, consisting of an intraoral camera and a computer, color liquid crystal display monitor, keyboard, and trackball, and the milling chamber, comprising 2 milling arms containing diamond instruments and a water reservoir. The acquisition unit records the cavity preparation digitally and designs the restoration; the milling chamber mills the final restoration according to the data obtained. The dental laboratory CEREC inLab system also has a milling chamber in which the cavity preparation is recorded from a die and the restoration is milled and a computer connected to the milling chamber that contains the CAD program used to design the restoration and direct the milling diamonds.

Analysis of Functions.—For the CEREC 3 system, the cavity preparation is similar to that for other bonded ceramic restorations, but the intraoral camera digitally records the cavity preparation, so no impression needs to be made. A virtual model of the cavity preparation is then available on the computer. Data used in creating the restoration come from the recorded cavity preparation and from a program-based anatomical dental database that proposes the restoration's design. Editing tools permit reproduction of the contours, anatomy, and contacts desired and can refine the occlusal relationships before milling. The full-contour restoration is created from a prefabricated block of ceramic or composite material, then tried in the cavity preparation; adjusted for fit, contour, and contacts; and either polished or glazed in a porcelain oven before cementing. When a conventional crown and bridge restoration is prepared with the CEREC inLab system, no model or wax-up of a crown is needed; a noncontact laser scanner records the cavity preparation from the die replica to the computer, where data are assembled into a graphic depiction. Recorded data and default settings are engaged to propose the design of the crown coping, and editing tools permit refinement. The computer processes the data and directs the milling diamonds to fabricate the coping. Restorative materials used with the CEREC 3 system include a highly homogeneous, fine-grained, feldspathic porcelain; a leucite-reinforced ceramic with a fine particle size; and a material with zirconia-silica filler particles 85% filled by weight with an average particle size of 0.6 mm. These materials are adhesively bonded to the cavity preparation with the use of a composite resin luting agent. Crowns can be conventionally cemented or adhesively bonded to the tooth. Fracture resistance depends on the material chosen. Advances have permitted a better marginal fit with the newer CAD/CAM devices than with their predecessors, but the material used also influences the marginal and internal fit of the milled crowns. A survey of 29 studies found that the survival rate of CEREC ceramic inlays was 97.4% over 4.2 years for restorations done between 1986 and 1997. In a 5-year study of the fine-grained feldspathic porcelain material, a 4.5% fracture incidence was found, and 84%, 97%, and 81% of the remaining inlays were rated excellent for color, surface, and anatomical form, respectively.

Conclusions.—Considerable flexibility in producing predictable all-ceramic restorations results with the use of CAD/CAM technology. The CEREC 3 system permits delivery of inlay, onlay, veneer, and full-coverage crown restorations in just 1 appointment without impressions or temporization. With the CEREC inLab system, single crowns and 3-unit fixed partial dentures with a reinforced ceramic core can be fabricated.

► CAD/CAM has sparked interest as an alternative to traditional restorative techniques. In the clinical setting, this method can provide an all-ceramic restoration in a single visit, with the use of an optical scan or "digital picture" of the preparation, a software program to assist in restoration design, and a milling unit that mills out the completed restoration in about 15 minutes. This restoration can then be fitted, adjusted, and polished for final cementation. A laboratory application with a modified procedure also exists.

The CEREC system for CAD/CAM restorations has been in use for more than 15 years. This article discusses the status of the current CEREC 3 and inLab systems. The 3-dimensional (3D) system now includes a 3D CAD program for designing the restoration, and a virtual model is generated from the optical scan of the prepared tooth. Anecdotally, several users have reported that the 3D modeling offers significant ease of use and control in the design process as compared with the previous CEREC 2 system. The technology is constantly undergoing improvements, and the 3D system represents the third iteration of the program with the added enhancements for 3D graphics.

Evidence is presented for the evaluation of CAD/CAM fracture resistance, fit, and restorative materials. There is a learning curve in producing these restorations, as the technique requires some changes from the standard restorative methods. For example, in place of the impression, the optical imaging process is an important step in the procedure because the computer will base its virtual model on this image. Training is also required to learn the various design techniques that allow the clinician to determine parameters for the restoration while taking into account the characteristics of the neighboring and occluding teeth. The evidence demonstrates that clinically acceptable and durable restorations with excellent color, surface, and anatomical form are possible with the use of this technology and that the newer version of the program performs better than the previous one. It should also be emphasized that proper technique is the key to successful restorations.

M. A. Robinson, DMD, MA

► Manufacturers are taking different approaches as they develop computer-assisted production processes. Some systems, such as the CEREC 3 described here, are designed for in-operatory fabrication of single-unit all-ceramic restorations, while others (Procera, Cerec In-Lab, Cercon) are aimed at digitizing 1 or more of the production steps for dental laboratories.

At this point, available laboratory CAD/CAM systems only produce single-component products, such as a ceramic inlay or zirconia frame, and cannot generate a multistratified—and hence more natural looking—restoration without the manual application of external layers by a dental technician. In its most popular laboratory application, CAD/CAM technology is currently complementing—and not replacing—the fabrication process by facilitating the production of all-ceramic and metal substructures for subsequent layering.

C. Moreno, CDT, MDT

Porcelain-Veneered Computer-Generated Partial Crowns

Denissen HW, El-Zohairy AA, van Waas MAJ, et al (Academic Ctr for Dentistry, Amsterdam)
Quintessence Int 33:723-730, 2002   15–5

Background.—Partial crowns preserve tissue and offer a conservative approach, as compared with a complete crown, which involves rebuilding a tooth with the use of core material. A partial crown can be fabricated from a uniformly colored, monolayered block of ceramic with the use of computer-aided design/computer-aided machining (CAD/CAM) technology, but the esthetics of natural teeth require a layered, lifelike ceramic. Grinding to produce such a restoration and designing the occlusion and articulation in the patient's mouth may achieve the esthetic result sought, but it is cumbersome. Ideally, a CAD/CAM system could be designed to fabricate a partial crown with a reduced occlusal table that can be layered with conventional porcelain veneer, thus obtaining a result that is esthetically acceptable, functional, and strong.

Methods.—Partial crown therapy was selected for 27 patients who had large defective resin composite or amalgam restorations in either maxillary or mandibular molars. In the partial crown preparation design, the occlusal surfaces were lowered 1.5 to 2.0 mm (Figs 3 and 4). Then a complete-arch hydrocolloid impression was obtained and poured in white stone; the master stone cast and stone cast were then mounted in an articulator. From this master stone cast, a partial hydrocolloid impression was obtained of the prepared molar and adjacent teeth, which was then poured in a brown reflective

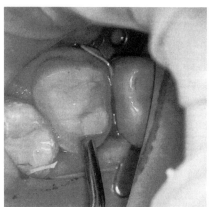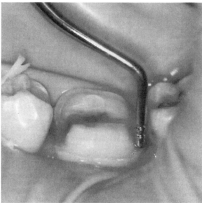

FIGURES 3 and 4.—Experimental preparation designs for CAD/CAM partial crowns on a maxillary first molar (**Fig 3**) and mandibular molar (**Fig 4**). The nonfunctional (buccal maxillary and lingual mandibular) cusps have broad occlusal shoulders of approximately 2.0 mm. The shoulder depth around the functional cusps (palatal aspect of the maxillary cusps and buccal aspect of the mandibular cusps) is 1.5 mm (indicated by the gauge on the maxillary molar). The proximal shoulders have a depth of 1.0 mm (indicated by the gauge on the mandibular molar). There are smooth transitions from the shoulder around the functional cusps to the shoulders in the proximal gingival margins. The proximal gingival shoulders continue smoothly into the occlusal shoulder on the nonfunctional cusps. (Courtesy of Denissen HW, El-Zohairy AA, van Waas MAJ, et al: Porcelain-veneered computer-generated partial crowns. *Quintessence Int* 33:723-730, 2002.)

stone. The porcelain on the adjacent teeth was color matched with the use of color guides; CAD/CAM partial crown samples were made of ProCAD Esthetic ceramic blocks or Vitapan 3D ceramic blocks. The block was then mounted in the spindle in the CAD/CAM system's milling chamber. The occlusal table thickness was determined on all sides with the use of calipers once the milling was completed. Next, the occlusal tables were veneered with porcelain, and occlusion and articulation contacts were determined. The porcelain-veneered partial crown was placed in acetone and treated ultrasonically for 5 minutes. Then its internal surface was cleaned with the use of phosphoric acid, rinsed, and dried before being placed in the patient's mouth. The prepared surface was covered with self-etching primer for 60 seconds, the Panavia F TC base paste and catalyst were mixed for 20 seconds, and the crown was seated within 40 seconds. A tapered fine diamond bur was used for final finishing of the margins of the partial crown.

Results.—Four Vitapan 3D partial crowns and 2 ProCAD partial crowns had a lowest occlusal thickness of 1.1 mm; 12 Vitapan and 14 ProCAD partial crowns had a lowest thickness of 1.2 mm; and 4 Vitapan and 2 ProCAD partial crowns had a lowest thickness of 1.3 mm. The porcelain veneer thickness at the thinnest occlusal CAD/CAM sites was 0.4 to 0.6 mm. The color samples provided proved useful in choosing appropriate ceramic blocks: specific hues, staining, and glazing gave a customized result. Over 1 to 4 years of follow-up observation, none of the partial crowns fractured.

Conclusions.—CAD/CAM technology was used to produce esthetically shaded partial crowns. Occlusal ceramic thickness was designed to prevent fractures, which it did, but should allow for porcelain veneering of the occlusal table. Optimal total occlusal thickness was between 1.5 and 2.0 mm for these partial crowns. All restorations demonstrated the feasibility of shoulder-type finishing lines wherein the gingival floor or occlusal surface meets the external and internal axial surfaces at a virtual right angle. In addition, oven glazing of these partial crowns produced significantly greater strength and higher resistance to loading than is achieved by surface polishing.

▶ CAD/CAM can be combined with conventional porcelain veneer techniques to create an optimally esthetic result as illustrated in this case study. The study focuses on 3 elements of partial crown restoration: tooth preparation, esthetics, and function.

- Tooth preparation: The case study suggests that the shoulder design is the "preparation of choice" for all ceramic CAD/CAM restorations in which a cylindrical bur is used for milling. It also recommends an occlusal table reduction of 1.4 mm above the preparation surface to allow for an adequate occlusal ceramic thickness of 1.5 to 2.0 mm.

- Esthetic color: To improve the uniform color of the restorative material blocks used in the CAD/CAM milling unit, the porcelain veneer technique included staining and glazing.

- Function: With appropriate tooth preparation, function was achieved through cusp–fossa relations designed into the porcelain veneering. Furthermore, improved strength was achieved with oven glazing.

The study demonstrates that conventional techniques and new technologies can work together to create a favorable outcome.

M. A. Robinson, DMD, MA

Digital Imaging Techniques

Influence of Displayed Image Size on Radiographic Detection of Approximal Caries

Haak R, Wicht MJ, Nowak G, et al (Univ of Cologne, Köln, Germany)
Dentomaxillofac Radiol 32:242-246, 2003   15–6

Background.—The detection of inaccessible approximal caries requires radiographs. Currently digital imaging systems are replacing conventional dental films, but it is important to know how to apply digital radiographic systems diagnostically. The degree of magnification of an image on-screen depends on various factors such as pixel dimension of the image, size of the monitor, and resolution setting of the display. Radiographs can only be magnified by the use of magnifying lenses, but zooming is a routine image processing tool used for digital radiography. The diagnostic advantages offered by zooming are not well documented. Detection of primary approximal caries was compared between radiographic images displayed on-screen at different sizes on a cathode ray tube (CRT) monitor and those displayed on a thin film transistor (TFT) monitor. It was anticipated that reduced image sizes would impair detection, that the TFT display would be better, and that dentinal lesions would be detected more accurately than all carious lesions.

Methods.—The extracted posterior teeth chosen for imaging had no restorations on the approximal aspect or any carious cavitations with a diameter exceeding 2 mm. The 160 teeth chosen comprised 20 pairs of upper and lower jaw quadrant blocks mounted with approximal tooth surfaces in contact. A polyether mask was used to simulate the gingival outline, and models were mounted in a modified jig. After the paralleling technique, the charge-coupled device full-size sensor was fixed at a focus–sensor distance of 30 cm. Radiographic images of approximal surfaces were reviewed by 5 university dentists (age range, 28-34 years) who routinely diagnosed with the use of digital radiographs for at least 2 years. A 6-point ordinal caries rating scale (ie, 0, no lesion; 1, the first half of enamel; 2, the second half of enamel; 3, the first quarter of dentine; 4, the second quarter of dentine; and 5, the inner half of dentine) was used to indicate the presence and penetration depth of lesions. The ratios were compared with the histologic extension of the lesions and were determined as the histologic presence of caries (validation threshold I) or dentine caries (II). In addition to sensitivity and specificity, observers' accuracy in detecting approximal caries was assessed with the use of nonparametric receiver operating characteristic analysis, with repeated measures analysis of variance to assess the type of display, the image size, and validation threshold.

Results.—The image size and validation threshold significantly affected detection rates, but the type of monitor display did not. When the image size ratio exceeded 1:1, there was pixelation with coarse-looking image details. Detection rates were not as good when the display of bitewing radiographs extended × 18 and × 30 that of conventional film. Only the pixel size increased above a 1:1 ratio, and visual data were dramatically reduced with ratios under 1:1. The image size of 1:7 had a lower detection rate because available radiographic data were not considered. Overall accuracy was significantly lower for the 1:7 ratio at both validation levels; no significant differences in accuracy were seen with 1:1 and 1:2 ratios. Slightly higher sensitivity and lower specificity were seen at threshold I, and reduced sensitivity was more notable at threshold I with the lowest image size.

Conclusions.—TFT and CRT monitors produced equally suitable images for detecting approximal caries; the TFT display's advantages in gray-scale perception in the middle of the gray-scale range did not optimize detection. Higher diagnostic validity was seen with image sizes in a display ratio of 1:1 and 1:2, which are, therefore, recommended.

▶ With the growing popularity of digital imaging in the treatment setting, considerations must be given to the diagnostic quality of images produced by these systems. Previous studies have compared conventional and digital radiographs.[1,2] Once the decision to go digital has been made, it is easy to be indecisive about the display options because visualization is so critical to disease detection.

This study used a charge-coupled device to capture digital radiographic images. This method is referred to as direct digital capture because the images from the sensor device are immediately displayed on the computer screen, as compared with indirect methods in which a "digital processing" step is required before the image becomes available for viewing. Once the image appears on-screen, several software tools are available to enhance the image by changing its size, contrast, brightness, and other features, thereby improving its diagnostic potential. The authors' hypotheses are based on popular knowledge that a liquid crystal display monitor provides a superior image display as compared with a CRT monitor and that enlarging the image will make it more diagnostic. Although there are several variables that affect the monitor's resolution and control screen quality, such as dot pitch and refresh rate, this study found that both the CRT and flat TFT monitors performed similarly for detection of approximal caries. Enlarging the image up to a certain point was found to assist caries detection, and optimal sizes were in the display ratios of 1:1 and 1:2.

Future studies may show the impact of other elements on image display. For now, it is important to use a suitable grade monitor and digital imaging software tool sets to obtain the best possible view of clinical images.

M. A. Robinson, DMD, MA

References

1. Syriopoulos K, Sanderink GC, Velders XL, et al: Radiographic detection of approximal caries: A comparison of dental films and digital imaging systems. *Dentomaxillofac Radiol* 29(5):312-318, 2000.
2. Berkhout WE, Sanderink GC, Van der Stelt PF: A comparison of digital and film radiography in Dutch dental practices assessed by questionnaire. *Dentomaxillofac Radiol* 31(2):93-99, 2000.

Comments on Noise and Resolution of the DenOptix Radiography System

Couture RA (Washington Univ, St Louis)
Oral Surg Oral Med Oral Pathol Oral Radiol Endod 95:746-751, 2003   15–7

Background.—The signal/noise (S/N) ratios of intraoral digital sensors have been reportedly relatively poor with the DenOptix Cephalographic Digital Imaging System (Gendex, Des Plaines, Ill), among others. Bony tissue images obtained are generally sharp, but gingival tissue images are poor. Because the S/N ratios obtained were inconsistent with those reported in recent articles, the S/N ratios were remeasured and more favorable results obtained. In addition, the likely cause of poor gingival tissue images was identified and a remedy suggested. Data for the DenOptix system were obtained with 2 different phosphor types and 2 pixel sizes, and measures were given for 3 x-ray sources and 2 scanner systems.

Methods.—An aluminum phantom was used to obtain S/N ratios, with noise determined by means of a step-wedge. A phosphor screen superimposed over a painted lead plate was used for in vitro radiographs. Radiograph scans were taken by means of a default photomultiplier tube setting of 650, yielding 8-bit rescaled data, and special software supplied by the manufacturer, giving 16-bit raw data using a pixel size of 84 µm (300 dots per inch).

True readings were obtained with the use of special software because the default software inverts and displaces the grayscale for both images. A second scanner system with default software and settings plus nine 16-bit raw data images of the same phantom was used for verification. The default intraoral screen type (30 × 40 mm [blue]), and the Fuji HR (white) were used. Data were compared with previously published findings.

Results.—The S/N ratios obtained were much higher than those reported for the DenOptix system and ranked among the best tested. S/N ratios of up to 13 at 2800 µGy and 17 at 5080 µGy were obtained by means of special software; default software yielded an S/N ratio of 15 at 3230 µGy. Digital clipping compromised the 8-bit images, which could not be used for S/N measurements. All pixel values in the hole and some background pixel values were clipped to 0 values, greatly reducing apparent contrast. Clipping occurs as a function of the distribution of brightness values in the complete image.

With a phantom covering only three fourths of the screen, clipping was absent and the same correct S/N ratios (13 at 2800 µGy) were obtained for 8-bit and 16-bit images. Several of the clinical 8-bit radiographs had clipping of part of the interproximal gingival tissue; usually clipping affects only soft tissue areas. Noise declines monotomically as exposure increases. Noise increased by about 25% with each decrease in pixel size.

Conclusion.—With the same screen type, comparable S/N ratios were obtained for the DenOptix and Digora (Soredex, Helsinki, Finland) systems. Those reported for the DenOptix were notably higher than previously measured. Detecting small-mass differences on a Rose-Burger phantom was judged subjectively superior with the DenOptix system and SR phosphor screens, except with low exposures. Good noise performance is required. The Digora system was inferior to the DenOptix system for resolution with either phosphor type using the 42-µm pixel size.

Better modulation transfer and subjective superiority in imaging small details (root canal spaces, root apices, and periodontal ligament spaces) were reported for the DenOptix system for both pixel sizes. The brightest and darkest 1% of the pixels in 8-bit images had digital clipping, which probably caused discrepancies between the S/N ratios here and in the literature; other causes were unlikely.

Clipping is not particularly noticeable on visual inspection but occurs often when the phantom covers the entire image area. Because the previously observed S/N ratios did not increase with exposure, a digital artifact may also be present. The 8-bit clipping algorithm was designed to handle clinical intraoral applications, so normal bony tissue images are unlikely to be clipped.

These findings indicate that the imaging of gingival tissues should not rely on 8-bit images, and gingival tissue imaging is likely to be worse with the more sensitive HR phosphor type, suggesting some images may be overexposed. The problem with clipping was not found in the 16-bit radiographs.

▶ Technically speaking, the S/N ratio is an important measure of the performance of a digital radiography system. Noise, or disturbances, are a component of all signal transmissions, including those present when exposing digital images. However, because noise negatively impacts radiographic interpretation by making it difficult to verify features of interest,[1] this parameter should be kept to minimum. Thus, digital radiography systems such as DenOptix or Digora (both photostimulable phosphors) will perform better if the S/N ratio is optimized such that the contribution of noise is lowered relative to the S/N combination.

In this study, the author investigates low S/N ratios associated with the DenOptix system and compares its performance to Digora. Higher S/N ratios are reported here as compared to previous studies, an effect that is explained by several causes of discrepancies, including digital clipping. DenOptix was also found to have higher resolution but higher noise as compared to Digora when the supplied receptors for each system were used.

M. A. Robinson, DMD, MA

Reference

    1. van Bemmel JH, Musen MA: *Handbook of Medical Informatics.* Heidelberg, Germany, Springer-Verlag, 1997, p 408.

Electronic Modeling

A New Technique for the Creation of a Computerized Composite Skull Model

Gateno J, Xia J, Teichgraeber JF, et al (Univ of Texas, Houston)
J Oral Maxillofac Surg 61:222-227, 2003   15–8

Introduction.—Computers are increasingly being used for surgical planning in orthognathic and craniofacial surgery. CT imaging is excellent for creating bone models, yet is not able to accurately represent the teeth. Despite this, current surgery planning still uses conventional dental model surgery to establish the occlusion and fabricate surgical splints. Plaster dental models remain the most accurate replicas of teeth. These models lack bony support. The limitation of conventional dental model surgery is that it is not possible to visualize the surrounding bony structures, which are essential in the treatment of complex craniofacial deformities. A computerized composite skull model using a combination of a 3-dimensional (3D) CT bone model with digital dental models was created and its accuracy was tested.

Methods.—A dry skull with intact dentition was used to develop a 4-step computerized technique as follows: (1) create digital dental models of the dry skull, (2) create a computerized 3-dimensional (3D) CT skull model from the dry skull, (3) incorporate the digital dental models into the 3D CT skull model, creating a computerized composite skull model, and (4) assess the accuracy of the computerized composite skull model. Fiducial markers were inserted into a radiolucent full-arch dental impression tray before dental impressions were made. The dental impressions with the 4 fiducial markers were scanned with a 3D laser surface scanner.

The dental impressions with fiducial markers were placed again into the maxillary and mandibular dental arch of the dry skull and underwent CT scanning. A 3D CT skull model with 4 fiducial markers was reconstructed by means of a divide-and-conquer technique, and the model was imported into custom computer software. The teeth of the CT skull model were removed. The fiducial markers remained in place. The digital dental models were incorporated into a 3D CT bone model (Fig 8). The accuracy of the composite skull model was evaluated by means of a digital Boley gauge by a single investigator on 3 different days.

Results.—No significant differences among the 3 measurements were observed, and they were thus averaged for each item. For the bone-to-bone measurements, the mean difference between the computerized composite skull model and the dry skull was 0.5 mm; it was 0.1 mm for the tooth-to-tooth measurements and 0.2 for the bone-to-tooth measurements.

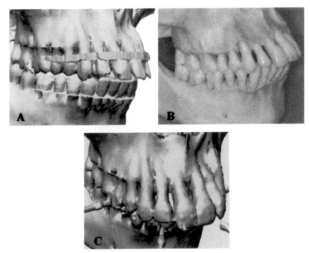

FIGURE 8.—The oblique views of the teeth from the computerized "composite skull model (**A**), dry skull (**B**), and 3-dimensional CT bone model directly reconstructed from CT scans (**C**). (Reprinted from Gateno J, Xia J, Teichgraeber JF, et al: A new technique for the creation of a computerized composite skull model. *J Oral Maxillofac Surg* 61:222-227, 2003. Copyright 2003, with permission from the American Association of Oral and Maxillofacial Surgeons.)

Conclusion.—The use of this computerized composite skull model could eliminate plaster dental model surgery. It may be that presurgical planning could be done entirely using the computer.

▶ CT is a very useful imaging modality that provides a 3D view of the skull but poor visualization of teeth. By using laser and optical scanning methods, digital dental models can be fabricated that are an excellent representation of teeth but fail to show its relationship to the skull. With technology, it turns out that these 2 methods can be combined to create a "super" CT scan that allows for visualization of both the skull and teeth.

Computerized surgical planning systems are an accepted modality of preplanning and are available for procedures such as implant placement and virtual osteotomies. However, the inability to combine the 3D skull image with a detailed view of the teeth often translates into additional planning steps with dental plaster models. While the techniques described here still require additional research, their accuracy in reproducing both bony skull structures and dentition shows promise for improving surgical planning and may have educational uses as well.

M. A. Robinson, DMD, MA

Accuracy of a System for Creating 3D Computer Models of Dental Arches
DeLong R, Heinzen M, Hodges JS, et al (Univ of Minnesota, Minneapolis)
J Dent Res 82:438-442, 2003   15–9

Background.—Diagnosis, treatment planning, and outcome assessment can all be facilitated by the use of 3-dimensional (3D) digital imaging once it is established that these images are accurately portraying the patient. A first step in determining image accuracy involves creating 3D computer models of simulated dental arches. The hardware and software tools of the Virtual Dental Patient (VDP) were evaluated for accuracy in this process.

Methods.—The 4 steps in creating 3D computer images of dental arches with the use of the VDP system were making tissue impressions, making stone casts from the impressions, scanning the casts, and processing the scan data. The standards against which the VDP system was measured were a "dental" steel standard and a quality stone cast of this standard, which mimics the traditional procedures in which the patient is the primary standard and the working cast the secondary one. The 11 impressions of the steel standard were fabricated in a 2-step process with the use of disposable impression trays, vinyl polysiloxane impression putty, and a scannable vinyl polysiloxane impression material. The stone cast having the fewest imperfections served as the stone standard, and the others were used to measure accuracy in the first 2 steps. The stone standard casts and impressions were scanned, then computer images were developed from the scan data once they had been filtered, aligned with individual views, and merged into a single data file. The computer model types created were mathematical (steel and stone mathematical models), stone standard (unprocessed and processed), impression, and cast. The average difference between the VDP measurement and the standard was considered to be the accuracy, and the SD of accuracy over repeated measures was considered to be the precision. Because the surface registration makes the average signed distance between the 2 surfaces equal to 0, absolute rather than signed distances between the computer and the mathematical models were used to determine accuracy.

Results.—The computer models and the standards differed to the same order of magnitude as the standards' intrinsic errors. The model creation process was found to be highly reproducible: processing SDs were less than 0.002 mm. The impression models' accuracy was 0.013 ± 0.003 mm, and the cast models' accuracy was 0.024 ± 0.002. The trends shown by center-to-center, offset, and point coordinate variables were the same as shown with the absolute distance variable. The accuracies of the 4 variables used were related through the law of propagation of errors, that is, the accuracy of the coordinates of a point on the surface of the model and the distance from that point to a known reference point depend on the accuracy of the computer model at that point.

Conclusions.—The accuracy of the cast computer models was close to the occlusal sensitivity of the average dental patient and equal to the thickness of commonly used contact marking films. That of the impression computer models was equivalent to the thickness of the shimstock used to identify contacts. Thus, computer models were accurate enough to be used clinically. However, the impressions were made without the biological factors and operator technique effects that influence impression quality in the clinical setting.

▶ As offices and clinics go paperless and increase the level of digital information available, technological advancements are making it possible for electronic counterparts to the dental arch model to become more usable. Electronic models have peaked interest because they alleviate the storage problems of traditional stone models and have the potential to provide information about the occlusion that can be used for diagnosis and treatment planning. Digitized information about the occlusion could also ultimately be analyzed with the use of computer algorithms, which would allow comparisons on a single patient or across a population of patients. Because accuracy is a prerequisite to the utility of these models, this article is timely in its measurement of image accuracy with 3D computer models.

A steel model, representing the patient, and a stone cast, representing the working cast, as "standards" were used in this study to demonstrate that 3D computer models can be produced that are acceptable for clinical use. The tools used to create and analyze the computer images from scanned data, including the scanning device and various software applications, are not all commercially available; however, a method for measuring accuracy is described. The result is that occlusal contacts can be indicated as accurately with the electronic models as in the traditional clinical setting. The authors note that the impressions used in the study were obtained under ideal conditions and that the clinical setting may introduce other variables, such as operator technique and tooth movement, that will have an unknown effect. Once accuracy is determined, 3D models can begin to become more mainstream.

M. A. Robinson, DMD, MA

Computer-Assisted Maxillofacial Prosthodontics: A New Treatment Protocol
Verdonck HWD, Poukens J, Overveld HV, et al (Univ Hosp Maastricht, The Netherlands; Rosmalen, The Netherlands)
Int J Prosthodont 16:326-328, 2003   15–10

Background.—The use of stereolithography (STL), which captures data for direct transfer to acrylic resin models of bony structures, has been a major step forward in prosthodontics. In addition, 3-dimensional (3-D) modeling of virtual medical models with haptic as well as visual feedback is also possible. A protocol combining existing techniques—such as CT, MRI, and surface scanning (photography or laser)—with software programs, termed CAMP, was used for a patient requiring prosthetic techniques.

Case Report.—Woman, 56, underwent surgical removal of a malignant tumor of the right eye. The defect was covered by skin but was judged to need an implant-retained silicone orbital prosthesis with magnet attachments. Data from the 3-D CT scan were converted into STL files and then imported and processed by Free Form Software, permitting real-time 3-D handling with the use of a haptic device. Virtual wax models of the eyeball and prosthesis were created by hand using mirror imaging from the contralateral side. The virtual wax models were then stored as separate STL files, and planning for implants was undertaken, moving data from the Free Form software and the original CT data into the Surgicase software.

The CT data allowed access to cross-sections at the various levels and in 3 directions, along with virtual 3-D head models on bone and skin levels. Bone availability and position of the virtual prosthesis were assessed to choose the best position for the 3 virtual implants, 2 in the superior and 1 in the inferior orbital rim. Rapid prototyping was used to translate virtual implants into an acrylic resin surgical stent with 3 metallic guiding cylinders for the pilot bur. The stent resembled a facial mask since its supporting surface was the skin. STL guides were applied manually, drilling was performed, and 3 Bonefit implants 6 mm long were placed.

Five months later, after osseointegration and placement of the abutment, implant positions were checked by CT scan, from which a new virtual 3-D facial model was made, reflecting anatomical changes after implant surgery. After converting CT data to an STL file and importing them into Free Form, virtual impression posts were placed to create space in the wax model for registration of the implant positions on the patient.

Adjustments to the previous virtual models of the prosthesis and eyeball were made to match the orbital defect and saved as STL files. Rapid prototyping was used to transfer the virtual wax models directly into real wax models, which were checked on the patient at the next office visit. The implant position was registered using impression magnet analogues; laboratory analogues were placed and plaster poured at the wax model's back side.

The eyeball model was converted to an acrylic resin model and placed in the prosthetic wax model. Magnets were placed and final fitting done, with traditional methods employed for finishing.

Conclusion.—The CAMP technique met expectations and provided good treatment for the patient. With further practice with other patients, it was possible to skip transferring the real wax model into silicone. The virtual wax model was translated directly into a transparent acrylic resin mold using rapid prototyping, and the intrinsic coloring was facilitated by the mold's transparency. In addition, a database of noses has been developed from CT and MRI data on file. Other modifications to be considered include using a photographic or laser surface scan rather than making a CT scan or MRI after placement of abutments.

▶ This case study describes a protocol for maxillofacial prosthodontics that combines several techniques to repair an orbital defect on a patient who has undergone surgical removal of a tumor of the right eye. Computer-based methods have several advantages for this case study, including reproducibility and the ability to draw from a database of facial features. The techniques employed are described below.

STL is a "rapid-prototyping" process that produces a physical, 3-D object or model from information captured by imaging. In this case, an acrylic resin model of the patient's bony structures is obtained from the imaging data. 3-D Modeling is made possible by use of a haptic arm and modeling software. Haptics are used typically in virtual reality systems to reproduce the sense of touch. This system provides both tactile and visual feedback for the operator.

The patient's soft and hard tissues of the skull are captured via the common techniques of CT, MRI, and/or surface scanning via photography or laser. Finally, the last technique involves presurgical planning software such as Simplant and Surgicase. These allow for surgical planning for implant placement preoperatively.

The above techniques were used to obtain a final prosthesis that was finished in the traditional manner. Although the authors do not explain in detail how this compares with the all-traditional methods, they state that the result met their expectations and that further work is needed.

M. A. Robinson, DMD, MA

Reliability and Validity of a Computer-Based Little Irregularity Index
Tran AM, Rugh JD, Chacon JA, et al (Univ of Texas, San Antonio)
Am J Orthod Dentofacial Orthop 123:349-351, 2003   15–11

Introduction.—Digital or dial calipers are typically used to measure dental casts in both research and clinical settings. A computer-assisted program for measurement with ImageJ software was examined and compared with a standard manual method (the Little irregularity index) to determine the reliability and validity of an alternative method for measuring mandibular incisor alignment.

Methods.—The mandibular casts of 30 patients with Class II malocclusion who were scheduled to undergo surgical mandibular advancement had measurements taken by a single examiner. Both the ImageJ and a digital caliper were used on 2 separate occasions 1 week apart. Test-retest reliabilities were estimated by means of the intraclass correlation coefficient. Validity was estimated by using correlating measurements obtained by both methods.

Results.—The mean index score for the digital caliper was 6.84 mm (range, 1.81-17.49 mm; standard deviation, 3.81). For ImageJ, the mean index score was 7.01 mm (range, 2.27-16.93 mm; standard deviation, 3.75). The intraexaminer test-retest reliabilities were 0.999 and 0.997 for the manual and computer-based methods, respectively.

Conclusion.—The ImageJ is a valid and reliable alternative technique for evaluating mandibular incisor alignment. The 2 methods described here may be used interchangeably. This is clinically and academically important since this is a convenient method that offers several benefits and advantages. Data from the ImageJ is portable and can easily be transferred to colleagues by e-mail or floppy or zip disk or posted on a Web page and made widely available. Measurements from ImageJ may be transferred directly to a database for documentation and manipulation. This would help decrease errors due to manual data transcription.

▶ Many of us use calculators, not always because of the difficulty of the mathematical equation but because the calculator is perceived as being faster, more accurate, and more reliable. Based on this principle, there is utility for computer-based methods in dental-related calculations such as tooth measurement. In orthodontics especially, measurements are made on a regular basis.

Although manual methods have been established that get the job done, this study demonstrates a computer-based method for measuring mandibular incisor alignment that equals the reliability of traditional techniques but has the added advantages of convenience, data portability, and improved data archiving and transfer. This method used the Little irregularity index, but the implication is that other measurement indices may also be amenable to digitization.

M. A. Robinson, DMD, MA

Educational Methodology

The Effectiveness of Computer-Aided, Self-Instructional Programs in Dental Education: A Systematic Review of the Literature
Rosenberg H, Grad HA, Matear DW (Univ of Toronto)
J Dent Educ 67:524-532, 2003   15–12

Background.—Among the methods of self-instruction available are computed-based self-instruction programs, which provide an accessible, interactive, and flexible means of learning. For health professions, the use of Computer-Aided Learning (CAL) has become popular as a way to share information between students, patients, and practitioners. The effectiveness of CAL in dental education, as compared with other methods of instruction, was evaluated.

Methods.—The published literature on CAL versus other learning methods was systematically reviewed. A total of 1042 articles were identified in broad terms. Of these, only 27 met the inclusion criteria of randomized controlled trials comparing CAL with any other method of instruction and using academically homogeneous samples of dental students or dental professionals plus objective outcome criteria. These criteria assessed performance, time spent, and attitudes. Twelve articles were finally identified, covering CAL in endodontics, orthodontics, oral anatomy, restorative dentistry, geriatric dentistry, and prosthodontics (Table 2).

TABLE 2.—Summary of Included Studies and Quantitative Results

Author/ Dental Field	Aim of Study	Participants	Study Groups (Randomly Allocated)	Outcomes Measured	Results
Bachman 1998/ Oral Anatomy Strength of Study: 7.5	To examine the difference in effectiveness between traditional instructional methods and computer-based instruction in teaching the anatomy of the permanent maxillary central incisors	85 first-year undergraduate dental students at the University of Minnesota, School of Dentistry	1. Group A (n=29) attended standard lecture only. 2. Group B (n=28) attended standard lecture and used computer program. 3. Group C (n=28) used computer program only. *No significant differences were found in pre-test scores among any of the three groups.	a. Performance on 20 multiple choice questions (MCQ) given pre- and post-intervention	a. No statistically significant differences among any of the three groups with respect to either pre-test or post-test scores (p-value not specified)
Clark 1997/ Orthodontics Strength of Study: 7.5	To compare the effectiveness of a Hypertext program versus conventional lectures to teach cephalometrics	52 first-year clinical undergraduate dental students	1. Computer group (n=26) 2. Lecture group (n=26) *No significant differences were found between the pre-test scores of the two groups.	a. Pre-intervention test (50 MCQ) b. Post-intervention test (150 MCQ including the 50 questions asked in the pre-test)	a. No significant difference between groups at start of study (p-value not specified) b. No significant difference between groups after tuition (p-value not specified)
Fouad 1997/ Endodontics Strength of Study: 8	To compare the effectiveness and efficiency of the computer simulation program with 1) a small-group problem-solving seminar and 2) no instruction to improve knowledge of endodontic diagnosis	101 third-year undergraduate dental students from 1995 to 1997 at the University of Connecticut, School of Dental Medicine	Assignment to each group based on pre-test scores in that the scores were sorted and students assigned to one of three groups in random order: 1. Simulation (n=34) 2. Seminar (n=32) 3. Control (n=24)	a. Effectiveness of program measured via a post-intervention test (20 MCQ) b. Efficiency measured by number of cases covered in unit time	a. The simulation group students improved significantly more from pre- to post-test than the seminar group (p=0.05) and the control group (p=0.0024). b. Students were able to cover more cases on average using the simulation program then were covered in the seminar (p=0.0001).
Hobson 1998/ Orthodontics Strength of Study: 7	To compare the effectiveness of CAL with traditional seminars to teach orthodontic diagnosis and the basic principles of treatment planning	59 fourth-year undergraduate dental students	1. CAL group (n=25) 2. Seminar group (n=24) *No significant differences were found between the pre-test scores of the two groups.	a. Performance on case-based written test	a. The seminar group had a greater improvement in test scores than the CAL group (p<0.0001).

(Continued)

TABLE 2. (cont.)

Author/ Dental Field	Aim of Study	Participants	Study Groups (Randomly Allocated)	Outcomes Measured	Results
Kay 2001/ Restorative Strength of Study: 8	To determine whether an educational intervention delivered by a computer-aided learning package improved the sensitivity and specificity of dentists' restorative treatment decisions	95 dentists	Using a Solomon three-group design: 1. Group 1 read radiographs pre- and post-CAL intervention. 2. Group 2 read the radiographs once, after the intervention. 3. Group 3 read the radiographs twice but received no intervention.	Dentists read 24 surfaces on each of 15 radiographs and made 360 decisions on how certain they were about restoring the tooth surface. Outcomes measured were: a. Sensitivity b. Specificity c. Area under ROC curves	There were no significant changes in sensitivity, specificity, or area under the curves caused by the intervention (p>0.05). There was no evidence that the level of agreement between dentists improved after the intervention.
Luffingham 1984/ Orthodontics Strength of Study: 7	To compare the effectiveness of a CAL program with traditional tutorial instruction in teaching orthodontic principles through case analysis	60 dental undergraduate students at the end of their first clinical year	1. Five groups (A) received tutorial instruction on Class III malocclusion and CAL on class II. 2. Five groups (B) received tutorial instruction on Class II malocclusion and CAL on class III.	a. Written test on the subjects covered	The CAL group scored significantly higher for both Class II instruction (p<0.02) and Class III instruction (p<0.01). *A comparison of the performance of groups A and B shows no significant difference between them.
Mullaney 1976/ Endodontics Strength of Study: 7	To compare CAL to instruction using a slide-tape presentation in teaching clinical endodontic problems	54 undergraduate dental students	Students were divided into nearly equal groups with high and low grade point standings and randomly assigned to: 1. Slide-tape group 2. CAL group	a. One-hour essay final examination consisting of ten problems in test selection or data gathering, diagnosis, and treatment planning of endodontic conditions	a. The CAL group of simulated clinical endodontic problems scored significantly higher in test selection (p=0.01) but not for diagnosis and treatment planning.
Mulligan 1993/ Geriatric Dentistry Strength of Study: 8	To compare the effectiveness of a computer-based program with a literature-based educational unit in teaching clinical decision making for the geriatric patient	20 third-year undergraduate dental students	Students were matched on grade point average and randomly assigned to: 1. Computer group 2. Literature-based group *No significant differences existed on outcome measures at pre-test (p>.05).	a. Clinical analogue (clinical roleplay) measuring seven outcome variables with a predetermined scoring system	a. Computer subjects outperformed the paper group on each of the seven measures; however, none reached statistical significance (.07<p<.61).

Study	Objective	Participants	Groups	Outcome Measure	Results
Plasschaert 1997/ Endodontics Strength of Study: 7	To compare the effectiveness of a CAL multimedia program with a more traditional approach consisting of written information, without interaction	28 fourth-year undergraduate dental students at the University of Kentucky	1. Multimedia group 2. Text-based group *No significant differences were found between the pre-test score of the two groups.	a. Performance on written post-test comprising the same two cases used in the pre-test	a. No significant differences were found between the post-test scores of the two groups (p>.05).
Puskas 1991/ Endodontics Strength of Study: 9	To compare the effectiveness of CAL with self-teaching booklets in teaching diagnostic testing	41 undergraduate dental students	Students were stratified according to their pre-test scores into quartiles and randomly assigned to: 1. Computer media group (n=21) 2. Self-teaching booklet group (n=20)	a. Performance on 30 MCQ	a. There were no statistically significant differences in post-test scores between the two groups (p=0.605).
Sandoval 1987/ Endodontics Strength of Study: 7	To compare the effectiveness of four different endodontic self-instructional review formats [slide-tape (ST), latent image (LI) simulation, computer-text (CTI) simulation, and computer-assisted video interactive (CAVI) simulation]	105 senior undergraduate dental students at the University of Texas, Dental School	1. Control (n=13) 2. Slide-tape (n=13) 3. ST-LI (n=13) 4. ST-CTI (n=13) 5. ST-CAVI (n=14) 6. LI (n=13) 7. CTI (13) 8. CAVI (n=13) *No significant differences were found between groups in each endo lab GAP, jr. year endo GPA, cumulative GPA, or pre-test scores.	a. Students' clinical endodontic performance measuring diagnostic and treatment error	a. Students in the study group made fewer diagnostic errors than those in the control group (p<.001), while the error reduction in clinical treatment was not significantly reduced between the two groups (p=.09). b. ST-CTI and ST-CAVI formats received the most favorable overall ratings by students.
Tira 1977/ Prosthodontics Strength of Study: 7	To compare the effectiveness of a CAL course with traditional classroom lectures in teaching the Applegate-Kennedy Classification system	93 undergraduate dental students	1. CAL group—randomly selected from volunteers 2. Lecture group—randomly selected from volunteers 3. Lecture group—randomly selected from nonvolunteers	a. Pre- and post-intervention written test	a. There were statistically significant differences in post-test scores between the CAL group and both group 2 (p<0.025) and group 3 (p<0.001).

Note: Included studies had to meet at least 7 of 9 criteria.
Abbreviation: CAL, Computer-aided learning.
(Courtesy of Rosenberg H, Gred HA, Matear DW: The effectiveness of computer-aided, self-instructional programs in dental education: A systematic review of the literature. *J Dent Educ* 67:524-532, 2003.)

Results.—Quantitative analysis showed significantly better scores with multiple choice tests, written tests, and clinical performance with CAL compared with other learning methods in 5 studies, similar outcomes in 6 studies, and worse outcomes with CAL than with seminar groups in 1 study. In comparison with seminar groups, groups studying with CAL were able to cover more cases on average and showed a significantly greater ability to diagnose and plan treatment between pretesting and posttesting. Qualitatively, 4 studies detailed positive responses of participants toward the CAL program, 5 showed no significant differences in participants' attitudes, and 2 did not evaluate participants' subjective experiences. Positive attributes cited for CAL included its innovative and interactive ways of presenting material, making it a useful adjunct to conventional teaching methods; its ability to motivate students by eliciting positive reactions; and its provision of multiple opportunities to review material.

Discussion.—CAL was shown to be positively received in about half of the studies and to offer no significant advantage in the other half. Its strengths include flexibility, interactive abilities, and accessibility.

▶ CAL has been popularized by the availability of computer hardware and software programs, the Internet, and an increasing number of trained professionals to create and implement such programming. In dentistry in particular, these systems serve as 1 method of self-instruction. Although CAL programs are available for several disciplines, access to certain subject areas in dentistry may be limited or require extensive searching. Anecdotally, a number of faculty state that they often do not know where to look for such programs for their specific courses. This systematic review examines the efficacy of CAL and makes recommendations for its use. Considering their guidelines, which recognize the positive effects of CAL, these programs should be more readily available to faculty as adjunct teaching tools. Increased use of these programs could also lead to the improved outcomes that the authors call for.

M. A. Robinson, DMD, MA

Evaluation of Educational Software
Schleyer TKL, Johnson LA (Univ of Pittsburgh, Pa; Univ of Michigan, Ann Arbor)
J Dent Educ 67:1221-1228, 2003   15–13

Background.—Applied to educational software, summative evaluation techniques can determine whether the expected outcomes or goals have been achieved. These techniques are used after a program has been implemented. The important issues operative in designing summative evaluation studies were outlined, along with barriers to and challenges for evaluation and an overview of the objectivist and subjectivist approaches to evaluation.

Challenges and Barriers.—Five major challenges faced in evaluating educational software were noted. First, the outcome must be defined and generally based on competencies in a clear, concise, precise, and unambiguous way. Second, educational outcomes must be measured. Methods include using standardized tests, oral examinations, assignments, direct observation, simulations, or competency examinations, among others. Difficulties in this area include independent measures that contradict one another and finding unexpected but significant outcomes only by chance.

Third, the effects of the delivery medium must be considered, with a distinction made between these and the effects of the educational method(s). This can prove difficult. Fourth, practical problems can arise with various study designs. For randomized experiments, the intervention is well understood and theories about causal effect can be formulated. Observational or exploratory studies may be more appropriate when new methods or media are first evaluated and may help in forming hypotheses to be assessed in more rigorous conditions. Among the problems are the study group's size, the options for stratification, contamination effects, confounding factors, and ethics questions.

Fifth, one must ask the correct research questions. Asking the wrong questions—such as whether computer-based instruction is "better" than traditional approaches—may lead one to choose an inadequate design providing inconclusive answers.

Approaches.—The objectivist approach to evaluation uses either comparison-based or objectives-based designs and focuses on how a resource meets designers' objectives. Its main concern is whether the resource is performing up to expectations rather than whether it outperforms what it replaced. Important factors in an objectivist approach are reliable and valid measures and measurement processes. If possible, the reliability and validity of measurements are checked in a measurement study so that readers can judge how confident they should be in the results.

In contrast, subjectivist designs fall into 4 categories: the quasi-legal, in which those for and against a program offer testimony and an independent jury makes a decision; art criticism, in which a single, experienced critic develops a formal evaluation that may be critiqued by other experts; professional review, wherein a panel of experts observes users as they work and identifies issues and immediately pursues answers; and responsive/illuminative, in which a program is evaluated from the end users' view, an approach especially useful in ethnographic or anthropologic studies.

The 2 types of skills evaluated in dental education are cognitive and psychomotor. They must be integrated to achieve excellent patient care. Examples of study designs using published educational software evaluations from dentistry and medicine include a combined subjectivist evaluation of a computer-based histology atlas, an objectivist comparison-based evaluation of computer-based simulations, and an objectivist comparison-based evaluation of a virtual reality–based simulator.

Conclusion.—Certain types of investigations are suggested that have the potential to promote better understanding of the use of and effects achieved with educational software in dental education. The various approaches were listed, challenges to achieving a good evaluation noted, and conceptual aspects outlined.

▶ In my comments on another article in this chapter (Abstract 15–12), I spoke briefly of locating computer-assisted learning (CAL) systems for use as adjunct self-instructional modules. That article described the efficacy of such systems, while the current publication examines evaluation methods for CAL.

Once a CAL intervention is implemented, its evaluation is challenging for several reasons discussed by the authors. The evaluation of computer-based systems can differ greatly in approach when compared with traditional evaluation methods. The discussion of basic concepts of evaluation as a topic demonstrates that many faculty may not be aware of established techniques for evaluating software.

The prior article focused on traditional clinical trials but recognized the need for other outcome measures. The techniques described here—including subjectivist evaluation and comparison-based objectivist evaluation—are all accepted means of conducting evaluations of the impact of information systems, including software and computer-assisted interventions. As the use of CAL increases, the need to adequately evaluate these systems becomes more significant. These methods are important for designers and creators of the systems as well as those who purchase and use them.

M. A. Robinson, DMD, MA

Teledentistry and Its Use in Dental Education
Chen J-W, Hobdell MH, Dunn K, et al (Univ of Texas, Houston)
J Am Dent Assoc 134:342-346, 2003   15–14

Introduction.—The Association of American Medical Colleges defines telemedicine as "the use of telecommunications technology to send data, graphics, audio, and video images between participants who are physically separate (ie, at a distance from one another) for the purpose of clinical care." This definition can also include oral health care and education. The Internet and broadband high-speed connections have greatly enhanced the abilities and uses of teledentistry. The Integrated Services Digital Network provides higher speed and information can travel in both directions simultaneously.

The next generation of teledentistry uses a combination of the World Wide Web for videoconferencing and the plain old telephone system. It does not necessitate a special network and is thus more cost effective. The Web-based network is of concern due to privacy and security factors. Teledentistry as it is used worldwide was discussed.

Uses of Teledentistry.—Formal online education is divided into 2 main categories: Web-based self-instruction and interactive video conferencing. A study of electronic mail–based oral medicine consultations revealed that face-to-face patient examinations are more accurate in determining a correct diagnosis for oral mucosal pathoses than is transmitted descriptive data alone. Interactive videoconferencing includes both a live interactive videoconference and supportive information.

An advantage of teledentistry is the ability to increase access to dental care, but users must be careful when providing consultation across state lines due to concerns about malpractice. The entire project may need to be discontinued if patient data are lost or stolen during transmission. For teledentistry courses, instructors need to have both teaching experience and computer knowledge.

Conclusion.—Teledentistry can be used to extend care to underserved patient populations at a reasonable cost. This technology provides an opportunity to supplement traditional teaching methods in dental education and will provide new opportunities for both dental students and dentists.

▶ While many practitioners have just become accustomed to e-mail, teledentistry opens the door to a new telecommunications technology for dental health care exchanges. Arising from its medical sister, telemedicine, this technology now provides a means for dental team members to interact with patients or other team members at a distant location for clinical care and education. This article focuses on the educational setting, the place that could help in the expansion of the use of teledentistry through instruction and continued research.

Communication for teledentistry requires high speed connections to the Internet that can be utilized for Web-based training or interactive videoconferencing. One of the barriers for institutions and those they connect to is cost for the installation and monthly fees for these lines. If these can be overcome (and several schools have already done so), teledentistry can provide an excellent method for connecting to rural populations, conducting screenings out in the field, providing learning experiences for distant learners, or providing assistance to understaffed satellite clinics. This technology has great potential once legal issues are understood, conformance to standards continues, and instructors who are skilled in distance learning can create course work and teach others.

M. A. Robinson, DMD, MA

16 Maxillofacial Imaging

The Accuracy of Dental Panoramic Tomographs in Determining the Root Morphology of Mandibular Third Molar Teeth Before Surgery
Bell GW, Rodgers JM, Grime RJ, et al (Cumberland Infirmary, Carlisle, UK; Newcastle Gen Hosp, Newcastle Upon Tyne, UK; Sunderland District Gen Hosp, UK; et al)
Oral Surg Oral Med Oral Pathol Oral Radiol Endod 95:119-125, 2003   16–1

Background.—The dental panoramic tomograph (DPT) is frequently used to obtain radiographic evaluation of the potential difficulty in removing a mandibular third molar tooth and the risk for injury to the inferior alveolar neurovascular bundle. The increased risk of injury to this region has been well established, and the preoperative radiographic assessment with the DPT allows the surgeon to advise the patient of the risks and possibly modify the surgical technique appropriately to lessen the risk of nerve injury. The accuracy of DPT was evaluated in the presurgical assessment of mandibular third molar teeth by correlation of the radiologic interpretation with surgical findings.

Methods.—The DPTs of 300 mandibular third molar teeth were evaluated by 9 staff oral surgeons for root morphology and proximity to the inferior alveolar neurovascular bundle. Detailed records were made at the time of surgery, and findings at surgery were compared with the preoperative assessment. Sensitivity and specificity values were calculated in relation to diagnostic accuracy for mesial and distal root curvatures and relation to the neurovascular bundle.

Results.—The sensitivity and specificity for observation of root curvatures ($\pm 15\%$) were 29% and 94%, respectively (Table 2). The sensitivity and specificity of determining an intimate relation between the root and the neu-

TABLE 2.—Reasons for Incorrectly Observing Root Curvatures

Failure to Observe Curvature	Predicting a Curve When None Present	Undermeasurement of Curvature (>15°)	Overmeasurement of Curvature (>15°)	Curve Identified but in Wrong Direction
739 (64%)	101 (9%)	189 (16%)	38 (3%)	88 (8%)

TABLE 3.—Correct and Incorrect Observations of 253 Individual Root Curvatures in Relation to Direction

	Mesial	Distal	Buccal	Lingual
Correct	42 (3%)	294 (24%)	28 (2%)	3 (0.2%)
Incorrect	168 (13%)	441 (34.8%)	252 (20%)	37 (3%)

(Reprinted by permission of the publisher from Bell GW, Rodgers JM, Grime RJ, et al: The accuracy of dental panoramic tomographs in determining the root morphology of mandibular third molar teeth before surgery. *Oral Surg Oral Med Oral Pathol Oral Radiol Endod* 95:119-125, 2003. Copyright 2003 by Elsevier.)

rovascular bundle were 66% and 74%, respectively (Table 3). Kappa analysis showed poor levels of agreement between radiologic interpretation and surgical findings when the number of roots was determined and when the roots were fused or separate.

Conclusions.—The use of DPTs for the assessment of mandibular third molar teeth before surgery does not provide adequate diagnostic accuracy in terms of anatomic form and structures.

▶ The authors have chosen a very practical topic to study and present. As panoramic units have populated the developed world they are increasingly being relied on for presurgical assessment of third molars. The gold standard for any imaging study is the "anatomic truth": that is, to display the anatomy as it exists in vivo. When an imaging technique alters the perception of the anatomic truth, then it may pose a clinical liability. This article provided a good description of the geometry associated with image formation. The authors stated that the line pair resolution decreased when the imaged objects were not centrally placed within the focal trough. In addition, I have found that the panoramic image created of objects moved buccal or lingual to the center of the focal trough changes the perception of object size, form, and position. Therefore, it could be very easy to misrepresent the spatial relationships between the mandibular canal and the adjacent third molar if these 2 anatomic structures occupy different buccolingual positions within the panoramic focal trough. The authors also noted that surgeons have managed quite well despite the limitations associated with panoramic projections. Emerging technology, including cone beam CT and standard tomography, may prove to be a valuable adjunct to panoramic techniques.

D. C. Hatcher, DDS, MSc

Landmark Identification on Direct Digital Versus Film-Based Cephalometric Radiographs: A Human Skull Study
Schulze RKW, Gloede MB, Doll GM (Johannes Gutenberg-Univ Mainz, Germany; Ludwig Maximilians-Univ, Munich)
Am J Orthod Dentofacial Orthop 122:635-642, 2002   16–2

Background.—Digital systems are increasingly replacing conventional film-based radiographic machines. Among the advantages of these digital systems over conventional radiographic equipment are instantaneously available image information, less radiation burden for the patient, lack of chemical development processes, simplified storage of images, and the ability to manipulate the image a posteriori for size or contrast. However, despite these advantages, the diagnostic performance of the new digital systems must be evaluated in comparison with that of the established film-screen combination. Differences in landmark identification on vertically scanned, direct digital, and conventional (18 × 25 cm) cephalometric radiographs were determined.

Methods.—Six landmarks were recorded twice on 3 digital and 3 conventional cephalograms obtained from 3 human skulls in a standardized fashion by 8 observers, all of whom were either orthodontists or postgraduate orthodontic students. The digital images were displayed on a 15.1-inch TFT monitor in 3:1 mode (20 × 26 cm). Recordings were transferred into standardized coordinate systems and evaluated separately for each coordinate. After correction for magnification, precision of the images was evaluated with Maloney-Rastogi tests, and intraobserver and interobserver reproducibility was calculated from squared differences.

Results.—The digital images had larger effective magnification. Significantly different precision was found between the 2 imaging modalities for nasion, posterior nasal spine, sella, supraspinate, and orbitale, but the average differences were entirely less than 1 mm. There were no significant differences in interobserver and intraobserver reproducibility between the 2 modalities. In both digital and film-based images the squared differences were largest for the posterior nasal spine and orbitale.

Conclusions.—The indication of these findings is that the digital imaging system and the film-based radiographic equipment evaluated in this study produced comparable errors in landmark recording. However, these results should be evaluated in the context of the specific display conditions for digital images because there is no general standard at this time.

▶ When I read the title and purpose of this article, I wondered if there could be any clinical value to the results. I initially assumed that the image formed by direct digital technique would be identical to the film-based technique because the beam geometry should be the same. As I read and understood the considerable differences in beam geometry between the 2 methods, I was ultimately surprised there was not a greater resulting difference between the 2 methods under study. This article provides a very intelligent discussion of the many factors related to the formation and display of the direction digital cephalometric image. The study fulfilled its mission but it left me wanting more information about the Sirona Orthophos DS Ceph.

Film-based cephalometric techniques use beam geometry collimated to a "pyramid" shape. The x (horizontal) and y (vertical) direction divergence angles are equal for the x-ray photons as they leave the focal spot, creating a simple projective geometry solution for determining magnification of objects differentially located in the z (transverse) direction. The Sirona Orthophos DS uses a beam collimated to a horizontal fan shape. That is, the beam diverges in the x (horizontal) direction and does not diverge in the y (vertical) direction. The y direction anatomic field of view is created by "scanning" the anatomy, thus sequentially imaging the skull by moving the fan shape x-ray beam and detectors in a vertical direction. The raw image data produced with this technique would have horizontal magnification similar to the film-based imaging but no vertical magnification. To get the results the authors of this article achieved, the software associated with the Sirona Orthophos DS must be applying a vertical (y) magnification correction factor. The vertical (y) correction factor would likely be computed to simulate the horizontal (x) magnification at transverse (z) distance midway between the ear rods. An image (correction factor applied) would have an x and y direction aspect ratio similar to film-based imaging for all points residing in a plane perpendicular to the constructed central ray (parallel to film plane) midway between the ear rods, but the aspect ratio would change for points residing in plane on either side of the midway plane. Theoretically, if a circular-shaped ring were placed midway on a rod suspended between the 2 ear rods, the resultant image of the ring would be circular. If this ring was moved on the rod to the ear rod closest to the film, the resultant image would create an oval-shaped ring with the longest axis of the oval being in a vertical (y) direction. Conversely, if the ring was moved to the ear rod furthest away from the film, then the resultant image of the ring would have an oval shape with the longest axis of the oval occurring in a horizontal (x) direction. Considering this theoretical experiment of moving the test object (ring) in a transverse direction (z), the resultant image would have a constant vertical (y) size equal to the raw data image size multiplied by the correction factor and horizontal (x) size variation directly proportional to the distance of the object from the film.

It is important to note when considering the results of this article that all the anatomic landmarks except orbitale were located on the plane midway between the ear rods; therefore, the potential differences between the 2 imaging methods may not have been fully revealed. Conventional film and direct digital resultant image comparison by imaging a gold standard object containing a swarm of surveyed points distributed throughout a volume equivalent to the size of a human head would be a good follow-on study to the present one.

I agree with the authors that direct digital imaging has the potential to reduce the operational costs and radiation and environmental burdens. However, the adoption of digital imaging introduces new issues to be considered. These new issues include the broad topic of workflow. With the film method the image might be stored in the patient chart and could be transported to any desired location for review; all that is needed is an illumination source. Digital images, however, are locked in the computer and computer program that acquired them. To view them elsewhere requires a computer/monitor to be located at each additional location. The images can be transferred to the additional work stations on storage media or by a network. In a dental office setting a network is preferred because the images can be stored on a central server and then distributed as needed. In the network scenario the archived images can be made available to other software programs and backed up with along with other data. A network also allows sharing of other resources, such as printing and the Internet.

D. C. Hatcher, DDS, MSc

Three-Dimensional Quantitation of Periradicular Bone Destruction by Micro-Computed Tomography

von Stechow D, Balto K, Stashenko P, et al (Harvard Med School, Boston)
J Endodont 29:252-256, 2003   16–3

Background.—The ability to monitor biologic changes in disease processes over time had become increasingly important in many areas of medicine, including dentistry, where inflammatory, osteolytic, and neoplastic processes can occur without detectable changes in the applied imaging methods. The detection of anatomic details can be challenging even after extraction of teeth, and precise anatomic analyses of teeth are only possible after the destruction of the specimen. It has been shown in previous studies that 2-dimensional, high-resolution, microcomputed tomography (micro-CT) is a rapid, reproducible, and noninvasive method for the measurement of periradicular bone resorption in mice and provides results virtually identical to histology. Whether a 3-dimensional (3D) volumetric quantitation of bone resorption could be obtained and whether this 3D quantitation would correlate with 2-dimensional (2D) measurements in a mouse model were determined.

Methods.—Periradicular lesions were induced in the lower first molars of mice by pulp exposure and infection, with unexposed teeth serving as controls. The mandibles were harvested on day 21 and subjected to 3D micro-CT imaging and conventional histology. A 3D model and semiautomatic contouring algorithm were used to determine 3D void volume, void surface, void thickness, and standard deviation of the thickness distribution.

Results.—A significant correlation was observed between lesion void volume and 2D lesion area by histology, and high correlations were observed between void volume and void thickness and standard deviation of the void thickness (Table 1). However, no relation with void surface was observed (Table 2)

Conclusions.—It would appear from these findings that 3D analysis of micro-CT images is highly correlated with 2D cross-sectional measurements of periradicular lesions. However, 3D micro-CT is useful in the assessment of additional microstructural features and subregional analysis of lesion development.

TABLE 1.—2-D Area Measurements Obtained by Histology and Micro-CT

Group	Histology	Micro-CT	Difference	P Value
Control ($n = 4$)	0.08 ± 0.02	0.08 ± 0.02	0.00 ± 0.02	0.63
Experimental ($n = 10$)	0.21 ± 0.08	0.22 ± 0.09	0.01 ± 0.08	0.15
Difference	0.13 ± 0.05	0.14 ± 0.06		
p value	<0.01*	<0.01*	<0.01*	

Note: Data are means ± SD. The 2-sample *t* test was used to evaluate differences between the control and experimental groups. Paired *t* tests were used to assess differences between histology and micro-CT measurements within each group.
*Statistically significant.
(Courtesy of von Stechow D, Balto K, Stashenko P, et al: Three-dimensional quantitation of periradicular bone destruction by microcomputed tomography. *J Endodont* 29:252-256, 2003.)

TABLE 2.—Group Differences for 2-D and 3-D Microtomographic Indexes

Index	Control	Experimental	Difference	P Value
2-D Area (mm2)	0.08 ± 0.2	0.22 ± 0.09	158%	<0.01*
3-D W (mm3)	0.13 ± 0.01	0.17 ± 0.04	28%	<0.01*
3-D VS (mm2)	5 ± 0.5	5.5 ± 0.6	10%	<0.05*
3-D VS/W (1/mm)	37.3 ± 4.6	33.4 ± 8	−11%	NS
3-D V.Th (mm)	0.07 ± 0.01	0.09 ± 0.02	26%	<0.01*
3-D V.Th.SD (mm)	0.01 ± 0.001	0.03 ± 0.02	118%	<0.01*

Note: Data are means ± SD. The 2-sample student *t* test was used to evaluate differences between the control and experimental groups.
*Statistically significant.
Abbreviation: NS, Not significant.
(Courtesy of von Stechow D, Balto K, Stashenko P, et al: Three-dimensional quantitation of periradicular bone destruction by microcomputed tomography. *J Endodont* 29:252-256, 2003.)

▶ Wow, I was very impressed with the quality of research presented in this study. The application of CT has not been widely used in the clinical dental practice because the image resolution (diagnostic value), study cost, and radiation dose have not been in line with expectations. The micro-CT unit presented in this article produces a volumetric image with a very small isotropic voxel of 17 μm in size and was able to demonstrate that volumetric imaging can accurately reveal normal and abnormal anatomy associated with periradicular and periapical tissues. I could envision many clinical applications using micro-CT if the study cost and radiation dose were acceptable. Emerging technology associated with multi-row detector spiral CT (fan beam) now has the ability to produce isotropic voxels of 600 μm dimension. Volumetric or cone beam CT optimized for the maxillofacial region has recently been introduced into the marketplace. The current generation of cone beam units will be able to produce an isotropic voxel as small as 100 or 125 μm. Cone beam CT can produce a study with a radiation exposure less than those produced with a fan beam CT and most likely at a cost more in line with usual dental investigations. Because of the emergence of cone beam CT for dentistry, 2D and 3D quantification studies are extremely important for validation.

D. C. Hatcher, DDS, MSc

Clinical Application of Spiral Tomography in Anterior Implant Placement: Case Report

Dixon DR, Morgan R, Hollender LG, et al (Univ of Washington, Seattle)
J Periodontol 73:1202-1209, 2002   16–4

Background.—Anatomic variations present one of the greatest challenges to a clinician in planning endosseous dental implant in edentulous areas of the anterior maxilla. Positioning of the implant is crucial in patients in whom high esthetic results are demanded but who have minimal ridge width or require augmentation. Recent advances in spiral tomography have facilitated more precise planning and placement of endosseous implants in these challenging areas. A series of clinical cases in which spiral tomography was used in the planning and placement of endosseous dental implants was presented.

Methods.—The cases of 2 patients are described. In both patients, initial spiral tomographic radiographs were used for implant planning and fabrication of the surgical guide. Postinsertion tomography was used to evaluate the results of implant position and inclination. The first patient was a 32-year-old student who presented for replacement of tooth 9. Past dental history included routine operative dentistry and orthodontic and surgical correction of a severe Angle's class III malocclusion. The patient was found to have apparently ideal dimensions for a single implant-supported prosthesis. The second patient was a 35-year-old man who presented for evaluation of tooth 7. Past dental history included a bicycle accident and trauma to teeth 7 and 8. An implant-supported prosthesis was planned for the area of tooth 7 in light of limited attachment over the facial aspect of tooth 7 with suppuration noted on the distal facial aspect and corresponding bone loss.

Results.—Preimplant spiral tomograms indicated that the initial prosthetic trajectory through the proposed incisal edge of each tooth replacement would result in a final osteotomy site, which would compromise the overall thickness of the facial cortical plate. After adjustment for magnification and distortion factors, new prosthetic/surgical trajectories were fabricated into the surgical guide, and these data were used in preparation of the final implant osteotomy site. The result of this adjustment was 2 mm of residual crestal facial bone postimplant insertion, which became wider at more apical measurements. These findings were verified on the postimplant serial tomograms.

Conclusions.—These cases were demonstrative of the use of spiral tomography in the treatment planning phases of endosseous dental implant placement, particularly in cases in which patients have minimal crestal width and high esthetic demands or in whom exact implant placement is critical for a successful outcome.

▶ The strategy associated with presurgical imaging of single tooth implant sites was very well presented. The imaging goals were perfectly presented in context of the prosthetic and anatomic considerations. The use of a radiographic template allowed for optimized planning of the implant trajectory and transfer of the radiographic plan to the mouth. I strongly advocate cross-sectional imaging, including tomography, for presurgical implant planning. I agree with the authors that complex motion tomography is better than linear tomography. The most difficult anatomic areas to image using tomography are the anterior regions of the maxilla and sometimes mandible, and this is associated with the curved arch form. To achieve the best tomographic results the tomographic plane needs to project through the jaw perpendicular to the tangent along the jaw curve.

D. C. Hatcher, DDS, MSc

The Use of Lipiodol in Spiral Tomography for Dental Implant Imaging

Siu ASC, Li TKL, Chu FCS, et al (Univ of Hong Kong)
Implant Dent 12:35-40, 2003   16–5

Background.—The treatment planning and successful placement of dental implants depends on preoperative radiographic assessment. For all but the most straightforward cases, tomographic examination with diagnostic radiographic templates is required. To date, the use of various radiopaque materials, such as barium sulfate and lead foil, has not provided satisfactory results. This study reports on the use of a new contrast medium, Lipiodol ethiodized oil, which can be mixed easily with the monomer of autopolymerizing acrylic resin. The resulting tomographic images are radiographically homogenous and demonstrate the contour of the future prosthesis, the angulation of the planned implant, and the thickness of the soft tissue.

Case Report.—Man, 20, presented with a request for replacement of his missing maxillary left canine that was extracted 2 years earlier because of a crown-root fracture. The edentulous ridge was observed to have mild resorption with adequate buccolingual bone width and interocclusal space. The mesodistal width was 9 mm, and the patient had a class I incisal relation and group function in lateral excursions. Full-arch impressions were made, and the Lipiodol template was fabricated as described for spiral tomography. The template was tried in the patient's mouth for an accurate fit. Tomograms were obtained and analyzed. The radiographic template was modified to become a surgical template by altering the position and angulation of the access hole. This surgical template carried the information regarding the proper implant position and angulation with regard to bone topography and planned prosthesis, and provided a precise guide for the guide drill and the first twist drill for the implant fixture. The planned implant was installed. After 6 months of healing, the surgical template was used for the second-stage surgery to locate the fixture position with ease. A working impression was taken at fixture level, and an abutment and crown were subsequently placed.

Conclusions.—There are several advantages to the use of Lipiodol as a radiographic contrast medium. It is chemically compatible with acrylic resin, and the resulting acrylic template is optically transparent, which facilitates good visibility. This transparent template can be further modified to registration of implant position at the time of surgery. This multipurpose template is inexpensive and simple to construct and is recommended for routine use in implant dentistry.

▶ This article advocated the value of radiographic template and introduced the use of an iodinated contrast, Lipiodol, as an opacifying agent to be mixed with acrylic resin during template fabrication. I agree with the rationale proposed for the use of the radiographic template and the manner in which it was used in the article.

D. C. Hatcher, DDS, MSc

Panoramic Radiographs: A Tool for Investigating Skeletal Pattern
Akcam MO, Altiok T, Ozdiler E (Ankara Univ, Turkey)
Am J Orthod Dentofacial Orthop 123:175-181, 2003   16–6

Background.—Panoramic radiography is an indispensable orthodontic screening tool and provides important information about the teeth, their axial inclinations, maturation periods, and surrounding tissues. Facial and mandibular asymmetries are of special interest in orthodontia. Previous studies regarding the intercondylar asymmetries of the temporomandibular joint and the interrelation of the mandibular condyle and its surrounding structures, as visualized on panoramic radiographs, indicate that a more definitive image is needed for evaluation of the temporomandibular joint. The possibility of enhancing the clinical versatility of the panoramic radiograph for evaluation of craniofacial characteristics was investigated.

Methods.—Lateral cephalometric and panoramic radiographs were obtained from 30 skeletal class II, dental class II division I patients, including 16 girls with a mean age of 11.7 ± 1.7 years and 14 boys with a mean age of 12.2 ± 0.9 years. All the subjects were in the "S" period of growth. Panoramic radiographs were obtained under standard conditions by a cephalostat with

TABLE 1.—Student *t* Test for Panoramic Radiograph and Cephalometric Measurements in Male (*n* = 14) and Female (*n* = 16) Subjects

Parameers	P	Test
FH/ANS (mean, R + L)	.79	NS
OMAND (mean, R + L)	.96	NS
FH/UOP (mean, R + L)	.49	NS
FH/LOP (mean, R + L)	.37	NS
UOCCL	.84	NS
LOCCL	.48	NS
OCOND (mean, R + L)	1.00	NS
OMID (mean, R + L)	.19	NS
ANB	.61	NS
SNA	.45	NS
SNB	.59	NS
S-N/N-ANS	.18	NS
Co-Go/Go-Me.	.90	NS
ANS-PNS/Go-Me	.87	NS
FH-U1	.11	NS
FH/ANS-PNS	.78	NS
Gonial angle	.38	NS
Go-Gn/S-N	.35	NS
FH/U6-U1	.54	NS
FH/L6-L1	.76	NS

Abbreviations: R, Right; *L*, left; *NS*, not significant.
(Reprinted by permission of the publisher from Akcam MK, Altiok T, Ozdiler E: Panoramic radiographs: A tool for investigating skeletal pattern. *Am J Orthod Dentofacial Orthop* 123:175-181, 2003. Copyright 2003 by Elsevier.)

the clinical Frankfort horizontal plane and midfacial planes corrected. A correlation test was performed between the parametric measurements, and the predictability level of the cephalometric measurements from the panoramic radiographs was determined by regression equations.

Results.—The equations indicated that the Go–Gn/S–N, ANS–PNS/Go–Me (palatal plane/mandibular plane), and Co–Go/Go–Me parameters could be predicted from panoramic radiographs within statistically significant levels. Their predictability levels were 20.6%, 15.6%, and 11.2%, respectively (Table 1). Statistically significant correlations and predictability levels were also determined for the cephalometric and corresponding panoramic parameters in which the Frankfort horizontal plane was used.

Conclusions.—It would appear from these findings that, although panoramic radiographs provide information regarding the vertical dimensions of craniofacial structures, they have low predictability percentages. Thus, clinicians should be extremely cautious when predicting skeletal cephalometric parameters from panoramic radiographs.

▶ It did not surprise me that a panoramic-based morphometric assessment of the craniofacial skeleton did not match those produced by a standard lateral cephalometric projection. A lateral cephalometric projection uses fairly rigid projection geometry protocols, whereas the same cannot be claimed for panoramic projections. The panoramic focal cannot be made to predictably match the patient's anatomy in such a way that the projection geometry is standardized. A mismatch between the panoramic focal trough and the patient's anatomy can result in an image showing a change in size, location, and shape of the imaged anatomy. The panoramic projection does allow for visualization of the right and left halves of the jaws separately, something a cephalometric projection cannot do.

D. C. Hatcher, DDS, MSc

A Comparison of a New Limited Cone Beam Computed Tomography Machine for Dental Use With a Multidetector Row Helical CT Machine

Hashimoto K, Arai Y, Iwai K, et al (Nihon Univ, Tokyo; Matsumoto Dental College, Nagano, Japan)
Oral Surg Oral Med Oral Pathol Oral Radiol Endod 95:371-377, 2003   16–7

Background.—The 3DX Multi Image Micro CT is a limited cone beam CT unit designed to be practical for use in dental settings. This device provides high-quality 3-dimensional images of the hard tissues of the maxillofacial, ear, and nose areas. The 3DX was compared with a multidetector row helical CT unit in terms of image quality and skin dose.

The 3DX Unit.—The 3DX machine uses a cone beam with a radiation field only 29 mm high and 38 mm wide at the center of rotation. Tube voltage is 80 kV, tube current 20 mA, and exposure time 17 seconds. The subject is seated in the center of the apparatus, which rotates to obtain data from 360°. Data are quantitated and reconstructed on a computer, which displays images parallel and perpendicular to the dental arch and perpendicular to the body axis.

Methods.—The 3DX and the Multidetector CT were used to obtain images of the right maxillary central incisor and the left mandibular first molar of an anthropometric phantom. Image quality in depicting various structures was compared by 2 experienced dental radiologists. Skin doses to the maxillofacial region were also compared for the 2 imaging units.

Findings.—For each of the structures assessed, image quality was rated significantly better for the 3DX than for the Multidetector CT. The mean skin dose per examination was just 1.19 mSv for the 3DX, compared with 458 mSv for the Multidetector CT.

Discussion.—The 3DX unit provides superior imaging of dental structures, compared with the latest CT multidetector. This improvement in imaging quality is obtained at a fraction of the radiation dose associated with the Multidetector CT.

▶ The results of this study are encouraging for dentistry and maxillofacial imaging. The ability to acquire a high-resolution CT scan of the teeth with a relatively low-dose technique is revolutionary. I can imagine the 3DX machine and other high-resolution cone beam CT units will have a wide diagnostic potential for all disciplines of dentistry. The image data volumes produced by cone beam CT have the ability to be viewed in any plane (x,y,z) slice by slice.

Conventional spiral CT scans still have a place in maxillofacial imaging because of their potential for a large field of view and their ability to display soft tissues.

D. C. Hatcher, DDS, MSc

Pathologic Findings in Orthodontic Radiographic Images
Kuhlberg AJ, Norton LA (Univ of Connecticut, Farmington)
Am J Orthod Dentofacial Orthop 123:182-184, 2003   16–8

Background.—Radiographic examinations are used by orthodontists to assess the skeletofacial characteristics of their patients and to refine their identification of pathologic processes and treatment plans. Cephalometric imaging can provide quantitative data concerning the dentoskeletal morphologic characteristics and its contribution to malocclusion, and cephalometric and dental images can provide qualitative data for the detection of hard and soft tissue pathologic features. The incidence of remarkable radiographic findings on commonly used orthodontic radiographs was determined.

Methods.—A total of 396 patients were included in this cross-sectional survey sample. All the patients were in active treatment or active retention at the beginning of the study. The radiographic examinations ranged from a lateral cephalogram and panoramic radiograph to a full orthodontic series, which consisted of a full-mouth series or panoramic radiograph, a lateral cephalogram, posteroanterior cephalogram, and left and right 45° lateral

TABLE.—Anatomic Location and Number of Positive Radiographic Findings
(*n* = 396 Patients)

Location	Finding	Number
Cranium and cranial base		
	J-shaped sella turcica*	1
	Osseosclerosis in mastoid region consistent with chronic inner ear inflammatory disease	1
Cervical spine		
	OS odontoidium	1
	Incomplete arcuate foramen	1
Paranasal sinuses		
	Mucous retention cyst	11
	Sinusitis	1
Maxilla and mandible		
	Taurodontism	1
	Complex odontoma	1
	Dentigerous cyst	3
	Benign fibro-osseous lesions of PDL	1
	Odontogenic cyst	1
	Ossifying fibroma/cemental blastoma	1
	Odontoma	1
	Condylar degenerative joint disease	1
Growth		
	Growth disorders (hand-wrist film indicates age >2 y difference from chronological age)	2
Total number of findings		28

*Sign of possible pathology or destructive lesion.

(Reprinted by permission of the publisher from Kuhlberg AJ, Norton LA: Pathologic findings in orthodontic radiographic images. *Am J Orthod Dentofacial Orthop* 123:182-184, 2003. Copyright 2003 by Elsevier.)

oblique views. The images were reviewed by oral radiologists for diagnoses of pathology or remarkable findings. Descriptions of malocclusion; decayed, missing, or filled teeth; periodontal disease; and endodontic findings were excluded. Reports of cleft palate or alveolus or other craniofacial disorders were also excluded.

Results.—Of the 396 sets of records examined, remarkable radiographic findings were reported for 26 (6.2%) patients, for a total of 28 specific lesions, conditions, or abnormalities (2 patients had multiple findings) (Table).

Conclusions.—This review of pathologic findings in orthodontic radiographs found that significant lesions, conditions, or abnormalities were present in 6% of patients. These findings are suggestive of a need by orthodontists to be aware of the potential for some of their patients to present with pathologic conditions on orthodontic radiographic imaging.

▶ This article presented a good topic. Orthodontic records include radiographic images of a major portion of the craniofacial skeleton and often from multiple view angles. Therefore, there is an opportunity to extend the benefit of the imaging study beyond fulfilling the routine orthodontic goals by detecting all abnormalities visible on the imaging study.

I have been quite impressed by how many radiographic abnormalities are detected by orthodontists on routine orthodontic records.

D. C. Hatcher, DDS, MSc

Anomalies of the Odontoid Process Discovered as Incidental Findings on Cephalometric Radiographs
Tetradis S, Kantor ML (Univ of California, Los Angeles; Univ of Medicine and Dentistry of New Jersey, Newark)
Am J Orthod Dentofacial Orthop 124:184-189, 2003   16–9

Background.—Cephalometric radiographs are standardized radiographs of the skull used for the evaluation of the development, growth, and morphometric relations of craniofacial and dental structures. Most orthodontic patients are young and healthy, but there have been reports of pathologic conditions or developmental abnormalities seen on cephalometric films. Two cases of cervical spine developmental anomalies detected as incidental findings on the cephalometric films of otherwise healthy, young orthodontic patients with chief symptoms of malocclusion were presented.

Case 1.—Boy, 11 years, was referred to an oral and maxillofacial radiology clinic for a lateral cephalometric radiograph to monitor his orthodontic treatment at the 2-year mark. The radiography demonstrated a separation of the odontoid ossicle from the body of the odontoid process by a 4-mm-wide radiolucent band. A diagnosis of os odontoideum was suspected. Lateral spine films demonstrated that the odontoid ossicle maintained a normal relation to the anterior arch of C1. The width of the spinal canal was 23 mm with the head in the neutral position, 16 mm in flexion, and 24 mm in extension, for a 7-mm anterior dislocation in flexion. The diagnosis was confirmed by these findings. The patient was physically active and asymptomatic and unaware of his condition. A neurosurgical examination confirmed the diagnosis, and the patient and his parents were advised that he should avoid contact sports. Yearly follow-up was recommended.

Case 2.—Girl, 12 years, presented for orthodontic treatment with a chief symptom of severe crowding. Her medical history was unremarkable. An initial orthodontic radiographic series was obtained, including lateral cephalometric films. The lateral cephalometric radiograph showed the absence of the odontoid process of C2. The posteroanterior cephalometric film depicted a severely hypoplastic odontoid process of the axis. The initial radiographic diagnosis was odontoid process agenesis. Lateral spine films in flexion and extension showed a severely hypoplastic odontoid process and hypermobility at C1–C2. The patient was referred for medical and neurologic evaluation. The medical history was significant for presumed migraine headaches between the ages of 5 and 10 years. At the time of examination, however, the patient was free of these symptoms. A complete neurologic examination was normal with the exception of absent or very hypoactive deep tendon reflexes throughout the upper and lower extremities. The patient had no cervical spine symptoms.

She was advised to avoid contact sports, and follow-up neurologic examination was recommended.

Conclusions.—Surgical stabilization of the anomalies of the odontoid process in these 2 patients was considered but was deferred because the patients were asymptomatic. Both patients were advised to avoid contact sports and strenuous exercise to protect them from head injuries. These 2 cases provide further evidence of the importance of evaluating head and neck structures visualized on cephalometric radiographs, independent of the customary morphometric analysis performed as part of orthodontic treatment.

▶ Cephalometric projections show a portion of the upper cervical spine. There are times when incidental observations associated with the cervical spine may be of clinical significance and warrant follow-up. This article describes 2 developmental anomalies of the odontoid process but touches on the larger topic of evaluating all anatomic structures visible on the cephalometric projection.

D. C. Hatcher, DDS, MSc

Correlating Carotid Artery Stenosis Detected by Panoramic Radiography With Clinically Relevant Carotid Artery Stenosis Determined by Duplex Ultrasound

Almog DM, Horev T, Illig KA, et al (Univ of Rochester, NY; Virginia Commonwealth Univ, Richmond)
Oral Surg Oral Med Oral Pathol Oral Radiol Endod 94:768-773, 2002   16–10

Background.—Stroke is the third leading cause of death in the United States and the leading cause of severe disability. Of the approximately 730,000 strokes annually, 15% are hemorrhagic and 85% are ischemic strokes. It is not possible to affect the incidence of hemorrhagic stroke, but it

TABLE 1.—DUS Results, Panoramic Positive Sides
(n = 26/40)

Results	No. of Sides
Percent stenosis	
1-15	9
16-49	4
50-79	9
80-99	3
Occluded	1
Total positive sides	26

Abbreviation: DUS, Duplex ultrasound.
(Reprinted by permission of the publisher from Almog DM, Horev T, Illig KA, et al: Correlating carotid artery stenosis detected by panoramic radiography with clinically relevant carotid artery stenosis determined by duplex ultrasound. *Oral Surg Oral Med Oral Pathol Oral Radiol Endod* 94:768-773, 2002. Copyright 2002 by Elsevier.)

TABLE 2.—DUS Results, Panoramic Negative Sides
($n = 14/40$)

Results	No. of Sides
Percent stenosis	
1-15	8
16-49	3
50-79	3
80-99	0
Total negative sides	14

(Reprinted by permission of the publisher from Almog DM, Horev T, Illig KA, et al: Correlating carotid artery stenosis detected by panoramic radiography with clinically relevant carotid artery stenosis determined by duplex ultrasound. *Oral Surg Oral Med Oral Pathol Oral Radiol Endod* 94:768-773, 2002. Copyright 2002 by Elsevier.)

may be possible to lower the incidence of ischemic stroke. It is believed that more than 50% of ischemic strokes are the result of atherosclerotic disease at the carotid bifurcation associated with embolization of atherosclerotic debris or a platelet-fibrin clot formed at the plaque surface. Carotid endarterectomy has been shown to significantly reduce the risk of stroke in both symptomatic and asymptomatic patients with significant lesions. Duplex US (DUS) is the current gold standard for the diagnosis of carotid artery stenosis (CAS); however, it is not cost effective unless the prevalence of significant disease in a large, symptom-free population is 4.5% or greater. The use of panoramic radiography as an adjunctive screening tool for the detection of significant asymptomatic CAS was assessed.

Methods.—A retrospective review was conducted of routine dental panoramic films of 778 patients aged 55 years and older at 1 center. The films were reviewed for calcifications around the carotid bifurcation, and patients with calcifications were referred for DUS. The goal was to correlate calcifications in the region of the carotid bifurcation on panoramic radiographs with clinically relevant CAS as documented on the DUS evaluation.

Results.—A total of 27 patients (3.5%) had suggestive radiographic calcifications on 1 or both sides (Table 1). Of these patients, 20 underwent DUS (Table 2). Clinically significant carotid stenoses (>50% luminal narrowing) were present in 50% of the sides with calcifications compared with 21% of

TABLE 3.—Percent Stenosis (<50% vs 50% or More)

	>50%	<50%	No. of Sides
Panoramic positive results	13 (50%)	13	26
Panoramic negative results	3 (21%)	11	14
Total Sides	16	24	40

$P = .08$, χ^2 test; $P = .10$, Fisher exact test.
(Reprinted by permission of the publisher from Almog DM, Horev T, Illig KA, et al: Correlating carotid artery stenosis detected by panoramic radiography with clinically relevant carotid artery stenosis determined by duplex ultrasound. *Oral Surg Oral Med Oral Pathol Oral Radiol Endod* 94:768-773, 2002. Copyright 2002 by Elsevier.)

the sides without calcifications (Table 3). Three patients had stenoses of >80% and underwent 4 carotid endarterectomies as a result of screening.

Conclusions.—It would appear from these findings that clinically significant stenoses may be present if calcifications are observed on panoramic radiographs. Incidental examination of this area would appear to be beneficial as a screening tool and has a minimal cost; however, definitive testing is necessary when calcifications are observed.

▶ Calcifications detected on panoramic projections located in the region of the carotid artery bifurcations were thought to be a predictor of carotid artery stenosis and a risk factor for cerebrovascular accidents.[1] From the early reports about these calcifications is was not clear what follow-up procedures would be of benefit. The present article recommends a reasonable follow-up strategy of DUS to identify or rule out carotid artery stenosis. Cardiovascular management protocols are then based on the results of the DUS.

D. C. Hatcher, DDS, MSc

Reference

1. Friedlander AH, Baker JD. Panoramic radiography: An aid in detecting patients at risk of cerebrovascular accident. *J Am Dent Assoc* 125:1598-1603, 1994.

Detection of an Early Ossification of Thyroid Cartilage in an Adolescent on a Lateral Cephalometric Radiograph

Mupparapu M, Vuppalapati A (Univ of Pennsylvania, Philadelphia)
Angle Orthod 72:576-578, 2002   16–11

Background.—Mineralization of the thyroid cartilage is a normal part of the aging process in adults. It has been found that the thyroid and cricoid undergo a greater frequency of ossification in women, but a higher degree of ossification has been noted in men. Early ossification of the thyroid lamina or the cornu is unusual in children or adolescents. A case of ossification of the thyroid cartilage detected on a routine lateral cephalometric film was presented and the clinical implications of this finding discussed.

Case Report.—Boy, 14 years, was referred for a routine preorthodontic lateral cephalometric radiograph. Two interesting anomalies were shown on the radiograph. The superior cornu of the thyroid cartilage, which is normally not radiographically apparent unless ossified, was clearly evident. In addition, an incidental limbus vertebra was found at the level of the fourth cervical vertebra. The patient had no history of significant medical problems, and the systems review was within normal limits; he was referred back to his orthodontist and primary care physician. The patient was schedule for a follow-up visit in 3 months to review reports from his physician. The primary care physician reported no clinical signs of hypercalcemia at the time of examination that would warrant additional imaging studies. The patient's serum calcium and phosphorus were found to be within normal limits, and serum parathyroid hormone was intact. The thyroid ossification was considered to be a physiologic variation, and no treatment was proposed.

Conclusions.—The mechanisms involved mineralization and ossification of human thyroid cartilage are not well understood. The degree of ossification of the thyroid and cricoid cartilages increases with age, beginning at age of 18 years to 20 years in both sexes. Metastatic calcinosis is usually the result of deposition of calcified product in otherwise normal tissues. This condition may be associated with several disorders, including end-stage renal disease and hyperparathyroidism, and may affect visceral organs and the eyes and skin. Clinicians should be alert to the various radiographic and clinical signs indicative of metastatic calcinosis when evaluating skeletal growth and development in patients before orthodontic treatment. In the absence of hyperphosphatemia, hypercalcemia, or increased serum parathyroid hormone, the early ossification of the thyroid cartilage, as described in this case, could be an anatomic variation.

▶ This article was a good review of the development of normal thyroid cartilage ossification. This information can be used to aid in evaluating cephalometric projections and to differentiate normal from abnormal findings.

D. C. Hatcher, DDS, MSc

Three-Dimensional Cephalometry Using Helical Computer Tomography: Measurement Error Caused by Head Inclination
Togashi K, Kitaura H, Yonetsu K, et al (Nagasaki Univ, Japan)
Angle Orthod 72:513-520, 2002   16–12

Introduction.—Cephalometric radiography offers valuable information for assessing craniofacial morphologic features to arrive at definite clinical diagnoses and treatment plans. Yet, ordinary 2-dimensional cephalographs are limited by problems of enlargement and distortion. The introduction of helical CT has improved conventional CT both in decreasing motion-associated artifacts and in the rapidity with which thin-sectioned images are produced. Three-dimensional (3D) linear measurements in the maxillofacial regions were performed to investigate errors caused by head rotation when 3D images with helical CT were reconstructed.

Methods.—Errors were assessed when the head positions were tilted with the 3D measurement. Helical CT was used to scan a dry skull, and data were used to reconstruct a 3D image. Eighteen points were plotted on the 3D images. The distance between 2 points was determined when points were expressed as coordinates. A dry skull was tilted by 10× from the reference position in 3 planes (horizontal, sagittal, and frontal planes), then was tilted in a combination of directions. Scanning was conducted with slice thicknesses of 1 mm, 3 mm, 5 mm, and 7 mm. The length between 2 points measured by 3D cephalometry was compared with the actual length ascertained by an antenna meter and a caliper and expressed as percentage errors of the actual length.

Results.—In all head positions, errors in all linear measurements on the images and the actual length measured on the skull were less than 5% when a slice thickness of 1 mm or 3 mm was used. When using a slick thickness of 5 mm or 7 mm, some linear measurements revealed larger measurement errors.

Conclusion.—A thickness of less than 3 mm was considered clinically appropriate because the accuracy of the measurements was not influenced by head rotation. Changing the slice thickness according to the purpose of cephalometry could decrease exposure dose.

▶ The profession of orthodontics has a long history of utilizing 2-dimensional cephalometric projections, primarily the lateral cephalometric projection, for the purpose of quantifying linear and angular relationships between anatomic and constructed points (landmarks). The lateral cephalometric projection, as the authors pointed out, differentially magnifies the craniofacial anatomy because of the projection geometry. In addition, there are additional limitations created by using only 1 point of view (lateral view), superimposing the right and left sides of the skull, and abstracting the 3D anatomy to points (landmarks). It has been the desire of the orthodontic profession to use the landmark data to determine the status of the craniofacial skeleton and occlusion, assess the potential for growth, plan treatment, and assess treatment and growth outcomes. These expectations with conventional lateral cephalometric projections have not been fully met because of the limitations of the method. It has been hoped that emerging 3D imaging technologies will supplement or replace conventional cephalometric techniques. The goal of the emerging technologies should be to acquire, display, and analyze the anatomy with an accuracy that approximates in vivo. CT scanners have the potential to acquire near-true size volumes, but there may be some difficulties associated with the analytical components. When the orthodontic profession goes forward, there will be the opportunity to continue with abstraction of the craniofacial anatomy into a 3D point cloud of landmarks, but I wonder if these 3D landmarks will adequately describe the variations in facial form. If the orthodontic profession chooses to do so, then it will throw away more than 99% of the available anatomic information collected during the imaging exam. The exercise of determining the accuracy of landmark detection with 3D techniques, as shown in this article, is good. In the end, the complete volume of anatomic image data is broken down into 3D subunits called volume elements (voxels), and when a landmark is selected in a 3D volume a single voxel is singled out and the x, y, and z coordinates of the landmark are recorded. The ability to navigate through a 3D volume with software visualization techniques allows the operator to visualize, identify, and select more accurately the desired anatomic features when compared with 2-dimensional cephalometry. The selected anatomic landmarks (points) can be resolved into a single voxel to correspond with each landmark. The dimension of the voxels can vary depending on attributes of the CT scanner and the parameters chosen to perform the study. The resolution and the accuracy of anatomic landmarking will improve with a reduction in voxel size. When performing a CT scan, there is the ability to vary the in-plane resolution by conforming the field of view (assignment of the pixel matrix) to the anatomy under study, and the out-of-plane resolution improves by keeping the slice thickness as small as possible. The smaller voxels reduce the effect of volume averaging, and thus the spatial correlation between the image and true anatomy improves. Some of the newer multirow detector spiral CT scanners have the ability to create near-isotropic voxels in the range of 0.5 to 0.6 mm. With this type of scanner, there should be no penalty for off-axis scanning. In addition, there has recently been the introduction of cone beam CT scanners optimized for the craniofacial skeleton and soft tissues. The newest generation of cone beam scanners produces 3D volumes that match the orthodontic areas of interest, produces an isotropic voxel size that ranges between 0.2 and 0.4 mm, has a 12-bit gray scale (4096 shades), and is associated with a relatively low dose and study cost. Wow, life is good.

D. C. Hatcher, DDS, MSc

Magnetic Resonance Imaging of Normal and Osteomyelitis in the Mandible: Assessment of Short Inversion Time Inversion Recovery Sequence
Lee K, Kaneda T, Mori S, et al (Nihon Univ, Chiba, Japan; Univ of Tokyo)
Oral Surg Oral Med Oral Pathol Oral Radiol Endod 96:499-507, 2003   16–13

Introduction.—Conventional radiographic modalities, including intraoral periapical radiography, occlusal radiography, panoramic radiography, x-ray CT, and bone scintigraphy with radiation, have been used to perform diagnostic imaging of mandibular osteomyelitis. The suitable MRI conditions for the short inversion time inversion recovery (STIR) sequence were assessed by phantoms to describe the signal characteristics of normal structures in the mandible and to assess the usefulness of STIR images in enabling the identification of mandibular osteomyelitis on conventional T1- and T2-weighted spin-echo images.

Methods.—Suitable mandibular STIR imaging conditions were ascertained by varying inversion time and repetition time in each sequence. The STIR MRIs of 162 healthy research subjects and T1- and T2-weighted spin-echo images of 21 persons with mandibular osteomyelitis were assessed.

Results.—For STIR imaging, the signal of oil was suppressed at an inversion time equal to 100 ms and a repetition time equal to 1500 to 3000 ms. In healthy research subjects, the mandibular marrow was demonstrated to have high signal intensities (100%). Cortical bone had no signal intensities (100%) on STIR images. In surrounding soft tissue, the submandibular glands had high signal intensities (100%); the parotid glands had intermediate to high signal intensities (100%); the sublingual glands had high (88.9%) and intermediate to high (11.1%) signal intensities; lymph nodes had high signal intensities (100%); and the masseter muscles had intermediate signal intensities (100%) on STIR images. The bone marrow lesions showed low (75%) and low to intermediate (25%) signal intensities (100%) on T1-weighted images and high (54%), intermediate to high (29%), and intermediate (17%) signal intensities on T2-weighted images. On STIR images, the signal intensities produced high (75%), intermediate to high (21%), and intermediate (4%) signal intensities.

Conclusion.—The STIR imaging is highly effective in assessing bone marrow and surrounding tissue in the identification of osteomyelitis in the mandible and in revealing inflammation spreading to soft tissue.

▶ Clinically, the diagnosis of osteomyelitis can, at times, be difficult. I can recall individual cases when osteomyelitis was present or suspected but the applied imaging modalities—including plane films, CT, and bone scintigraphy—neither confirmed nor ruled out the condition of osteomyelitis. MRI has relatively good spatial resolution and has the ability to image bone marrow; thus, MRI is potentially a good tool to employ for the investigation of troublesome cases of suspected osteomyelitis. MRIs are complicated instruments that need to be matched or tuned to the clinical task. The selection of scanning parameters is where the magic of MR imaging occurs. This article describes strategies or protocols (STIR) used to fulfill the clinical objective of identifying osteomyelitis.

D. C. Hatcher, DDS, MSc

Magnetic Resonance Imaging Diagnosis of the Temporomandibular Joint in Patients With Orthodontic Appliances
Okano Y, Yamashiro M, Kaneda T, et al (Nihon Univ, Matsudo, Chiba, Japan)
Oral Surg Oral Med Oral Pathol Oral Radiol Endod 95:255-263, 2003   16–14

Introduction.—If magnetic substances are present in the oral cavity when MRI is performed, metal artifacts may interfere with diagnostic imaging. The accuracy of MRI diagnosis of the temporomandibular joints (TMJs) was assessed in patients with orthodontic appliances with a 0.5 Tesla MRI unit for images of the TMJs with and without orthodontic appliances.

Methods.—The mean age of 10 men and 2 women with no metal artifacts in their oral cavity (20 TMJs) was 25.2 years (range, 23-36 years). These research subjects underwent MRI before and after insertion of 6 types of orthodontic appliances (types 1-6); MRIs were compared.

Results.—In terms of disc position, the diagnostic accuracy was 80%, 75%, 70%, 70%, 65%, and 60%, respectively, from type 1 through type 6. The distribution of stages for the evaluation of condylar configurations was 80%, 55%, 40%, 40%, 20%, and 10% in order from type 1 through type 6. No significant alterations were detected in the condylar head marrow signals.

Conclusion.—The MRI diagnosis of temporomandibular disorders in orthodontic patients can be performed, preferably by using ceramic brackets in the front teeth and direct bonding tubes in the molar teeth while removing arch wires.

▶ It is not uncommon for patients undergoing orthodontic treatment with metallic orthodontic appliances to require an MRI examination of the TMJs. The request for a TMJ MRI exam can create a dilemma; do the orthodontic appliances need to be removed before exam to prevent artifact formation, thus reducing the quality of TMJ investigation? Before seeing the results of this article, I did not realize the potential for subtle magnetic field distortions that changed the recording of the disk/fossa/condyle size, form, and position. This study used a 0.5 Tesla field strength magnet, but the most commonly used magnet has a field strength of 1.5 Tesla, and it not clear if the conclusions acquired on a 0.5 Tesla machine directly apply to all other field strengths. Without consideration of the field strength, a good take-home message is to remove as much metal as is reasonably achievable before a scan. It is easy to request removal of orthodontic appliances, but I suspect that is easier said than done. Perhaps just removal the arch wire would be a good compromise, that is, relatively easy to remove before the scan and replace after the scan.

D. C. Hatcher, DDS, MSc

Artifacts From Dental Casting Alloys in Magnetic Resonance Imaging
Shafiei F, Honda E, Takahashi H, et al (Advanced Biomaterials, Tokyo; Tokyo Med and Dental Univ; Univ of Tokushima, Japan)
J Dent Res 82:602-606, 2003   16–15

Introduction.—MRI artifacts linked with a metallic object depend primarily on the inhomogeneity of the magnetic field and the magnetic susceptibility of the specific materials used to make the object, along with the amount of metal, shape, orientation, and position of the object in situ. The effects of alloy composition on the magnitude of artifacts on MRI were examined by using 11 kinds of dental casting alloys or implant materials.

Methods.—The dental casting alloys and implant materials were imaged with a 1.5 Tesla MRI apparatus with 3 different sequences. The mean and standard deviation of water signal intensity around the sample in the region of interest (1200 m^2) were calculated. The coefficient of variation was compared for assessment of the homogeneity of the signal intensity.

Results.—A variety of artifacts with various magnitudes was observed. Only 1 of the samples that was composed primarily of palladium, indium, and antimony demonstrated no artifacts in all imaging sequences.

Conclusion.—The selection of specific dental casing alloys according to their elemental compositions could minimize the metal artifacts during MRI. Titanium alloys are problematic with respect to producing MRI artifacts.

▶ Metallic magnetic susceptibility artifacts play a significant role in degrading the quality of MRI studies. The authors suggest that the potential for magnetic susceptibility artifacts be considered when selecting dental materials. This article also illustrates the artifact pattern, which can be a useful pattern to recognize clinically. Small metallic fragments remaining in the tissues after surgery may create the magnetic susceptibility artifacts yet not be visible on plain films.

D. C. Hatcher, DDS, MSc

Radiation Absorbed in Maxillofacial Imaging With a New Dental Computed Tomography Device

Mah JK, Danforth RA, Bumann A, et al (Univ of Southern California, Los Angeles; Univ of California, San Francisco)
Oral Surg Oral Med Oral Pathol Oral Radiol Endod 96:508-513, 2003   16–16

Introduction.—The use of CT has increased dramatically during the past 2 decades in both the medical and dental fields. There are surprisingly few data available concerning the amount of radiation absorbed and the risk linked with a maxillofacial CT examination of the jaw. The tissue-absorbed dose and the effective dose for the NewTom 9000, a new generation of CT devices designed specifically for dental applications, were measured.

Methods.—Comparisons were made with existing reports on dose measurement and effective dose estimates for panoramic examinations and other CT modalities for dental implants. Thermoluminescent dosimeters were implanted with a tissue-equivalent humanoid phantom at anatomic sites of interest. Absorbed dose measurements were obtained for single and double exposures. The averaged tissue-absorbed doses were used to determine the whole-body effective dose.

Results.—The effective dose for imaging maxillomandibular volume with a NewTom 9000 machine is 50.3 μSv (Tables 1, 2, and 3).

Conclusion.—The effective dose for the NewTom 9000 machine is significantly below that achieved with other CT approaches and is within the range of traditional dental imaging modalities.

▶ The rate of adoption of imaging devices for clinical use is associated with a balance among availability, clinical value, patient cost per study, and patient risk per study. One goal is to keep the radiation dose as low as reasonably achievable. When cone beam CT became available for clinical use in the United States in May 2001, the balance among clinical value, cost, and risk had not been established, and this information void was the basis for undertaking the present study. The results of the Mah et al study showed that the NewTom 9000 cone beam CT, when using the widest possible field of view, produced an absorbed dose in the range of other dental studies and significantly less than newer-generation conventional CT scans. This was great news. The next gen-

TABLE 1.—Mean Tissue Absorbed Dose (Average Absorbed Dose in Microgray) From an Oral Maxillofacial Examination With the NewTom 9000 Machine and Other Modalities Used in Previous Studies

Modality	Bone Marrow			Salivary Glands			Thyroid	Sella	Eyes
	C-Spine	Mandible	Calvaria	Parotid	Submandibular	Sub-Lingual			
NewTom 9000	975 ± 25	1064 ± 424¶	56 ± 44	1300 ± 100	1400 ± 82	1350 ± 100	783 ± 24	450 ± 71	400 ± 0
Panoramic*	198	311 / 369	0	291	183	104	41	9	0
CT of the mandible†	NA		912 (avg)		30,907	3560	3776	NA	1756
CT of the mandible‡		18,807 (R) / 17,127 (L)	375 (avg)	9641 (R) / 10,763 (L)	5862 (R) / 17,809 (L)	NA	1673	1257	622 (R) / 601 (L)
CT of the mandible	15,500 (C2) / 700 (C6)	18,229 (avg)		33,900 (R) / 31,500 (L)	6800 (R) / 9500 (L)	NA	1400	1500	NA
CT of the mandible‖	12,849 ± 4122	28,323 ± 14,417	NA	35,912 ± 27,086	NA	382	3459 ± 887	3709 ± 690	NA
CT of the maxilla‡	NA	1041 (R) / 1297 (L)	1007 (avg)	6460 (R) / 8538 (L)	623 (R) / 930 (L)	NA	243	1237	680 (R) / 883 (L)
CT of the maxilla§	2300 (C2) / 200 (C6)	1557 (avg)	700 (avg)	2400	1200 (R) / 1200 (L)	NA	400	1200	NA
CT of the maxilla‖	3279 ± 493	8602		6845 ± 2045	NA	NA	806 ± 278	7921 ± 1568	NA

*Planmeca PM 2002 CC Proline machine operated by using the same dosimetry phantom.
†GE 9800-Quick CT, 40 axial scans acquired by using the same dosimetry phantom.
‡GE 9800 CT, 36 slices of the mandible and 23 slices of the maxilla.
§Picker IQ CT, 2 contiguous 1-cm slices of the maxilla, 4 contiguous 1-cm slices of the mandible.
‖Elsinct Excel 2400 CT, 29 and 33 axial scans of the mandible, 23 and 26 scans of the maxilla.
¶Overall mean value for symphysis (1450 ± 50), mandibular body (1450 ± 108), ramus (1183 ± 131), coronoids (688 ± 85), and temporomandibular joints (550 ± 71).
Abbreviations: NA, Data not available; R, right; L, left; ave, average; C2 and C6, second and sixth cervical vertebrae, respectively.
(Reprinted by permission of the publisher from Mah JK, Danforth RA, Bumann A, et al: Radiation absorbed in maxillofacial imaging with a new dental computed tomography device. *Oral Surg Oral Med Oral Pathol Oral Radiol Endod* 96:508-513, 2003. Copyright 2003 by Elsevier.)

TABLE 2.—Comparisons of Equivalent Dose (in Microsieverts) per Tissue With the NewTom 9000 Machine

Modality	Bone Marrow	Salivary Glands	Thyroid	Sella	Eyes
NewTom 9000	53.6*	1335	782.5	450	400
Panoramic radiography	11*	237	41	9	No dose detected
CT of the mandible	369*	30,907	3776	NA	NA
CT of the mandible	244†	9901	1673	1257	NA
CT of the mandible	600	20,000‡	1400	1500	NA
CT of the mandible	2124§	21,125†	3459	3709	6115
CT of the maxilla	27†	4685	243	1237	NA
CT of the maxilla	100	1800‡	400	1200	NA
CT of the maxilla	3695§	4026¶	806	7921	7815

Order of machines tested same as in Table 1.
*Sum of bone marrow in calvaria (D_T [average absorbed dose] × 11.8%), mandibular (D_T × 1.3%), and cervical spine (D_T × 3.4%).
†Does not include values for cervical spine.
‡Submandibular and parotid glands only.
§0.165 × (average D's of mandibular marrow + cervical spine + condyles).
‖Parotid gland only.
(Reprinted by permission of the publisher from Mah JK, Danforth RA, Bumann A, et al: Radiation absorbed in maxillofacial imaging with a new dental computed tomography device. *Oral Surg Oral Med Oral Pathol Oral Radiol Endod* 96:508-513, 2003. Copyright 2003 by Elsevier.)

eration of cone beam CT scanners has passed through Food and Drug Administration clearance and will have a higher diagnostic value and most likely a lower absorbed dose.

D. C. Hatcher, DDS, MSc

TABLE 3.—Effective Dose (E; in Microsieverts) per Tissue/Organ From an Oral Maxillofacial Examination With the NewTom 9000 Machine

Modality	Bone Marrow	Bone Surface*	Thyroid	Remainder†	Total E
NewTom™ 9000	6.43	2.49	39.1	2.25	50.27
Panoramic radiography	1.3	0.5	2.0	0.045	3.85
CT of the mandible	44.3	17.2	188.8	NA	250.3
CT of the mandible	29.3‡	11.3‡	83.7	0.6	124.9
CT of the mandible	71	67	72	4	214
CT of the mandible	255	99	173	1.4	528.4
CT of the maxilla	3.2‡	1.3‡	12.5	0.6	17.6
CT of the maxilla	13	7	19	3	42
CT of the maxilla	443	171	40	2.9	656.9

Order of machines tested same as in Table 1.
*Calculated bone surface dose = bone marrow dose × 4.64.
†Results do not include salivary glands.
‡Does not include values for cervical spine.
Abbreviation: NA, Data not available.
(Reprinted by permission of the publisher from Mah JK, Danforth RA, Bumann A, et al: Radiation absorbed in maxillofacial imaging with a new dental computed tomography device. *Oral Surg Oral Med Oral Pathol Oral Radiol Endod* 96:508-513, 2003. Copyright 2003 by Elsevier.)

Analysis of the Morbidity of Submerged Deciduous Molars: The Use of Imaging Techniques
Cobourne MT, Brown JE, McDonald F, et al (King's College, London)
Oral Surg Oral Med Oral Pathol Oral Radiol Endod 93:98-102, 2002   16–17

Introduction.—Submerged deciduous molars can be challenging to manage in regard to disruption of the developing occlusion. Presented is a patient with a Class I occlusion on a Class I skeletal base with a retained and submerged deciduous molar causing impaction of the second premolar.

> *Case Report.*—Boy, 13 years, with a Class I molar and incisor relation found during routine referral to an orthodontic practitioner had no evidence of the mandibular right second premolar intraorally. He was not aware of any problems. Overall, his oral hygiene was good and caries were few. A routine panoramic radiographic view was obtained to assess the development of the occlusion and illustrate the submergence of the second deciduous molar. The lower second premolar had not erupted and was lying close to the medial root of the first permanent molar and close to the lower border of the mandible. It seemed to be in close proximity to the inferior dental canal. Cross-sectional tomograms through the region of the permanent first molar revealed the structural weakness that could arise if this molar were extracted. The path of the inferior dental canal was not clear because an obvious cortical outline to the canal was not visible. MRI was performed with a T1-weighted scanning protocol to visualize clearly the soft tissues of the inferior dental neurovascular bundle. The parasagittal sections were taken along the length of the mandible. The observation of the proximity of the submerged tooth to the neurovascular bundle of the inferior dental canal influenced the decision to leave the tooth in situ and continue with follow-up.

Conclusion.—Three potential surgical risks in the treatment of submerging teeth are damage to the mental foramen, damage to the inferior dental canal, and risk of possible mandibular fracture after removal. The position of the inferior dental canal and mental foramen in relation to the tooth has to be determined, making MRI a useful adjunct in evaluating the risks of surgery in patients for whom the inferior dental canal is not able to be clearly visualized on conventional radiographic and tomographic images.

▶ Imaging modalities are tools to be used to solve specific clinical problems. Clinical problem solving is a dynamic process that begins with defining the goals or expectations of the imaging, choosing the appropriate imaging tools, and then applying the imaging tools appropriately. The authors of this article presented a very solid imaging strategy to solve clinical problems associated with submerged deciduous molars. They defined the clinical goals, including spatially localizing the submerged teeth, mandibular canal, mental foramen, and the buccal and lingual cortices of the mandible. There was a thoughtful assessment of the value of various imaging tools, including panoramic, tomography, and MRI. I was happy to see MRI mentioned because of its unique ability to show contrast between the contents of the neurovascular bundle and surrounding bone. Clinically, there are times when there is not enough bone adjacent to the mandibular canal for tomography or CT scans to define the mandibular canal adequately, and MRI would be a useful alternative imaging technique.

D. C. Hatcher, DDS, MSc

17 Temporomandibular Disorders

Condylar Erosion and Disc Displacement: Detection With High-Resolution Ultrasonography

Emshoff R, Brandlmaier I, Godner G, et al (Univ of Innsbruck, Austria)
J Oral Maxillofac Surg 61:877-881, 2003   17–1

Background.—In patients with osteoarthritic changes at the temporomandibular joint (TMJ), evaluation must include a determination of the nature, location, and extension of the osseous changes and detection of any associated disk displacements. The use of MRI is currently favored for diagnosing TMJ pathology, but sonography has reported accuracy in detecting disk disorders, especially disk displacements. A prospective evaluation was performed to determine the accuracy of sonography in identifying condylar erosion and associated disk displacements.

Methods.—Ninety-six joints in 48 consecutive patients with TMJ disorders were assessed with a 12.5-MHz array transducer. Both condylar erosion and disk displacement were sought and the findings compared with those obtained by MRI.

Results.—Condylar erosion was identified in 44 cases by sonography, but MRI confirmed only 15. MRI revealed that 14 of the others had normal condylar morphology, 8 osteophytes, and 7 osteophytes plus surface irregularities. A condylar erosion was interpreted as surface irregularity, condylar flattening, and normal condylar morphology in 3 patients, respectively, but MRI revealed interruption of the cortical lining. Eighteen TMJs had condylar erosions. Sonography had a sensitivity of 83%, specificity of 63%, accuracy of 67%, positive predictive value of 34%, and negative predictive value of 94% for detecting condylar erosions. MRI found disk displacements occurring with condylar erosion in 16 (89%) of the 18 cases, and all were disk displacements without reduction. Sonography detected 14 of the 16 disk displacements without reduction that were linked to condylar erosion. Sixteen (37.2%) of 43 disk displacements without reduction were associated with a condylar erosion, whereas 2 (6.3%) of 32 TMJS that did not have disk displacement had a condylar erosion. The presence of condylar erosion was significantly correlated with the type of internal derangement. Disk displacement without reduction was found with an accuracy of 93%, whereas disk displacement without reduction concomitant with condylar erosion was found with an accuracy of 80%.

Conclusions.—The assessment of disk displacement without reduction was reliably handled by sonography, but this technique was insufficient for detecting condylar erosion.

▶ The ultimate imaging technology would provide the desired diagnostic information and have a low risk and low cost. High-resolution US has been associated with low risk and cost, but this article showed that the diagnostic value was not sufficient to recommend it for routine use in detecting condylar erosions and disc position. When reviewing the US images included in this article, there was significant noise, thus making the etiology of the observations ambiguous. It would also seem that the morphology of the TMJs would not lend themselves to a detailed inspection by US. The combination of bone and soft tissue surfaces does not have the potential for a homogeneous interaction with sound. In addition, the curvature of the articular surfaces it seems would not allow US access to the medial sides of the joints.

The range of clinically valuable findings discovered with MRI for TMJ studies goes beyond determining disc position and identifying or ruling out degenerative joint disease (osteoarthrosis), thus allowing the clinician to consider a broad differential diagnosis.

D. C. Hatcher, DDS, MSc

Volume and Shape of Masticatory Muscles in Patients With Hemifacial Microsomia

Takashima M, Kitai N, Murakami S, et al (Osaka Univ, Japan; Univ of Copenhagen)
Cleft Palate Craniofac J 40:6-12, 2003   17–2

Background.—Aural, mandibular, and dental development can be adversely affected by hemifacial microsomia (HFM), which may be mild to severe and unilateral or bilateral. Establishing diagnostic criteria has been difficult because of the wide variety of presentations. Various hypotheses concerning HFM were evaluated, including the following: (1) in a comparison with the unaffected side, the volumes of the masseter, lateral and medial pterygoid, and temporal muscles are reduced on the affected side; (2) the degrees of right-left disproportion in the 4 masticatory muscles are significantly different; (3) the masticatory muscles circumferential shapes are more irregular on the affected than the unaffected side; and (4) the severity of the right-left disproportion of the masticatory muscles is related to the degree of ear, mandibular, or dental anomalies on that side.

Methods.—Facial photographs, dental casts, cephalometric and panoramic radiographs, helical CT scans, and a 3-dimensional reconstruction technique were used to evaluate 10 preadolescent patients with HFM. Measures included the volumes of the masseter, lateral and medial pterygoid, and temporal muscles on both sides; muscle volume disproportion (volume disproportion index [VDI]); and muscle circumferential irregularity, expressed as the ratio between the total circumferential length and the corresponding cross-sectional area (circumferential irregularity index [CII]).

Results.—Compared with the unaffected side, the mean volumes for the masticatory muscles on the affected side were significantly smaller, although the VDI values of the 4 masticatory muscles showed no significant differences. Significantly higher mean CII values were obtained on the affected side than on the unaffected side, which indicated that the shape irregularity of the masticatory muscles on the affected side was greater. The mean CII values for the masseter and medial pterygoid muscles on the affected side were 3 times the values found on the unaffected side. For the lateral pterygoid and temporal muscles the mean CII values were only twice as great on the affected side compared with the unaffected side. The mean VDI values of the patients with mild/severe ear anomaly, mild/severe mandibular anomaly, and normal/abnormal dental dentition status exhibited no significant differences.

Conclusions.—The principal findings included significantly reduced volumes of the masticatory muscles on the affected sides; no significant differences in the degree of disproportion of the 4 masticatory muscles; greater irregularity of shape in the masticatory muscles on the affected side; and no significant relation between ear anomalies and the degree of masticatory muscle disproportion, between degree of mandibular hypoplasia and degree of masticatory muscle disproportion, or between degree of dental anomaly and masticatory muscle disproportion. Thus, the severity of the masticatory muscle disproportion cannot be predicted by the degree of anomaly found in ear, mandibular, or dental structures.

▶ Maxillofacial imaging has primarily involved imaging of the hard tissues of the jaws. Descriptions of mandibular and facial asymmetries have almost always been limited to the skeleton, dentition, and external facial soft tissues without attention to the masticatory muscles. Therefore, treatment strategies do not primarily involve the masticatory muscles. This article quantifies the involvement of masticatory muscles in patients with HFM and presents methods for imaging muscles. In addition, this study showed that the hard tissues changes could not be used to predict the degree of muscle involvement. When considering the functional interactions of the jaws, muscles, and dentition in patients with HFM, there is the possibility that chewing and speech efficiencies are maintained by functional adaptations by the involved tissues. These adaptations may include the 3-dimensional positions of the occlusal plane; temporomandibular joint; and muscles and muscle volume, length, and vectors.

D. C. Hatcher, DDS, MSc

Morphologic Changes in the Unloaded Temporomandibular Joint After Mandibulectomy

Hamada Y, Kondoh T, Sekiya H, et al (Tsurumi Univ, Yokohama, Japan)
J Oral Maxillofac Surg 61:437-441, 2003   17–3

Background.—The temporomandibular joint (TMJ) bears mechanical loads constantly, with intra-articular pathologic changes linked to abnormal mechanical loads. Releasing the TMJ from any mechanical load should produce changes, but the nature of those changes is undefined. Seventeen of 60 TMJs from 30 patients who had long-term mandibular continuity defects resulting from mandibulectomy including the condyle or segmental mandibulectomy were assessed. These were identified clinically as unloaded TMJs, thus not influenced by any muscles other than the lateral pterygoid. The intra-articular conditions found in these TMJs were assessed by MRI and arthroscopy.

Methods.—Eleven of the 17 were classified as "without condyle" (WOC), having had the condyle removed but the disk and superior joint compartment preserved (Fig 1). Six joints were classified as "with condyle" (WC), and the TMJs were connected to the condylar process (Figs 2 and 4). MRI analysis focused on the disk configuration, any bony changes, and the presence of joint effusion. Eight joints underwent arthroscopic evaluation. The disk configurations were divided into biconcave type, enlargement of posterior band type, even thickness type, or biconvex type. The data obtained for the WOC and WC groups were compared, and a relation between arthroscopic results and joint effusion was sought.

Results.—Four of the disks in the WOC group and all those in the WC group exhibited the biconcave configuration. The biconvex type was found in 1 WOC joint and the even thickness type in 6 WOC joints. A significant difference in the frequency of the presence of deformed disks was noted be-

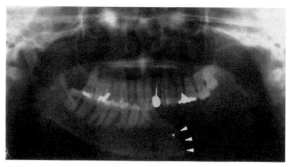

FIGURE 1.—Panoramic radiograph of a patient who underwent mandibulectomy including the left condyle. Left TMJ is classified into the WOC group. *Arrowheads,* Border of the residual mandibular fragment. (Reprinted from Hamada Y, Kondoh T, Sekiya H, et al: Morphologic changes in the unloaded temporomandibular joint after mandibulectomy. *J Oral Maxillofac Surg* 61:437-441, 2003. Copyright 2003, with permission from the American Association of Oral and Maxillofacial Surgeons.)

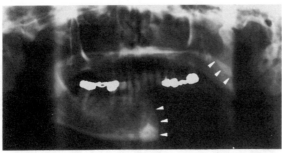

FIGURE 2.—Panoramic radiograph of a patient who underwent segmental mandibulectomy. Left TMJ is only connected to the condylar process and is classified into the WC group. Condyle is dislocated anteriorly out of the glenoid fossa. *Arrowheads*, Borders of residual mandibular fragments. (Reprinted from Hamada Y, Kondoh T, Sekiya H, et al: Morphologic changes in the unloaded temporomandibular joint after mandibulectomy. *J Oral Maxillofac Surg* 61:437-441, 2003. Copyright 2003, with permission from the American Association of Oral and Maxillofacial Surgeons.)

tween the 2 groups. None of the joints in either group displayed evidence of bony changes. Fifteen had evidence of joint effusion, with the 2 not showing effusion belonging to the WOC group. Joint effusion was found with equal frequency in the 2 groups. Seven of the 8 joints undergoing arthroscopy had various types of fibrous adhesion; the frequency did not differ between the WC and WOC groups. No other osteoarthritic changes were present. One WC joint had normal findings on arthroscopy. Fibrous adhesions were not linked significantly to MRI evidence of joint effusion, but joint effusion was found in 6 of the 7 joints that had fibrous adhesion.

Conclusions.—Nearly 64% of the patients in the WOC group had disk deformities. The altered relation between the disk and the condyle appeared to be more important in initiating disk deformation than in altering loading conditions on the disk. Articular degeneration was apparently brought on by the disturbance in synovial fluid metabolism, but bony conditions were not affected, even in the presence of fibrous adhesion and joint effusion.

▶ It seems reasonable that biomechanical consequences of function or lack of function would alter the form of the TMJ disk. The presence of joint effusion in nonfunctioning joints was a unique observation supporting the contention that that inflammation is not a prerequisite for fluid accumulation.

D. C. Hatcher, DDS, MSc

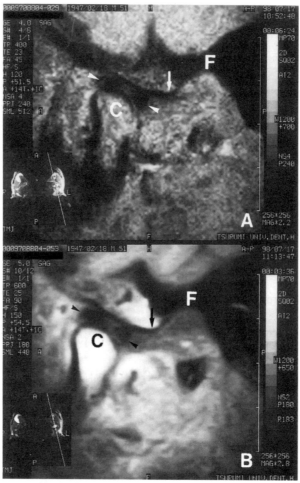

FIGURE 4.—**A,** Sagittal closed-mouth T1-weighted MRI of TMJ in the WC group. Disk and condyle (*C*) are displaced anteriorly out of glenoid fossa (*F*), while maintaining their normal relation. **B,** Sagittal open-mouth T1-weighted MRI of same TMJ. Disk and condylar position have not changed. *Arrow,* Summit of articular eminence. *Arrowheads,* Anterior and posterior ends of disk. (Reprinted from Hamada Y, Kondoh T, Sekiya H, et al: Morphologic changes in the unloaded temporomandibular joint after mandibulectomy. *J Oral Maxillofac Surg* 61:437-441, 2003. Copyright 2003, with permission from the American Association of Oral and Maxillofacial Surgeons.)

Experimentally Induced Unilateral Tooth Loss: Expression of Type II Collagen in Temporomandibular Joint Cartilage

Huang Q, Opstelten D, Samman N, et al (Univ of Hong Kong)
J Oral Maxillofac Surg 61:1054-1060, 2003   17–4

Background.—In temporomandibular joint (TMJ) cartilage, collagens are important elements, with type II collagen, although present in lesser

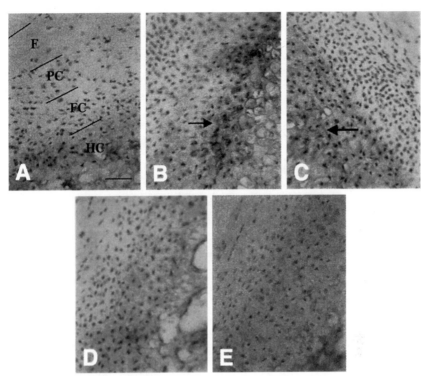

FIGURE 2.—Photomicrographs of anti–type II collagen antibody binding to condylar cartilage. **A,** Normal rabbit; **B,** nonfunctional side and **C,** functional side, 3 weeks after unilateral removal of teeth; **D,** nonfunctional side and **E,** functional side, 6 weeks after unilateral removal of teeth. *Arrows,* Intensity levels of antibody binding at 3 weeks are dramatically higher than normal (immunostaining; original magnification, ×200.) *Abbreviations: F,* Fibrous layer; *PC,* prechondroblast layer; *FC,* functional chondroblast layer; *HC,* hypertrophic chondroblast layer. (Reprinted from Huang Q, Opstelten D, Samman N, et al: Experimentally induced unilateral tooth loss: Expression of type II collagen in temporomandibular joint cartilage. *J Oral Maxillofac Surg* 61:1054-1060, 2003. Copyright 2003, with permission from the American Association of Oral and Maxillofacial Surgeons.)

quantities than type I collagen, playing a role in biomechanical properties, handling both compressive and tensile forces. It was hypothesized that abnormal TMJ loading caused by the unilateral removal of teeth would disturb the synthesis and degradation rates of type II collagen, which would then alter its amount and pattern. Alterations should differ between the functional and nonfunctional sides of the TMJ. The expression and spatial distribution of type II collagen were evaluated in rabbit TMJs after teeth were removed unilaterally.

Methods.—Twelve rabbits underwent extraction of mandibular teeth and were then killed 3 or 6 weeks later. Three other rabbits with no extraction served as control subjects. The TMJ blocks obtained from these 15 animals were evaluated for presence and distribution of type II collagen by using an immunoperoxidase technique. In the semiquantitative assessment, the extracellular matrix (ECM) was assessed, focusing on the territorial matrix (TM), or that seen in the immediate vicinity of the cells or cell clusters, and

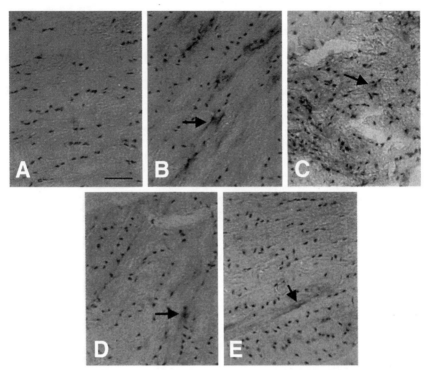

FIGURE 3.—Photomicrographs of anti–type II collagen antibody binding to TMJ disk. **A**, Normal rabbit; **B**, nonfunctional side and **C**, functional side, 3 weeks after unilateral removal of teeth; **D**, nonfunctional side and **E**, functional side, 6 weeks after unilateral removal of teeth. *Arrows*, Anti–type II collagen antibody binding was shown in the experimental rabbits. (Immunostaining; original magnification, ×200.) (Reprinted from Huang Q, Opstelten D, Samman N, et al: Experimentally induced unilateral tooth loss: Expression of type II collagen in temporomandibular joint cartilage. *J Oral Maxillofac Surg* 61:1054-1060, 2003. Copyright 2003, with permission from the American Association of Oral and Maxillofacial Surgeons.)

the interterritorial matrix (ITM), or the rest of the ECM. Staining intensity levels were judged by a scale ranging from no staining (0) to very strong staining (6).

Results.—Because the negative control sections exhibited no brown staining, all that found in test sections was interpreted as specific anti–type II collagen antibody binding. Fibrous and prechondroblast layers showed no distinction between the TM and ITM areas, so the entire ECM was considered. In condylar cartilage, type II collagen staining was found mostly in the ECM of the hypertrophic chondroblast layer, and the ITM stained more abundantly than the TM (Fig 2). Slight staining in the ITM and sparse staining in the TM were found in the functional chondroblast layer, and sparse staining was noted in the ECM of the articular disks. Anti–type II collagen antibody binding occurred at a greater that normal level 3 weeks after tooth extraction, with the functional and nonfunctional sides differing in quantity. A low but detectable level was found in the ECM of the nonfunctional side of the TMJ; no statistical difference with the findings in the control subjects was noted. The TM bound the antibody significantly more strongly in the hypertrophic chondroblast layer than in normal subjects, and the nonfunctional side had a greater increase than the functional side. Both the functional and nonfunctional sides had greater degrees of staining of the disk than did normal sections. In addition, the central region was the most prominently stained, with part exhibiting a pattern of slightly wavy, fibril-like staining (Fig 3). Antibody binding intensity varied considerably 6 weeks after tooth extraction and differed from the patterns noted after 3 weeks. The differences were significant compared with normal or 3-week rabbit sections. The staining in the disk was greater than normal on both sides of the TMJ, with the same slightly wavy, fibril-like staining as noted in the 3-week samples.

Conclusions.—In samples obtained 6 weeks after the unilateral removal of teeth, anti–type II collagen antibody binding increased and the pattern of staining in the TMJ cartilage was altered. The condylar cartilage and disk thus adapt to the imbalance through chondrocyte repair processes that include collagen II expression.

▶ There is a functional biomechanical relationship among the occlusion, masticatory muscles, and the TMJs. A change in the occlusion may alter the joint loading characteristics and induce changes in joint tissues. Numerical models (static equilibrium, finite element and dynamic) have shown that alteration of the occlusion, including the simulation of removing posterior teeth, may alter mechanics of mandibular function and produce bilateral changes in the resultant joint-loading magnitudes and direction. In addition, there have been reports in the literature that a loss of posterior teeth in humans is associated with degenerative joint disease. Therefore, the premise of this article is very good: that the loss of posterior teeth alters the joint loads and induces a soft tissue response. It makes sense that joints would have the capacity to dynamically adapt to changes in their biomechanical environment.

D. C. Hatcher, DDS, MSc

Specific Expression in Inducible Nitric Oxide Synthase in the Synovium of the Diseased Temporomandibular Joint
Takahashi T, Homma H, Nagai H, et al (Kyushu Dental College, Kitakyushu, Japan; Akita Univ, Japan; Tohoku Univ, Sendai, Japan; et al)
Oral Surg Oral Med Oral Pathol Oral Radiol Endod 95:174-181, 2003   17–5

Background.—Overloading that produces microtrauma is being explored for its role in the pathophysiology of temporomandibular joint (TMJ) diseases. Both internal derangement (ID) and osteoarthritis (OA) may be caused by direct mechanical injury and hypoxia-reperfusion mechanisms, with oxidative stress possibly leading to an accumulation of free radicals that damage TMJ tissues. Nitric oxide (NO), a gaseous free radical, regulates various immunologic and inflammatory functions. NO is a potent vasodilator, increases vascular permeability, stimulates angiogenesis, inhibits collage and proteoglycan synthesis, and combines with superoxides to produce peroxynitrite, which is implicated in tissue injury. Activation of the inducible nitric synthase (iNOS) pathway is involved in the pathogenesis of inflammatory arthritides. The expression of iNOS in arthroscopically derived specimens from the TMJ was evaluated to determine the role of NO in the pathogenesis of TMJ synovitis and degenerative changes.

Methods.—Fifteen patients with symptomatic ID or OA of the TMJ were the source for synovial biopsies of 18 TMJs; 8 control TMJs were also assessed by immunohistochemical techniques to determine iNOS expression. Findings were compared with the results of clinical, arthroscopic, and histologic evaluations.

Results.—On arthroscopy, most TMJs from symptomatic patients showed hypervascularity, hyperemia, or synovial hyperplasia; 11 had moderate or pronounced synovitis, and 15 had varying degrees of fibrous adhesion. In 2 cases, perforations occurred at the junction between the posterior attachment and the disk. Control TMJs had no evidence of synovitis or osteoarthritis, although 3 of 4 TMJs with mandibular condyle fractures showed hypervascularity and hyperemia. Disk perforations and fibrous adhesions were absent in control joints. Definite or intense iNOS staining was present in the synovial lining and endothelial cells of all TMJs with symptomatic ID or OA, with weaker staining of synovial fibroblasts. Control specimens had neither intense nor definite iNOS staining. The iNOS expression in the synovium correlated significantly with arthroscopic evidence of synovitis; none of the TMJs that were negative for synovitis showed intense or definite iNOS expression (Table 2). No statistically significant correlation was found between iNOS expression and arthroscopic evidence of degenerative changes. The iNOS expression and histologic grade of synovial lining cell layers were significantly related, and all TMJs that had synovia with moderate to pronounced hyperplasia were positive for iNOS; however, 5 patients with normal synovial lining cell layers were also positive for iNOS (Table 3). No significant associations were found between iNOS immunohistochemical reactivity and any arthroscopic or histologic findings among symptomatic TMJs or between iNOS reactivity and clinical values for maximum mouth opening or scores for joint pain.

TABLE 2.—Relation Between iNOS Expression and Arthroscopic Findings

| | Arthroscopic Findings | | | | | |
| | Synovitis (Score)* | | | Degenerative Changes (Score) | | |
iNOS Staining (Score)	0	1	2	0	1	2
0	4 (0)	3 (0)	1 (0)	7 (0)	1 (0)	0 (0)
1	0 (0)	3 (3)	8 (8)	3 (3)	2 (2)	6 (6)
2	0 (0)	4 (4)	3 (3)	3 (3)	2 (2)	2 (2)
Total	4 (0)	10 (7)	12 (11)	13 (6)	5 (4)	8 (8)

Note: Nonparenthetical numbers are number of TMJs. Numbers in parentheses are number of TMJ diseases (ID or OA).

*Synovitis: $P < .05$. Degenerative changes were not significant.

(Reprinted by permission of the publisher from Takahashi T, Homma H, Nagai H, et al: Specific expression in inducible nitric oxide synthase in the synovium of the diseased temporomandibular joint. *Oral Surg Oral Med Oral Pathol Oral Radiol Endod* 95:174-181, 2003. Copyright 2003 by Elsevier.)

TABLE 3.—Relation Between iNOS Expression and Histologic Findings

iNOS Staining (Score)	Synovial Lining Cell Layers (Score)			
	0	1	2	3
0	6 (0)	2 (0)	0 (0)	0 (0)
1	4 (4)	4 (4)	2 (2)	0 (0)
2	1 (1)	2 (2)	4 (4)	1 (1)
Total	11 (5)	8 (6)	6 (6)	1 (1)

Note: Nonparenthetical numbers are number of TMJs. Numbers in parentheses are number of TMJ diseases (ID or OA).
$P < .05$.
(Reprinted by permission of the publisher from Takahashi T, Homma H, Nagai H, et al: Specific expression in inducible nitric oxide synthase in the synovium of the diseased temporomandibular joint. *Oral Surg Oral Med Oral Pathol Oral Radiol Endod* 95:174-181, 2003. Copyright 2003 by Elsevier.)

Conclusions.—The synovia of TMJs from patients with symptomatic ID or OA expressed iNOS, whereas control TMJs with asymptomatic ID had no or only weak iNOS staining. Control subjects with arthroscopic evidence of synovitis also had weak or marginal iNOS expression. Thus, iNOS expression correlated with arthroscopic degree of synovitis, meaning that NO is produced locally by iNOS in diseased TMJs and probably plays a significant role in the pathogenesis of TMJ synovitis and osteoarthritic changes.

▶ This was a good article to read. Joint damage and repair or adaptation is a fascinating topic but difficult to study or clinically assess. Many of the clinical assessment tools involve imaging, and they can only record macroscopic changes; but the real action is occurring at a microscopic or biochemical level. Identifying regulators associated with apoptotic, immunologic, and inflammatory processes involving synovial joints, such as OA and rheumatoid arthritis, is a large step toward developing improved clinical assessment and management capabilities. Free radical production, including iNOS, following mechanical stress was proposed in this article as being associated with joint pathology.

D. C. Hatcher, DDS, MSc

Expression of Matrix Metalloproteinases in Articular Cartilage of Temporomandibular and Knee Joints of Mice During Growth, Maturation, and Aging

Gepstein A, Shapiro S, Arbel G, et al (Technion, Haifa, Israel; Carmel Med Ctr, Haifa, Israel)
Arthritis Rheum 46:3240-3250, 2002   17–6

Background.—The integrity of cartilage depends on maintaining balance between the synthesis and degradation of the extracellular matrix. Changes in this homeostatic steady state quickly influence cartilage function and produce excessive degradation. The matrix metalloproteinases (MMPs) are important components of extracellular matrix remodeling and are divided into collagenases, stromelysins, and gelatinases based on their substrate specificity. The messenger RNA levels of MMPs were monitored, and the activity and expression of MMPs that participate in the turnover of extracellular matrix were evaluated in the articular cartilage of joints belonging to neonatal, young, matured, and aged mice.

Methods.—Zymography was used to assess the activity of MMP-2 and MMP-9, which are gelatinases, by using homogenates of intact tibial plateau, femoral condyle, and temporomandibular joint (TMJ) condyle cartilages from mice aged newborn to 18 months (1 day, 2 days, 1 week, 2 weeks, 1 month, 4 months, and 18 months, specifically). Semiquantitative reverse transcription–polymerase chain reaction was used in assessing the mRNA expression of MMPs 1, 2, 3, 9, and 13 in tibial plateau cartilage. MMPs 2, 3, 9, and 13 were localized in knee joints and TMJ by immunohistochemical means.

Results.—The zymography of 1-month-old mice showed that both MMP-2 and MMP-9 were expressed, with distinct differences between the TMJ condyle, femoral condyle, and tibial plateau. The femoral condyle had the highest MMP-9 expression, which was at least 5-fold higher than in the TMJ cartilage and 1.5-fold higher than in the tibial plateau cartilage. The latent form of MMP-2 was expressed most in the tibial plateau cartilage, whereas the active form was found in highest quantities in the TMJ cartilage. Expression patterns varied with age, with the profiles in the tibial plateau and femoral condyle similar in neonatal, mature, and aging animals, that is, gradually increasing with age, but different from the expression in the TMJ cartilage, where it gradually declined with maturation and aging. MMP-3 and MMP-13 mRNA expression was very low until age 1 month, then increased to age 18 months; MMP-2 mRNA expression peaked at age 2 weeks and declined somewhat thereafter, as did MMP-9 expression. MMP-1 was not expressed at any time period. On immunohistochemical analysis, MMP-13 was found to be constitutively highly expressed at 1 day, 2 weeks, and 18 months and was localized mainly in articular surfaces and chondroblastic zones, hypertrophic cells, and at the joint's resorption front. In the knee joint, MMP-13 expression increased from newborn to 2 weeks, then gradually declined with age. All age groups had positive MMP-3 staining in the TMJ; MMP-3 was only found in hypertrophic cells and the resorption front in newborns, along the articular surface in the chondroblastic zone and surrounding matrix at 2 weeks, and in chondrocytes in all regions of the cartilage at 18 months, with an expression pattern in the knee similar to that of MMP-13. Similar patterns were noted for MMP-2 and MMP-9.

Conclusions.—The expression and activity of MMPs in articular cartilage are evidence of their role in the developmental processes of growth, maturation, and aging. The differences seen in temporospatial expression between the various joints assessed seem to indicate that load and function influence MMP activity.

▶ The biochemical consequences on the extracellular matrix of biomechanical components of joint function were a theme of this article.

D. C. Hatcher, DDS, MSc

Tomographic Assessment of Temporomandibular Joint Osseous Articular Surface Contour and Spatial Relationships Associated With Disc Displacement and Disc Length

Major PW, Kinniburgh RD, Nebbe B, et al (Univ of Alberta, Edmonton, Canada; Calgary, Canada)
Am J Orthod Dentofacial Orthop 121:152-161, 2002   17–7

Background.—Internal derangement of the TMJ is a common condition in adolescent patients. The associations of TMJ osseous morphology and joint space relations with disk displacements have been reported in adults, but this information is not directly applicable to adolescent patients because their articular tissue provides for growth and thus their adaptive response could be different. Whether there are associations between osseous TMJ characteristics and TMJ internal derangement in adolescents was examined.

Methods.—Axially corrected tomographic radiographs and MRIs of 335 TMJs in 175 subjects (106 female and 69 male) between 7 and 20 years of age (mean, 13 years of age) were used in this study. Nine tomographic variables were measured from pretreatment tomograms, and tomographic data were cross-referenced with MRI data. Male and female samples were evaluated separately.

Results.—On stepwise linear regression, associations were seen between disk displacement and reduced superior joint space, increase posterior joint space, increased anterior joint space, and reduced articular eminence convexity, with a R^2 value of 0.41 for male patients and 0.38 for female patients. The associations between reduced disk length and condylar position and eminence flattening were weaker, with an R^2 value of 0.16 for male patients and 0.32 for female patients.

Conclusions.—Internal derangement of the TMJ in adolescent patients is associated with functional osseous adaptation within the joint.

▶ Tomography is a much more commonly used TMJ imaging assessment method than MRI; therefore, it is beneficial to know if tomography is a good screening tool for disk position. A tomographic image cannot show the disk position, but if the superior joint space is narrowed or the posterior slope of the articular eminence has lost its convexity, then there is an increased probability of a displaced disk. There is a caution about overinterpreting the superior joint space because a narrowed superior joint space without a disk displacement can also be observed in individuals with a thinned disk or with a skeletal Class III.

D. C. Hatcher, DDS, MSc

Magnetic Resonance Imaging of Temporomandibular Joint Synovial Fluid Collection and Disk Morphology

Huh J-K, Kim H-G, Ko J-Y, et al (Yonsei Univ, Gyeonggi, Korea)
Oral Surg Oral Med Oral Pathol Oral Radiol Endod 95:665-671, 2003   17–8

Background.—High signal intensity within the TMJ space, or joint effusion, is easily observed on T2-weighted MRI. However, the relation of high signal intensity to joint inflammation is controversial, and the presence of joint effusion in the painless joint has not been fully explained. The features of synovial fluid, the shape of the disk, and the presence of disk displacement without reduction (DDsR) of the TMJ were determined.

Methods.—A total of 612 bilateral temporomandibular MR images of 306 patients were reviewed. The mean age of the patients was 30 years, with

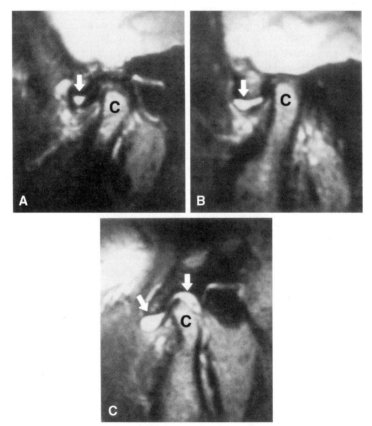

FIGURE 1.—High signal intensity within the superior joint space is observed on T2-weighted MR images. A small amount (A), a moderate amount (B), and a large amount (C) of synovial fluid was collected, respectively (*arrows*). *Abbreviation:* C, Condylar head. (Reprinted by permission of the publisher from Huh J-K, Kim H-G, Ko J-Y: Magnetic resonance imaging of temporomandibular joint synovial fluid collection and disk morphology. *Oral Surg Oral Med Oral Pathol Oral Radiol Endod* 95:665-671, 2003. Copyright 2003 by Elsevier.)

a range of 13 to 80 years. Of the 306 patients, 224 (73%) were female. The status of the TMJ was categorized as normal disk position, disk displacement with reduction, acute DDsR, subacute DDsR, and chronic DDsR. The shape of the disk was categorized as biconcave, cup-shaped, flattened, eyeglass-shaped, amorphous, or discontinuous. The amount of synovial fluid was divided into 4 categories as not observed, small, moderate, or large (Fig 1).

Results.—Synovial fluid was not evident in 90% of the normally shaped disks. However, synovial fluid was visible in 93.7% of the cap-shaped disks and in 91% of the cup-shaped disks (Fig 3). A moderate amount of synovial fluid was also observed more frequently in the folded disks (18.1%) than in any other disk shapes (Table 2).

Conclusions.—This T2-weighted MRI study found that synovial fluid collection is more frequent in the early stage of disk displacement without

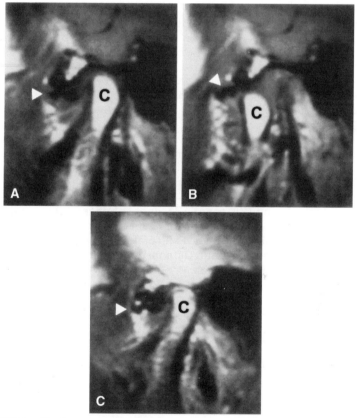

FIGURE 3.—Closed-mouth (**A**) and open-mouth (**B**) T1-weighted MR images reveal chronic disk displacement without reduction. The disk (*arrowheads*) is eyeglass shaped. **B**, Few morphologic changes in the disk are present on opening. **C**, Synovial fluid collection is not remarkable on the T2-weighted MR image. *Abbreviation:* C, Condylar head. (Reprinted by permission of the publisher from Huh J-K, Kim H-G, Ko J-Y: Magnetic resonance imaging of temporomandibular joint synovial fluid collection and disk morphology. *Oral Surg Oral Med Oral Pathol Oral Radiol Endod* 95:665-671, 2003. Copyright 2003 by Elsevier.)

TABLE 2.—Frequency of Synovial Fluid Collection Distributed in Terms of Joint Status

Status of Joint	No. of Joints (Left/Right)	Not Observed	Amount of Synovial Fluid Small Amount	Moderate Amount
Normal	192 (98/94)	178 (92.7%)	14 (7.3%)	0 (0.0%)
DDcR	236 (109/127)	162 (68.6%)	66 (28.0%)	8 (3.4%)
Subacute DDsR	124 (68/56)	17 (13.7%)	85 (68.5%)	22 (17.7%)
Chronic DDsR	60 (31/29)	47 (78.3%)	11 (18.3%)	2 (3.3%)
Total	612 (306/306)	404 (66.0%)	176 (28.8%)	32 (5.2%)

Abbreviation: DDcR, Disk displacement with reduction.
(Reprinted by permission of the publisher from Huh J-K, Kim H-G, Ko J-Y: Magnetic resonance imaging of temporomandibular joint synovial fluid collection and disk morphology. *Oral Surg Oral Med Oral Pathol Oral Radiol Endod* 95:665-671, 2003. Copyright 2003 by Elsevier.)

reduction. On MR imaging, the high signal intensity within the disk space should be viewed as a simple matter of fluid collection. However, when an extremely large amount of synovial fluid is observed in the upper or lower joint space without osteoarthritis on MRI, other pathologic states, such as synovial chondromatosis, should be considered.

▶ The etiology of a synovial fluid joint effusion has been controversial. Is the fluid accumulation secondary to an inflammatory process, or does it accumulate to fill a dead space? The authors devised a method of subgrouping disc displacement without reduction cases into acute, subacute, and chronic states to better understand when and where synovial fluid accumulates. This was a very good noninvasive approach to study the problem.

D. C. Hatcher, DDS, MSc

Does Joint Effusion on T2 Magnetic Resonance Images Reflect Synovitis? Part 2. Comparison of Concentration Levels of Proinflammatory Cytokines and Total Protein in Synovial Fluid of the Temporomandibular Joint With Internal Derangements and Osteoarthrosis

Segami N, Miyamaru M, Nishimura M, et al (Kanazawa Med Univ, Uchinada, Japan; Kyoto Univ, Japan)
Oral Surg Oral Med Oral Pathol Oral Radiol Endod 94:515-521, 2002   17–9

Background.—Joint effusion (JE) as visualized on T2-weighted MR images is commonly viewed as representative of hypertrophic synovium and exudation from inflamed tissue not only in the TMJ but also in other joints. Thus, JE is thought to reflect intra-articular pathosis. However, there is a need for more scientific evidence to confirm this view. In a previous study, it was shown that a significant correlation exists between the amount of JE and the severity of synovitis detected arthroscopically. The nature of JE on T2-weighted MR images of the TMJ was clarified by analysis of the synovial fluid in the superior compartments of patients with internal derangements of the TMJ and osteoarthrosis.

Methods.—A total of 110 symptomatic TMJs in 100 patients, including 65 internal derangements and 35 osteoarthroses, were scanned with MR imaging. The synovial was sampled on the same day. The amount of JE was evaluated on a scale of 0 to 3, with grades 0 and 1 indicating an absence or only a negligible amount of JE, respectively, and grades 2 and 3 indicating the presence of JE. Correlation was evaluated among the amount of JE and the concentrations of the total protein and interleukin-1β (IL-1β), IL-6, IL-8, and tumor necrosis factor-α in the synovial fluid.

Results.—On MR imaging, JE was absent in 40 joints (17 joints at grade 0 and 23 joints at grade 1) and present in 60 joints (31 joints at grade 2 and 29 joints at grade 3). The joints with effusion had significantly higher concentrations of total protein (1675 μg vs 714 μg) and IL-6 (42.9 pg vs 10.6 pg) than joints without effusion. There were also significant correlations between the grade of JE and the concentrations of the total protein, IL-6, and IL-8. The detection ratio of cytokines among the presence-absence groups of JE was indicative of a significant difference in tumor necrosis factor-α (68.3% vs 47.5%) and IL-6 (86.7% vs 67.5%).

Conclusions.—JE may contain the released products when there is pronounced synovitis, and the JE is likely composed of high concentrations of total protein with inflammatory cytokines. IL-6 and IL-8 are important in the pathogenesis of JE in TMJ disorders.

▶ This study determined the proinflammatory cytokine content in patients with combinations of painful TMJ, JE, displaced disks, and osteoarthrosis. In patients with painful joints a JE is associated with higher levels of proinflammatory cytokines and protein concentration.

D. C. Hatcher, DDS, MSc

Does Joint Effusion on T2 Magnetic Resonance Images Reflect Synovitis? Part 3. Comparison of Histologic Findings of Arthroscopically Obtained Synovium in Internal Derangements of the Temporomandibular Joint
Segami N, Suzuki T, Sato J, et al (Kanazawa Med Univ, Japan)
Oral Surg Oral Med Oral Pathol Oral Radiol Endod 95:761-766, 2003   17–10

Background.—It has been suggested in previous studies that joint effusion detected by T2-weighted MRI may be a reflection of intra-articular pathologic processes in symptomatic TMJs. These reports have been limited to comparisons of clinical signs and symptoms, synovial fluid analysis, and histopathologic findings of extirpated disks. The relation between the volume of joint effusion, as visualized on MRI, and microscopic findings of synovial inflammation was evaluated in internal derangement of the TMJ to determine whether joint effusion is a sign of synovitis.

Methods.—MR images were obtained in 53 patients with symptomatic TMJs associated with painful hypomobility in an effort to evaluate the degree of joint effusion on a scale of 0 to 3. Within 2 months after MRI, biopsy specimens obtained by arthroscopy were quantitatively assessed (by

Gynther's grading system) for severity of hyperplasia of synovial lining cell layers, vascularity, and the presence of inflammatory cells. The synovitis scores were compared among the 4 joint effusion grades and between effusion present (grades 2 and 3) and effusion absent (grades 0 and 1).

Results.—Joint effusion was found to be distributed as grade 0 in 14 joints, grade 1 in 9 joints, grade 2 in 19 joints, grade 3 in 11 joints. There were significant relations between the grades of joint effusion and scores of synovial lining cell layers as well as between the grades of joint effusion and scores of presence of inflammatory cells. The joints with effusion had significantly higher scores for synovial lining cell layers than the joints without effusion. No statistically significant correlation was evident between the scores of vascularity and joint effusion.

Conclusions.—Evidence of joint effusion on MRI would appear to be correlated with synovial inflammatory activity. These findings provide confirmation of the common consensus that joint effusion is likely a reflection of synovitis, particularly when synovial hyperplasia has a key role in the pathogenesis of joint effusion.

▶ In patients with painful joints, joint effusion is most likely associated with a synovitis.

D. C. Hatcher, DDS, MSc

The Effects of Mechanical Strain on Synovial Fibroblasts
Sambajon VV, Cillo JE Jr, Gassner RJ, et al (Univ of Pittsburgh, Pa)
J Oral Maxillofac Surg 61:707-712, 2003   17–11

Background.—Studies of arthritic conditions in recent years have suggested that inflammatory mediators and proteinases may have a role in the pathogenesis of conditions such as rheumatoid arthritis and osteoarthritis. Recent clinical evidence from physical therapy and other therapeutic regimens has shown a significant decline in TMJ symptoms in patients with early disease. The effect of mechanical strain on the production of mediators of inflammation by synovial fibroblasts, including prostaglandin E_2 (PGE_2) and proteinases, was examined.

Methods.—An established synovial fibroblast cell line (HIG-82) was grown to confluency in modified Eagle's medium supplemented with 10% fetal calf serum. The monolayer of fibroblasts was then subjected to mechanical strain by the Flexercell Strain Unit at 3 cycles/min, with 10 seconds of elongation to 24% and 10 seconds of relaxation. PGE_2 levels were measured by radioimmunoassay with a commercially available product and measured in nanograms per milliliter of supernatant. Collagenase, gelatinase, and stromelysin were measured by H3 radioactive labeling of acidic anhydride to the specific substrate. Enzymatic proteolysis of the radiolabeled substrate was measured in supernate, and all results were analyzed by student *t* test.

TABLE 1.—Values of Metalloproteinase and PGE_2 Levels for Control and Experimental Conditions

	Control Condition	Experimental Condition
Collagenase (U/mL)	4.27 ± 1.5	3.99 ± 1.9
Gelatinase (U/mL)	4.62 ± 0.11	4.02 ± 0.9
Stromelysin (U/mL)	0.11 ± 0.012	0.12 ± 0.0
Prostaglandin E_2 (ng/mL)	58.0 ± 9.17	18.1 ± 13.4

(Reprinted from Sambajon VV, Cillo JE Jr, Gassner RJ, et al: The effects of mechanical strain on synovial fibroblasts. *J Oral Maxillofacial Surg* 61:707-712, 2003. Copyright 2003, with permission from the American Association of Oral and Maxillofacial Surgeons.)

Results.—The PGE_2 level of mechanically activated cells was 18.1 ± 13.4 ng/mL compared with control levels of 59 ± 9.2 ng/mL—a statistically significant decrease between strained and unstrained cells ($P < .05$) (Table 1). In the control cells, proteinase activity that degrades collagen, gelatin, or casein was 4.27 ± 1.5, 4.62 ± 0.11, or 0.11 ± 0.01 U/mL, respectively. For mechanically strained cells the levels were 3.99 ± 1.90, 4.02 ± 0.90, and 0.12 ± 0.012 U/mL, respectively. These findings are an indication of a significant decline in PGE_2 levels of synovial fibroblasts undergoing mechanical strain. The proteinases examined in this study demonstrated no difference in levels between mechanically activated fibroblasts and their controls.

Conclusions.—The findings that PGE_2 production in synovial fibroblasts during mechanical strain may facilitate the understanding of the mechanism by which physical therapy leads to a decline in inflammatory mediators in the TMJ.

▶ Mechanical stress and strain on the articular cartilage of the TMJs are necessary for growth, development, and maintenance of those tissues. Stress is a mechanical term indicating force/area and strain is the deformation of the tissues induced by force (change in length/original length). Strain rates and strain quantity may be important factors when understanding tissue and biochemical responses. Physical therapy and continuous passive motion may produce small repetitive strains and influence fluid mechanics associated with joint lubrication and nutrition resulting in a beneficial tissue response. Conversely, excessive strains may activate tissue degradation.

D. C. Hatcher, DDS, MSc

18 Modeling and Biomechanics

Structure and Function of the Temporomandibular Joint Disc: Implications for Tissue Engineering
Detamore MS, Athanasiou KA (Rice Univ, Houston)
J Oral Maxillofac Surg 61:494-506, 2003   18–1

Introduction.—The TMJ disk is a poorly understood structure that is associated with several pathologic disorders. Tissue engineering approaches are needed to address the pathophysiologic characteristics of the TMJ disk. A clear understanding of the structure-function relation needs to be developed, particularly because they are related to the regeneration potential of the tissue. The biochemical content of the TMJ disk was correlated with mechanical behavior to determined what this correlation infers for tissue engineering investigations of the TMJ disk.

Findings.—The TMJ disk has a somewhat biconcaval shape. It is thicker in the anterior and posterior bands and thinner in the intermediate zone. The disk is an anisotropic and nonhomogeneous tissue and is composed nearly entirely of type I collagen with trace amounts of type II and other types. Collagen fibers in the intermediate zone generally seem to run primarily in an anteroposterior direction and in a ringlike fashion around the periphery. Collagen orientation demonstrated higher tensile stiffness and strength in the center anteroposteriorly versus mediolaterally and in the anterior and posterior bands versus the intermediate zone mediolaterally. Tensile tests have established that the disk is stiffer and stronger in the direction of the collagen fibers. Elastin fibers generally are seen along the collagen fibers and most likely function in restoring and retaining disk form after loading. The 2 primary glycosaminoglycans of the disk are chondroitin sulfate and dermatan sulfate; their distribution is not clear. Compression trials are conflicting. There is evidence that the disk is compressively stiffest in the center.

Conclusion.—Only a few tissue engineering investigations of the TMJ disk have been performed so far. Tissue engineering trials need to take advantage of existing information for experimental design and construct validation. More research is required to characterize the disk to create a clearer understanding of goals for tissue engineering of the TMJ disk.

▶ This is a good review article describing the structure of the articular disk, functional properties of the disk, and the correlation with function. Not only is this information valuable for tissue engineering, but it will also help computer modeling of the jaws and all forms of TMJ reconstructions. There have been numerous instances of joint replacement materials failing, in part, because of an incompatibility between the functional demands and material properties.

D. C. Hatcher, DDS, MSc

Biomechanics of the Human Temporomandibular Joint During Chewing
Naeije M, Hofman N (Academic Ctr Dentistry Amsterdam (ACTA))
J Dent Res 82:528-531, 2003   18–2

Background.—Currently, no data document the mechanical loading of the human TMJ during chewing and chopping, but joint loading is estimated with the use of biomechanical models. It has been suggested that during chewing, when the opening and closing condylar movement traces coincide, the TMJ is compressed during the closing stroke. However, no compression or only slight compression is present when these traces do not coincide. Loading of the TMJ during chewing and chopping was investigated by means of a latex-packed food bolus on the right or left side of the mouth.

Methods.—Ten healthy subjects (ages 21-32 years) participated in this study of mandibular movements. The distances traveled by the condylar kinematic centers were normalized in conjunction with the distance traveled with maximum opening. Coincidence of closing and opening condylar movement traces was approximated.

Results.—No difference was noted during chopping, but the distance traveled by the condylar kinematic centers was shorter on the ipsilateral side than on the contralateral side during chewing. The kinematic centers of all contralateral joints coincided during chewing and chopping. Significantly fewer joints with a coinciding movement pattern were noted on the ipsilateral than on the contralateral side.

Discussion.—The results line up somewhat with the predictions of biomechanical models. The ipsilateral joints are less heavily loaded than the contralateral joints during chewing and chopping actions. This finding may help explain why patients who have joint pain claim to have less pain when they chew on the painful side.

▶ These authors proposed a novel and interesting method to estimate in vivo bilateral dynamic loading conditions within the TMJs. The kinematic approach for estimating joint loads raises a question in my mind. Could the vertical position of the condylar surface be a function of joint compression and/or thickness of interpositional tissues located between the osseous components of the condyle and opposing eminence? This article assumes that the sagittal tracing path is a function of compressive force within the TMJ, but I wonder if it is possible to have a difference in opening and closing condylar paths with or without variations in joint loads by a relative changes in disk position? During the mandibular opening and closed movements, the disk-condyle spatial relationships change, but I am not sure it the opening and closing cycles of the mandible if the disk-condyle spatial relationships are symmetrical.

D. C. Hatcher, DDS, MSc

Dynamic Shear Properties of the Temporomandibular Joint Disc

Tanaka E, Hanaoka K, van Eijden T, et al (Hiroshima Univ, Japan; Academic Centre for Dentistry Amsterdam (ACTA); Osaka Univ, Japan; et al)
J Dent Res 82:228-231, 2003   18–3

Introduction.—The TMJ disk is subject to various types of loading that can usually be divided into compression, tension, and shear components. Shear stress may be an important factor linked with fatigue failure and damage of the TMJ disk. Few data are available concerning the dynamic behavior of the disk in shear. The dynamic shear properties of the porcine disk were examined over a wide range of loading frequencies. Because the disk is anisotropic and viscoelastic in structure, the effects of frequency and direction of the applied load on these properties were assessed.

Findings.—Shear stress was introduced in both anteroposterior and mediolateral directions. The dynamic moduli rose as the loading frequency increased. The dynamic elasticity was significantly greater in the anteroposterior test than in the mediolateral test; the dynamic viscosity was similar for both tests.

Conclusion.—It appears that nonlinearities, compression/shear coupling, and intrinsic viscoelasticity affect the shear material behavior of the disk, which may have important implications for the transmission of load in the TMJ.

▶ The TMJs are loaded during function with the loads being transmitted through the disk. Joint loads are necessary for maintenance of the joint tissues, but excessive loads or loads that exceed the adaptive capacity of the tissues may contribute to joint failure, including disk displacement. Understanding of the load-bearing characteristics of the disk, that is, types of loads (compressive, tensile, and shear stress), load rate, load direction, and load quantity contribute to understanding of the balance between joint health and failure in the clinical population. The anisotropic properties of the disk being related to the internal structure of the disk may create an unfavorable scenario when the disk starts to displace. That is, it is not uncommon for a disk to be partially displaced by rotating on its horizontal axis so that lateral portion of the disk is anterior to the medial portion. This may change the loading pattern on the disk so that the condyle translates along the central portion of the disk oblique to the central collagen fibers.

D. C. Hatcher, DDS, MSc

Human Masticatory Muscle Forces During Static Biting

Nickel JC, Iwasaki LR, Walker RD, et al (Univ of Nebraska, Lincoln; Univ of Manitoba, Winnipeg, Canada; Univ at Buffalo, NY)

J Dent Res 82:212-217, 2003   18–4

Introduction.—The mix of muscle forces during mastication determines the magnitude and direction of TMJ loads. This is of clinical importance, particularly because the likelihood of degenerative joint disease rises with increased TMJ loads. Data from living research subjects were compared with numerical model predictions of muscle forces determined from the 3-dimensional geometry of the individual and an objective function of minimization of joint load (MJL) or minimization of muscle effort (MME).

Findings.—Numeric model predictions with data from 6 research subjects (1 female; 5 male; age range, 23-32 years) were compared. Biting tasks that produced moments on molar and incisor teeth were modeled, with MJL or MME as the basis. The slope of predicted versus electromyographic data for each participant was compared with a perfect match slope of 1.00. Predictions based on MME had the closest match with electromyographic activity for molar biting (slopes, 0.89-1.16) (Table). Predictions from either or both models corresponded with EMG results for incisor biting (best-match slopes, 0.95-1.07).

Conclusion.—Muscle forces during isometric biting seem to be consistent with objectives of MJL or MME, depending on the individual participant, biting location, and moment.

TABLE.—Slopes and R^2 Values for the Relation Between Predicted and Measured Masseter and Anterior Temporalis Muscle Outputs for Equivalent Biting Moments

	Model vs. Measured Muscle Outputs for:				
	MJL Model		MME Model		Number of
Subject	Slope	R^2	Slope	R^2	Data Points
	Molar Biting				
m1*	1.88	0.33	1.03†	0.96	6
m2	6.10	0.74	0.93†	0.96	12
m3	10.20	0.69	0.92†	0.91	17
f1	1.60	0.96	0.89†	0.92	12
m4	0.19	0.52	0.92†	0.92	12
m5	2.30	0.52	1.16†	0.94	12
	Incisor Biting				
m1*	0.95‡	0.58	0.95‡	0.58	6
m2	1.04‡	0.63	0.79	0.76	12
m3	0.10	0.09	1.00‡	0.73	12
f1	0.95‡	0.78	0.95‡	0.78	12
m4	0.20	0.07	0.96‡	0.51	12
m5	1.07‡	0.73	0.69	0.65	12

*Data from biting task session before facial trauma.
†‡Best-match model results with experimental data.
(Courtesy of Nickel JC, Iwasaki LR, Walker DR, et al: Human masticatory muscle forces during static biting. *J Dent Res* 82:212-217, 2003.)

▶ Three-dimensional modeling is emerging as a useful way to analyze structural and functional interactions in the masticatory system. Computer modeling to simulate function can be used to examine the biomechanical relationships between anatomic form and function. Computer modeling starts with anatomic reconstructions that include muscles, jaws, dentition, and TMJs. Clinically useful simulations and predictions depend on accuracy of the modeling, including the reconstructions and assumptions used to mimic the biomechanical events. Modeling the human masticatory muscles, muscle recruitment strategies, and model validation are extremely important but very difficult. Nickel et al, in this paper and prior work, have contributed to our understanding of computer modeling.

D. C. Hatcher, DDS, MSc

The Transfer of Occlusal Forces Through the Maxillary Molars: A Finite Element Study
Cattaneo PM, Dalstra M, Melsen B (Univ of Aarhus, Denmark)
Am J Orthod Dentofacial Orthop 123:367-373, 2003   18–5

Introduction.—Distal displacement of the maxillary molars is a commonly used modulus in the treatment of patients with Class II malocclusions. The form-function balance appears to be disregarded when displacing molars forward and backward in the maxilla during treatment. It seems appropriate to examine the effect of these displacements on the load transfer during occlusion. The finite element (FE) method has previously been applied to the evaluation of load transfer through the skull. An FE analysis permits simulation of the displacement of a molar in relation to the well-defined morphologic features of the maxilla. An FE analysis of the stress/strain distribution of the maxillary complex during normal function was evaluated with the molars in a neutral position and displaced both mesially and distally with respect to the infrazygomatic crest.

Findings.—Three-dimensional unilateral models of a maxilla from a skull with skeletal Class I and neutral molar relations were created on the basis of CT scan data. The maxillary first molar was localized for the contour of the mesial root to continue into the infrazygomatic crest. When the molar was loaded with occlusal forces, the stresses were transferred, primarily through the infrazygomatic crest. This was altered when mesial and distal displacements of the molars were simulated. In the model with mesial molar displacement, a greater portion of the bite forces was transferred through the anterior part of the maxilla. This resulted in the buccal bone being loaded in compression. In the model with distal molar displacement, the posterior portion of the maxilla was deformed through compression, producing higher compensatory tensile stresses in the anterior portions of the maxilla at the zygomatic arch.

Conclusion.—This distribution of the occlusal forces may contribute to the posterior rotation frequently described as the orthopedic effect of extraoral traction. This 3-dimensional FE analysis of the transfer of occlusal forces in mesially and distally displaced molars has deepened the understanding of both the orthopedic changes in relation to sagittal displacement of molars and the strong tendency of a molar to regain its original position below the infrazygomatic crest.

▶ Biomechanical manipulations of the maxillofacial anatomy, combined with an understanding of the relationships between form and function, are an integral part of the orthodontic profession. Unresolved forces following treatment or misdirected forces may lead to relapse or tissue injury. Modeling, as shown in this article, allows the clinician to test the biomechanical relationships between form and function. In the future, there may be the ability to have patient-specific anatomic models to test the biomechanical consequences of various treatment options. In this study, I particularly enjoyed the visualization technique used that segmented the anatomy based on stress distribution. Methods of visualizing quantitative information are important for conveying complex information.

D. C. Hatcher, DDS, MSc

Removal of Osteosynthesis Material by Minimally Invasive Surgery Based on 3-Dimensional Computed Tomography–Guided Navigation
Schultes G, Zimmermann V, Feichtinger M, et al (Univ Hosp Graz, Austria)
J Oral Maxillofac Surg 61:401-405, 2003   18–6

Introduction.—The introduction of 3-dimensional (3D) CT-based navigation has made it possible to transform precise preoperative planning into the intraoperative situation without the need for mechanical aids. Described is minimally invasive surgery for removal of osteosynthesis material with 3D CT-guided navigation.

    Case Report.—Man, 19, with a fracture of the left mandibular condyle underwent osteosynthesis by a submandibular approach. The 2 fragments were stabilized with a normal 4-hole miniplate. Soon after osteosynthesis, oral movement was completely restored. The patient had pain, reduced mouth opening, and paresthesia after healing. At 6 months after osteosynthesis, the plate and the 3 caudal screws were removed by the same submandibular approach. The cranial screw was not detected and could not be adequately reached with the screwdriver. Because the patient was not informed concerning the possibility of a preauricular approach, the screw was left within the condyle and the plate was destroyed. The patient continued to have limited mouth opening (25 mm), paresthesia, and pain in the left zygomatic arch during oral movement. The exact location of the screw was identified by CT-generated data. A dental acrylic splint with embedded miniscrews was manufactured to ascertain the exact preoperative and intraoperative repositioning of the mandible to the skull. Two surgical approaches were calculated by 3D reconstruction. A horizontal approach was used for better instrumental adjustment. To avoid the preauricular approach, minimally invasive surgery was performed by CT-guided navigation. A head frame was used to fix the patient's skull during surgery. The mandible was fixed in the same position as during CT scanning, and the screw was removed under visual control with a screwdriver. There were no complications and the patient has been free from pain and his mouth opening has been normal since reoperation.

Conclusion.—The CT-guided navigation system appears to be useful in removing very small foreign bodies within the mandible.

▶ This article illustrates the value of computers to enhance images so they can be used assist the surgeon with surgical navigation by using a minimally invasive technique. A 3D CT volume is a spatially accurate volume that can be used to aid in diagnosis, localization, and treatment planning. In the typical clinical scenario, the CT volume is analyzed by the clinician and a navigation route to retrieve a foreign body is mentally formulated by the surgeon. In other words, the CT image will stay on the computer and the surgeon has to memorize the relevant findings and mentally transfer the information to the patient. The alternative scenario would be to use computers to spatially register the CT volume to the patient and then use the computer to guide the surgeon as planned. Using computers to assist with navigation allows the procedure to be performed with minimally invasive techniques.

The use of computers to assist with many components of patient care will increase in the next several years. Computers are assisting with imaging, including 2-dimensional images, CT scans, cone beam CT scan, and MRI. Computers will be used to assist our vision; to create virtual patients (anatomic reconstructions) for research, treatment simulations, and treatment planning; and ultimately to assist with treatment, as shown in this article. If we can create an accurate 3D reconstruction of the patient with imaging as the source data and create a 3D simulation of the proposed treatment on the reconstructed model, then the computer has the information needed to assist with treatment.

D. C. Hatcher, DDS, MSc

19 Dental Education

Introduction

This chapter covers a variety of topics and issues that were significant in dental education this year. Included is a discussion of the challenges ahead for dental education, particularly in the areas of dental student debt loads and recruitment and retention of dental school faculty members. Distance learning continues to be a topic of great interest in dental education. Diversity in dental schools and in the profession, and the need to produce clinicians who are equipped to provide culturally sensitive care, were also important topics. Finally, the need to produce well-trained clinical researchers, and possible strategies for doing so, is discussed.

Kristin A. Zakariasen Victoroff, DDS

Dental Education Summits: The Challenges Ahead
Bailit H, Weaver R, Haden K, et al (Univ of Connecticut, Farmington)
J Am Dent Assoc 134:1109-1113, 2003   19–1

Introduction.—The financial pressures facing US dental schools threaten their ability to maintain the high quality of American dental education. In 2001 and 2002, the American Dental Association held summit meetings on challenges facing dental education, including the costs of dental education, the high debts carried by dental students, and recruitment of dental school faculty. Major findings from these summits are summarized.

Cost Issues.—During the 1990s, state and local revenue support for dental schools decreased by 22%. Dental schools tried to make up the difference through tuition increases and other means, largely unsuccessfully. At the same time, growing discrepancies between the income of practicing versus academic dentists made it more difficult to recruit and retain dental school faculty. New federal legislation will allow dental schools to receive graduate medical education funding for some residents and graduate studies, although the impact of these funds remains unclear. With current budgetary crises on the state level, state support for dental schools will likely decrease still further.

Debt Issues.—As tuition increases, so does dental student debt, which averaged approximately $69,000 for graduates of public institutions to $114,000 for those from private schools. This is in addition to preexisting debt from undergraduate studies. High indebtedness has been linked to a reduction in minority dental school graduates and restrictions on career choices. At the same time, the quality of applicants to dental schools remains high.

Faculty Issues.—The problem of recruiting qualified dental school faculty is likely to worsen in the years ahead, with hundreds of new positions becoming open in the next decade. Such shortages, particularly acute in the dental specialties, are likely to compromise dental schools' educational and research capabilities.

Possible Responses.—Summit participants proposed various options for dealing with the problems of rising expenses and falling revenues. Clinics are an important target for expense reduction, which may be achieved by having trainees spending more time in community clinics. In addition to their cost-saving potential, community-based education will provide students with valuable experience in providing high-quality, efficient care. Other options include developing regional dental schools and using technology to share resources. From the revenue standpoint, efforts are needed to maximize state support. Lobbying efforts will seek new forms of federal support, including special initiatives to provide care to low-income populations. The participants also urged creation of an endowment to support dental education.

Conclusions.—Dental education faces difficult financial challenges in the years ahead. Sustained efforts will be needed to reduce expenses while seeking more government support for dental education. These and other measures are essential to keep dental schools open and to maintain the high quality of US dental education and research programs.

▶ This article speaks for itself—dental education currently faces significant and serious financial challenges. As the authors note, creative solutions to these problems are needed. Some of these solutions may be out of the box, very different than what has been done in the past, and these new approaches are likely to push educators and others out of our comfort zone. The dental education system in the United States has historically been successful in producing very well-trained dentists, and we may be uncomfortable making radical changes in a system that worked for us. As the process of meeting these new challenges unfolds, we will need to keep in mind that the goal is not to preserve a particular way of doing things, but to preserve the desired outcome—skilled, capable, well-prepared dentists.

K. A. Zakariasen Victoroff, DDS

Meeting the Demand for Future Dental School Faculty: Trends, Challenges, and Responses
Haden NK, Weaver RG, Valachovic RW, et al (American Dental Association, Washington, DC)
J Dent Educ 66:1102-1113, 2002   19–2

Objective.—Recruitment and retention of faculty are becoming urgent problems for US dental schools. Even as enrollment continues to increase, so does the average number of vacant faculty positions. A survey of dental schools regarding vacant faculty positions is reported, along with a review of future challenges.

Survey Findings.—All 54 US dental schools responded to a 2001 to 2002 American Dental Education Association survey regarding vacant, budgeted faculty positions. The total number of vacant positions was 344, representing a 4% decrease from the previous year. Seventy-nine percent of the vacancies were in full-time positions, mainly in the clinical sciences. By primary discipline, the greatest number of vacancies was in general/restorative dentistry. Ninety-six of the reported vacancies were new positions. No current search was in progress for 27% of the reported vacancies, and most positions had been vacant for 4 months or longer. The dental schools reported a total of 1011 faculty separations, nearly 3-fold more than in the previous survey. Where the information was available, 53% of the departing faculty members were going into private practice.

Discussion.—The survey results suggest a continued trend toward an increasing number of unfilled dental faculty positions. The data on vacancies with no active search suggest that some positions are being lost because of budget cuts or other reasons. The shortage of dental faculty is likely to continue into the future, for reasons including the growing gap in income for private versus academic dentists, increasing student debt, a large number of upcoming retirements, increasing research expectations, and the national economic situation. Possible responses are summarized in this and previous American Dental Education Association reports.

▶ This article provides more detail regarding the current shortage of dental school faculty in the United States. The faculty shortage is attributable to a variety of factors, and efforts on many fronts will be required to solve the problem. The involvement and concern of a variety of constituents—organized dentistry, dental educators, NIDCR—are encouraging. In my own discussions with students, heavy debt loads seem to be a major concern. While many express an interest in being involved in dental education "down the road," few feel able to pursue that path immediately following graduation, given the magnitude of their educational debt and relatively low faculty starting salaries. Should greater flexibility in career paths be considered? For example, could there be greater opportunities to re-enter the academic track after having spent time in private practice? In addition, whether academics is actively promoted to students as a desirable and important career path remains unclear.

Do students have adequate experiences in which they could discover if teaching or research is of interest to them?

K. A. Zakariasen Victoroff, DDS

Distance Education in the U.S. and Canadian Undergraduate Dental Curriculum
Andrews KG, Demps EL (Univ of Texas, San Antonio)
J Dent Educ 67:427-438, 2003   19–3

Objective.—In dental education, as in other areas, there is interest in the potential uses of distance education. Several approaches have been suggested for using computers and communication technologies to provide online learning opportunities. North American dental schools were surveyed regarding their uses of distance education.

Methods.—A paper questionnaire regarding distance education was sent to 64 academic deans of US and Canadian dental schools. In addition, faculty members at the schools were asked to respond to an Internet survey. Responses were obtained from 38 of the deans and from 448 faculty members.

Findings.—Fifty-two percent of the deans reported that their schools were currently using Web-based and distance learning technologies for predoctoral education, whereas another 21% were planning or considering implementing such programs. Distance learning technologies were used for graduate medical education at 33% of schools and for continuing dental education at 45%. Web-based programs were much more frequently used than video or audio conferencing. Ninety percent of respondents reported positive experiences with distance learning. When asked about barriers to distance learning, the respondents most commonly cited a lack of incentives and rewards, lack of faculty development opportunities, and the lack of personal contact with students.

In the faculty survey, approximately one third of respondents said they used Web-based learning in their courses, whereas another 44% said they planned to do so in the future. The main components of Web-based learning were e-mail communication, posted syllabus and course objectives, lecture slides and handouts, images and radiographs, and web resources. More than 80% of faculty members reported a satisfactory experience with Web-based learning.

Discussion.—Survey results suggest that distance learning technologies are commonly used by North American dental schools and that the use of such technologies is likely to increase in the future. Dental schools must provide the necessary infrastructure to support faculty's use of distance education, including faculty development programs. Future studies should examine the ways in which online learning affects the role of the teacher.

Interdisciplinary, Web-Based, Self-Study, Interactive Programs in the Dental Undergraduate Program: A Pilot

Cohen HB, Walker SR, Tenenbaum HC, et al (Univ of Toronto)
J Dent Educ 67:661-667, 2003   19–4

Purpose.—With Internet technology, flexible learning programs can be developed to provide anytime access for students. An important capability of these programs is the ability to provide horizontal and vertical integration among disciplines. Readily created with the use of hypertext markup language, cross-references can facilitate collaboration among the overlapping fields involved in dental education. The development and initial evaluation of a series of prototype self-study modules for dental students are described.

Methods and Results.—Existing programs such as FrontPage and Photoshop were used to create pilot modules, called StudyWeb, in the areas of histology, pharmacology, prosthodontics, and radiology. The developers intentionally used low-end technologies to maximize capability with individual users' equipment and access. The 4 prototype modules were evaluated in terms of functionality, usability, and ease of navigation. The histology module included an image map showing a sagittal view of an embryonic palate, with "clickable" links allowing students to check their accuracy in identifying key histologic features. The pharmacology module provided case examples and a prescription-writing exercise, and the prosthodontics module included a simple animation of mandibular movements. The radiology module included case histories and radiographic images along with questions and answers pertaining to the illustrated cases. On extensive testing, the StudyWeb modules showed good compatibility with various browsers, computer systems, and Internet connections.

Conclusions.—The development and initial evaluation of a series of Web-based instructional modules for dental education were described. Further evaluations will focus on the instructional effectiveness of the StudyWeb modules. This process will focus on the goals of horizontal and vertical integration, beginning with the pharmacology module.

▶ These 2 articles (Abstracts 19–3 and 19–4) focus our attention on the issue of the use of information technology in dental education. The overarching question in both articles is: How can information technology be utilized to help meet our educational goals? Dental educators must thoughtfully consider ways in which online learning resources can (1) meet needs of learners that are not being met through the traditional curriculum, (2) make learning more efficient, and (3) free up face-to-face interaction time between faculty and students for higher level tasks (questions, synthesis of information, problem-solving activities) instead of transfer of basic information. As on-line resources are added to dental curricula, we must be conscious of both (1) what is potentially gained through the use of on-line learning (eg, flexibility, efficiency) and what is potentially lost (face-to-face interactions with faculty and peers, in which role-modeling and professional development occurs).

The second article (Abstract 19–4) challenges educators to think about creative possibilities for the use of on-line learning and to consider how on-line learning can be used to add unique value to the educational process. Specific examples, such as posting an interactive prescription-writing activity on-line, are given to stimulate thought. The authors make the very good point that because the structure of the Web allows for easy cross-referencing through links, on-line resources may be a great tool for emphasizing integration across subject areas. This may be an important value-added feature of on-line learning.

K. A. Zakariasen Victoroff, DDS

Why Practice Culturally Sensitive Care? Integrating Ethics and Behavioral Science

Donate-Bartfield E, Lausten L (Marquette Univ, Milwaukee, Wis; Univ of Missouri, Kansas City)
J Dent Educ 66:1006-1011, 2002   19–5

Background.—There is a growing emphasis on providing health care services in a culturally sensitive manner. Reasons supporting this approach include facilitation of dental care and respect for patient autonomy. To understand the latter reason, the practitioner must be aware of some key principle of ethics and reasoning. Ethical and behavioral issues involved in providing culturally sensitive dental care are reviewed.

Ethics of Culturally Sensitive Care.—Culture affects people's perceptions of the world, with important affects on attitudes, beliefs, and assumptions. Culturally sensitive care acknowledges these differences and their effects on health care delivery in a nonjudgmental way. Different cultures are diverse in a broad range of areas, including diet, dress, motivations, and beliefs and values, as well as behaviors affecting disease and health. Making treatment and preventive recommendations in ways that are relevant to the patient's culture will increase the likelihood of compliance with those recommendations.

In addition to improving patient outcomes, culturally sensitive care is important because it promotes the ethical principles of autonomy, beneficence, and justice. Teaching students the ethical obligation to provide culturally sensitive care helps provide them with the reasoning ability needed to negotiate compromises that respect differing cultural values. Under the principle of autonomy, the dentist must respect the patient's decisions. However, this does not mean being obligated to provide inappropriate care. A culturally sensitive view of care means accepting patient differences in a nonjudgmental way, communicating about culture differences, negotiating valued practices in the patient-dentist relationship, and respecting patients' rights to make treatment decisions. The ethical and behavioral issues involved in culturally sensitive care are illustrated in fictional vignettes in which the patient's and dentist's ideas about appropriate care come into conflict.

Conclusions.—Understanding of ethical principles is an important aspect of providing culturally sensitive dental care. Providing care in a way that respects patients' cultural values not only enhances the outcomes of treatment, it promotes the key ethical principles of dentistry.

▶ This article highlights 2 very important topics in dental eduction today—cultural sensitivity and ethics. Given the diversity of patient populations and the complexity of decision-making in clinical practice, students need to be well prepared in both these areas. While these subjects are often taught as separate topics, the authors make a strong case for integrating the 2 topics, making the links explicit for students. This type of integration across topics is exactly what we should be striving for.

K. A. Zakariasen Victoroff, DDS

Creating an Environment for Diversity in Dental Schools: One School's Approach
Formicola AJ, Klyvert M, McIntosh J, et al (Columbia Univ, New York)
J Dent Educ 67:491-499, 2003   19–6

Introduction.—There is a call for increased diversity in the dental and medical workforce. Numbers of female and Asian dental students have increased substantially over the years, but enrollment of Hispanic students lags behind and the number of African American students has decreased. Special programs to increase diversity in one dental school are described, along with complementary efforts promoting a climate of diversity.

Diversity Programs.—The authors review a number of programs introduced to promote enrollment of minority students at the Columbia University School of Dental and Oral Surgery. Under the DDS Minority Admissions Program, acceptance criteria were broadened to include attributes other than grades and test scores, including recommendations, interviews, extracurricular activities, and personal circumstances. The initiative included a summer enrichment program for enrollees with less-than-average preparation. Other types of programs were considered essential to make the dental school more attractive to minority students. A Postdoctoral Minority Admissions Program was instituted to enroll minority students in residency programs at Harlem Hospital, with tuition waivers for trainees who agreed to remain on staff for a certain period. The result has been expansion of dental services and training available at the hospital, with high levels of achievement by trainees. Other programs have included a Science and Technology Entry Program for middle school and high school students and a "Zero" Tuition Dental Assisting Training Program for minority students.

At the same time, complementary efforts were made to foster a climate of delivery at the school. Efforts to consider candidates from all racial/ethnic groups in search processes helped to correct the problem of minority underrepresentation on the faculty. A Multicultural Affairs Committee was formed to undertake a climate study to learn about the experiences of the newly diverse student body at the dental school. The results of the study suggested that the environment was not equitable for all students, leading to recommendations for leadership training, staff development, and other programs emphasizing cultural pluralism. A follow-up survey suggested that, although there was still room for improvement, conditions improved significantly after these measures were taken.

Conclusions.—One dental school's efforts to promote cultural diversity are reviewed. A comprehensive plan is essential, especially in terms of attracting African American and Hispanic students. Key components of the successful effort include involving leadership at all levels, recruiting input from minority faculty, and taking steps to avoid the perception of favoritism.

▶ The need for a health care workforce that is representative of the race/ethnicity of the population being served has been well articulated. Efforts to create such a workforce are ongoing in both dentistry and medicine. This article highlights the fact that both (1) recruitment of a diverse student body and (2) provision of a positive and supportive educational environment are vitally important aspects of these efforts. This article provides a detailed description of one school's efforts in this area. Of particular interest in this article is the climate study conducted by the school to determine how the diverse student body perceived the school's educational environment. Members of the dominant racial/ethnic group—faculty, staff and/or students—may be unaware of issues faced by minority group students. A climate study can provide important information and insights. This technique could be used effectively at other schools.

K. A. Zakariasen Victoroff, DDS

Goals, Costs, and Outcomes of a Predoctoral Student Research Program
Rosenstiel SF, Johnston WM (Ohio State Univ, Columbus)
J Dent Educ 66:1368-1373, 2002   19–7

Introduction.—Dental faculty recruitment and retention are of great concern to the future of dental education due to the increasing number of vacant budgeted faculty positions. The goals and costs of the Ohio State University College of Dentistry program were reviewed. The career choices and financial donations of dental alumni who received student research experience were compared with those of the class as a whole.

Findings.—The identity of participants in the student research program were determined by review of college records. Outcome data on student researchers from 1991 to 1994 were collected by telephone survey. Survey responses were compared with recent alumni surveys from the classes of 1992 and 1994 and mathematically corrected to generate an estimate for non-research participants. A student research program that involves approximately one fourth of the class currently costs over $100,000. Yet the benefits of student research programs were considerable. Compared with the class as a whole, after 7 to 10 years, student researchers were 3.5 times more likely to complete specialty education (50% vs 15%), about 5 times more likely to become full-time faculty members (5% vs 1.1%), and 32% more likely to become donors (42% vs 32%).

Conclusion.—Compared with their class as a whole, student researchers were over 3 times more likely to complete specialty education, about 5 times more likely to become full-time faculty members, and 32% more likely to be financial donors to the school.

Capacity for Training in Clinical Research: Status and Opportunities
Gordon SM, Heft MW, Dionne RA, et al (NIH, Bethesda, Md; Univ of Florida; Univ of Pennsylvania)
J Dent Educ 67:622-629, 2003   19–8

Introduction.—The shortage of clinical researchers is widespread among the health professions. It may be felt more acutely in dentistry due to decreased numbers of graduating dentists, the rising cost of dental education and increasing debt loads, and the economic promise of private dental practice. Dental schools have less than half the faculty needed to offer a strong research environment. The growing chasm between research opportunities and numbers of educated clinical researchers has been recognized in medicine and resulted in the creation of training initiatives that are opportunities and models for dentistry. Opportunities for clinical research in the dental profession were discussed.

Opportunities for Clinical Research.—The Nathan Report (committee chair, David G. Nathan) was prepared by a 1995 panel convened by the National Institutes of Health to examine the crisis in clinical research threatening to hinder the translation and clinical application of biomedical discovery. Many of the issues identified in the Nathan Report have specific relevance to the missions of dental schools, including the need to strengthen partnerships among the academic health centers, research foundations, and the pharmaceutical and managed care industries for the conduct of clinical research. The current clinical research training environments include academic health centers, National Institutes of Health intramural training programs, and other clinical research training environments, including multiple funding sources to support clinical research and education (pharmaceutical industry, contract research organizations, fellowships or rotation in the US Food and Drug Administration, and third party payers).

Conclusion.—By increasing clinical research education throughout several environments, it is possible to have scientists, academicians, faculty, and students working toward common goals for clinical research and problems within the dental profession. This form of cooperation will ultimately make contributions to new preventive and therapeutic options to improve patient care.

▶ The first of these articles (Abstract 19–7) describes a predoctoral student research program. Since the students who participated in the program were self-selected, no conclusion can be drawn about the impact of participation in student research on subsequent career choices. As the authors note, it is quite likely that students who were already planning to specialize and/or pursue an academic career were more likely to participate in student research. Hence, the need to assess the impact of student research programs on students' career choices remains.

As reported in the second article (Abstract 19–8), there is concern that the number of dentists trained to conduct clinical research is insufficient. In addition, the article reports that some clinical research training opportunities for dentists are underutilized. While certainly financial considerations—including substantial student debt and relatively greater average incomes in private clinical practice than in full-time academics—are relevant, it seems that other factors may be at play, too. Is a culture shift in dental education needed? How can we significantly enhance students' interest in both the process and products of dental research? Do we need to more effectively send the message that clinical research and an academic career are as valid and important career paths as clinical patient care?

K. A. Zakariasen Victoroff, DDS

Subject Index

427

Author Index